Attachment-Based
Yoga *&* Meditation
for Trauma Recovery

Attachment-Based Yoga & Meditation

for Trauma Recovery

Simple, Safe, and Effective Practices for Therapy

Deirdre Fay

Foreword by Christopher Germer

W. W. Norton & Company
Independent Publishers Since 1923
New York • London

Note to Readers: Standards of clinical practice and protocol change over time, and no technique or recommendation is guaranteed to be safe or effective in all circumstances. This volume is intended as a general information resource for professionals practicing in the field of psychotherapy and mental health; it is not a substitute for appropriate training, peer review, and/or clinical supervision. Neither the publisher nor the author(s) can guarantee the complete accuracy, efficacy, or appropriateness of any particular recommendation in every respect.

For information about permission to reproduce selections from this book, write to Permissions, W. W. Norton & Company, Inc., 500 Fifth Avenue, New York, NY 10110

For information about special discounts for bulk purchases, please contact W. W. Norton Special Sales at specialsales@wwnorton.com or 800-233-4830

Manufacturing by Sheridan Books
Production manager: Christine Critelli

Library of Congress Cataloging-in-Publication Data

Names: Fay, Deirdre, author.
Title: Attachment-based yoga & meditation for trauma recovery : simple, safe, and effective practices for therapy / Deirdre Fay ; foreword by Christopher Germer.
Other titles: Attachment-based yoga and meditation for trauma recovery
Description: First edition. | New York : W.W. Norton & Company, [2017] | "A Norton professional book." | Includes bibliographical references and index.
Identifiers: LCCN 2016036770 | ISBN 9780393709902 (hardcover)
Subjects: | MESH: Mind-Body Therapies | Wounds and Injuries—therapy | Object Attachment
Classification: LCC RC489.M53 A88 2017 | NLM WB 880 | DDC 617.1/062—dc23
LC record available at https://lccn.loc.gov/2016036770

W. W. Norton & Company, Inc., 500 Fifth Avenue, New York, N.Y. 10110
                    www.wwnorton.com
W. W. Norton & Company Ltd., 15 Carlisle Street, London W1D 3BS

3 4 5 6 7 8 9 0

To all of us who have ever been in pain:
May all who suffer, find peace.
May pain give rise to kindness and equanimity.
May our intimate contact with suffering bring forth a world of compassion and love.

May we remember our true nature,
welcoming in the spectrum of qualities that make us uniquely ourselves,
allowing ourselves to be guided from within, turning toward nourishment,
replenishing ourselves to live the life we want to live.
May we have the grace to know that mistakes arise to guide us, allowing us
        to course-correct, generating new avenues for relational repair.

Contents

Foreword

IT IS INDEED an honor to contribute a foreword to this book. In these pages, Deirdre Fay offers a unique, new vision for understanding and treating trauma. Her insights are the result of deep personal inquiry and years of clinical practice, exploring the intersection of attachment-based psychotherapy, yoga, parts psychology, mindfulness, and self-compassion. Individually, each of these approaches may be considered cutting-edge in the trauma field, but together they have profound significance for how we can assist trauma survivors on the path to healing. The more we learn about trauma, the more we understand how the traumas of everyday life contract the heart and limit our capacity to live fully. I found that reading this book brought new insight not only to my work with traumatized patients, but to psychotherapy in general.

The basic premise of the book is that everyone needs a safe, secure base from which to explore the world, especially in times of stress. When we don't find a secure base as children—when our efforts to connect with caregivers are painful or confusing—our need for safety and connection goes underground. This may come out later in uncomfortable and bewildering ways, such as becoming angry when we feel sad or distancing ourselves from others when we long for closeness. Sometimes an event as simple as a compliment from a friend is enough to trigger fear and suspicion rooted in childhood.

For therapists, attachment theory is a compassionate lens through which we can see our clients' wounds more clearly and learn to be with them in corrective ways. The hope is that, over time, the therapy relationship rubs off on our clients and they internalize the sense of security and the benign, supportive conversation. In other words, the compassionate self-to-other relationship gradually becomes a compassionate self-to-self relationship. Fortunately, the therapy relationship can also be rendered more portable by teaching specific skills to clients that can be practiced between sessions—skills that clients can use to grow, beginning with a secure base.

A unique feature of this book is how the author draws from many sources, both ancient and modern, to help clients cultivate a secure base. For example, yoga philosophy offers up the True Self—an unconditioned essence that cannot be wounded and is infinitely wise and compassionate. This notion is very comforting to trauma survivors who cannot imagine a self beyond their abuse or neglect. The Self is also central to the Internal Family Systems (IFS) model of Richard Schwartz. IFS assumes that everyone consists of parts that hold burdens from the past. Our parts are willing to gradually relinquish their burdens when they are compassionately engaged by the compassionate Self.

Yoga provides many other healing opportunities for trauma survivors, including stabilizing attention by concentrating on the breath or by standing with one's spine against a wall, breaking out of loneliness by breathing *So Hum* (I am that), and learning to untangle body sensations from thoughts and feelings by distinguishing the physical body (*annamaya kosha*) from the mental body (*manomaya kosha*). Many of the yoga-inspired practices in this book are creative new applications that deserve to be in the toolbox of every therapist who works with trauma.

After establishing a safe base, so much of trauma therapy is learning to live in the present moment—facing our past so that it doesn't unwittingly intrude into the present. This is where mindfulness comes in—slowing down and opening to the present moment—*this* moment. However, when a traumatized person is triggered, the present moment is sometimes impossible to bear. Skillfully applied, mindfulness offers a soft landing into the present moment. This can be as simple as saying, "Oh, I'm being triggered!" or "this hurts!" and choosing a healthy response rather than being condemned to repeat painful cycles of thought (unworthiness), feeling (shame), and behavior (self-harm).

One healthy response to emotional pain is self-compassion—treating ourselves as we would treat someone we truly love. This might mean drinking a cup of tea or petting the dog when we suffer, fail, or feel inadequate, or it might be more complicated, such as loving-kindness meditation. Sometimes, however, even *thinking* of being kind to oneself can trigger an emotional storm in a person with early childhood trauma who doesn't feel deserving of kindness. That's backdraft, and it's the primary reason why people have fear of compassion. When we give ourselves unconditional love, we discover the conditions under which we were unloved. It's a challenge for traumatized people to take the medicine they so desperately need—compassion.

A common question is, "What can we do when backdraft occurs?" This book answers that question. It fills an important gap in the trauma and self-compassion literature by showing how to help clients create a safe inner space. The process of opening up with compassion, experiencing backdraft, and then learning to respond to backdraft by returning to a secure base can be deeply transformative for trauma survivors.

With a secure base, we can also step back from our relentless quest for life to be other than it is. Just consider how it feels when you are struggling and a trusted friend puts his or her arm around you, listens carefully, and understands your plight. Perhaps nothing else in your life changes, but you feel much better. You stop resisting your moment-to-moment experience. Curiously, most of the suffering in our lives is due to resistance—the countless ways we argue, complain, ruminate, and blame ourselves (or others) for our misfortune.

Mindfulness is the opposite of resistance—opening to the way things are, moment-to-moment. However, when we're caught in the grip of intense emotions, such as flooded with shame or dread, it's impossible to be mindful. In such moments we need compassionate connection with others, need to return to a place of inner safety and refuge, before we can observe what's happening in our lives and take appropriate action. Discovering the importance of a safe base, and learning how to cultivate that state of mind, is therefore an important contribution to mindfulness practice. Anchoring mindfulness practice in the web of our relationships—in our attachment patterns—also provides rich material for self-inquiry. Without this foundation, meditation and mindfulness may be unwittingly practiced as a way of avoiding our experience rather than clear seeing.

The message of this book is radically positive. The model honors and engages the client's personal history while simultaneously offering the promise of emotional freedom by cultivating a new, more accepting relationship to one's suffering and to one's self. As long as we're alive, there is always hope. It is never too late to change our relationship to pain and to our wounded parts. Furthermore, as Deirdre Fay concludes in this book, the flow of energy in our bodies (*prana*) moves inexorably toward wholeness and integration. Every obstacle we encounter on the healing path is an opportunity to recognize our deepest needs, meet them with kindness and understanding, and live a fuller, more authentic, life.

The model of trauma treatment presented in this book is deep and multidimensional. Readers will probably want to return to it again and again, as I have, for insight, inspiration, and most especially for the compassionate tone that it conveys. When back in their offices, readers will surely see their clients through new eyes, know how to engage them more compassionately and effectively, and have new tools by their side to help their clients reclaim their wise and compassionate selves.

—Christopher Germer, PhD
Faculty, Harvard Medical School
Author, *The Mindful Path to Self-Compassion*
Co-editor, *Mindfulness and Psychotherapy*

Preface

I WAS TO BRING just one book? For weeks of traveling and hiking in Nepal? That's the guideline my friend Umesh Baldwin gave me as I got ready for a trek in the Himalayas that he was leading with his wife Vasanti. This was in the 1990s, before the days of Kindle or tablets. The prospect of only one book was causing me quite a bit of turbulence. I always traveled accompanied by a bag of books. Learning that my bag would be carried on the backs of Nepalese Sherpas up and down the Himalayas helped me rigorously reject my tendency to travel with an overpreponderance of books. Umesh and Vasanti, my friends and guides, were taking me along on a trip to Nepal, and made it clear—one book. So after a great deal of deliberation, I realized the only book that I wanted to delve into, one that would engage me on every level for weeks, would be Taimni's commentary on Patanjali's Yoga Sutras. I had no idea then that that book would form the backbone into the inquiry of this book so many years later.

That trip happened at the tail end of six and a half years of living at Kripalu Center for Yoga & Health in Lenox, Massachusetts. The years of yoga, meditation, and community immersed me in a rigorous ashram lifestyle, providing the safe holding in which my own traumatic history erupted, changing everything. I went from an active life of working as a resident, engaged in yogic practices (*sadhana*) of asana, breathing (*pranayama*), and meditation, and a lifestyle of daily swimming, cycling, running—to having my trauma history explode into consciousness. I wanted to hide in my room, curl into my duvet, alternatingly terrified and numb. The whole thing was confusing. How did I go from getting up at 4:15 a.m. every morning (well, almost every morning) to do morning *sadhana*, to wanting to shut down, numb out? I grappled with the extreme before-and-after existence, wondering how I had so easily been in my body before, whereas now, with the advent of this traumatic material exploding inside, being in my body felt impossible. It didn't make sense. I wanted all the pieces to fit together. I didn't want to be alone in the mess of it and I also knew that I didn't want anyone else to have to go through the confusing, disorienting mess either, certainly not by themselves.

In the midst of that cauldron, seemingly out of nowhere, some determination arose within me, fiercely pushing me to explore the intersection of yoga, meditation, and trauma. If the yogic teachings said the body was the temple of the soul, which I had clearly experienced before, how come it was lost to me now? The bliss and clarity that I knew before was something I wanted again. That inquiry has lasted over thirty years, driving me to leave the ashram, get my social work degree at Smith College, intern at McLean Hospital—where I taught meditation and yoga in the evenings on the dissociative units—and to find my way into the remarkable tutelage of Bessel van der Kolk and the incredible team he had assembled around him.

The Becoming Safely Embodied™ Skills I developed rose from the ashes of my history as I explored integrating the ancient practices of yoga and meditation with contemporary trauma and attachment treatment. Central to my exploration was how each person can embody and remember their own wisdom, and allow that internal wisdom to guide them on their way to a more satisfying and nourishing life. It was in staying close to this tenet that I found the importance of yogic philosophy. The external practices of yoga postures (*asana*), breathing practices (*pranayama*), and meditation are critical. Yet those practices rest on more foundational practices of ethical and characterological development (*yamas* and *niyamas*), which allow the person to have internal energy and character riverbanks to protect their unfolding journey. Yoga in this way is a practice of remembering, awakening to the true spirit and nature of our own being. Attending to the life force as it moves within, we channel *prana*, as it is known in yoga, while it pushes, urges, cajoles, and reminds us of our true nature.

Inevitably, when any of us opens the door to our unintegrated life, we encounter what keeps us comfortable on an old familiar path, even if it means we're stuck in ways that no longer feel good. In working with trauma and attachment wounding over the past twenty-plus years, it became increasingly clear that simple adages didn't help people navigate their disorganized inner worlds. They needed, as I had needed, concrete, practical tools that pointed out ways to organize the ricocheting disruption. Key to this are the practices of mindfulness and concentration that are foundational to all wisdom traditions. To traverse the exploding inner world, a person needs to be able not only to name what's going on but to cultivate themselves to be present with whatever shows up, learning over time how to welcome the discord. Michael Stone writes: "What we find after our initial foray or honeymoon period is a matrix of psychological and physical holding patterns that have captured our minds and bodies within tightly conditioned parameters" (2008, p. 3).

These are the disruptions that drive our clients into our offices. They want symptom relief. They want the problem to go away. Who can blame them? We all want that to happen. As therapists, our first step is to reduce the immediate pain. In terms of trauma treatment that means to reduce the burning fire of their symptoms. Treating the immediate symptoms creates a psychobiological space inside. We also need to juggle our client's need for immediate symptom relief while exploring with them the underlying patterns and history that resulted in these particular symptoms arising. The goal of this book is not primarily to accomplish symptom relief, although some clients might find the practices do ease the symptoms. Instead this book is about identifying, repairing, and remapping the patterns that generated the symptoms.

Both yogic psychology and attachment address the fire of disruption that shows up in a primordial protest: "This isn't right!" or "It shouldn't be like this!" Attachment treatment remaps the relational templates to walk the person into an earned secure status. Yogic psychology looks at the disruptions as the burning away of what isn't, so that what is can generate new options and possibilities. One of the great metaphors of my teenage years was Michelangelo's carving of the statue *David*. After finding a beautiful, yet flawed block of marble, Michelangelo saw something wanting to be expressed. It was through his carving and sanding away that which wasn't David that the beautiful sculpture we know emerged.

That is the metaphor of becoming that is inherent in trauma and attachment healing. Difficult histories encrust our being, making it hard to remember who we were before the heavy protections enveloped our psyche and altered our somatic awareness. Yet, the life force of *prana* that yoga illuminates is relentless. The great yogic sages tell us that this life force only knows the path home to itself, to unity consciousness or as Don Stapleton (2004) calls it the "multi-dimensional experience." Integrating yoga, meditation, and trauma and attachment treatment gives us a healing prescription that honors the deeply painful wounds, while urging us to remember that is not all that we are. Having an attachment perspective in trauma treatment includes the relational component, what Diana Fosha (2000, 2011) has called a Transformational Other, the person who knows the path forward and can partner with another walking toward a more integrated life. Therapists with contemplative perspectives enter tender ground, one in which there is nobody to fix, nothing to change. Yet, our clients desperately need support and guidance. With attachment wounding, people need to be able to reach out to another, need to be able to learn to ask for support, for guidance, for direction, and even advice. We become partners on the road, together curious about the client and how they are unique and special. This book explores weaving yogic philosophy and practices with the important contemporary treatment of trauma and attachment, partnering with the client as she remembers her way home to herself.

Chapter 1 outlines the rich tradition of attachment theory with a beginning description of yogic philosophy. Chapter 2 deals with the crippling effects of shame and the importance of cultivating compassion as a force field to buffer the somatic shocks imprinted by shame. It's at that point, in Chapter 3, that we explore the practices of entering the body, describing the path in concrete, practical terms. Once the foundation is there to enter the body, Chapter 4 forays into the vast topic of dissociation. In this book I've begun an inquiry into dissociation from an attachment perspective, which is then followed up in Chapter 5 with an exploration of the triggers that formed in and through attachment. Chapter 6 introduces boundaries that come from a warped Self/Other distinction. It's then in Chapter 7 that we look into what's possible, trusting *prana* to access individual wisdom as a means of secure internal attachment and to find each particular person's path home to their Self.

The first six chapters are replete with practices with which to experiment. It's absolutely clear to me that there is no right way to do this. After a great deal of reflection, I decided to offer a spectrum of practices, from psychoeducational to yoga and meditation, as I've found over the years that I need a large toolbox to seamlessly respond to individual clients. It is in being present to myself while simultaneously entering the intersubjective matrix (Stern, 2004) that we meet in a field ripe with potential for transformation. With a humble bow to the teachings of yoga and meditation, I've learned that wisdom arises from each individual encounter with the present moment. This bottom-up practice comes from being in the "sloppy" (Stern, 2004) mix of encountering another human being. Or as Georg Feuerstein (2013) declares, it's through practicing that we gather and learn from the teachings of yoga.

Every client needs to have the space and freedom to explore their body, their experience. Each of the practices in this book can be adapted to meet the individual needs of the people you work with. I trust you'll find adaptations and interesting angles. Enjoy them, especially as you give the client the permission to explore the experience in their own way. When these practices become intriguing to the client, they'll want to try them often. That's the most important part: providing a corrective experience of positive exploration of body, mind, and heart, which is one of the foundations of building secure attachment. Doing this, the client begins to safely explore their own native intelligence and guidance. We're helping the client to light up the parts of the brain that help us notice, witness, and observe experience. Perhaps it helps to think of it as mind training.

Attachment-Based
Yoga *&* Meditation
for Trauma Recovery

Introduction

HAFIZ, THE SUFI POET, writes, "I know the way you can get when you have not had a drink of Love: Your face hardens, your sweet muscles cramp." (Ladinsky, 1996, p. 42). We know this intuitively. Without kindness, affiliation, warmth, and safety, faces tighten, close off. People feel empty and lost, even if presenting differently to the world. Those suffering from unresolved trauma or attachment issues hold this internal conflict in their eyes, in the muscles of their face and body, and in how their physical and psychological structures conform to protect against further harm.

Every child should have had the gift of safety from birth onwards. In that state of grace, a child flourishes, steps out beyond their comfort zone, makes mistakes, reaches for reassurance, learns and grows from mistakes without shame. Returning to a safe haven after stretching out into the world, the child finds out from others that they'll be okay despite anything untoward that happened. In this cocoon of care, a child naturally develops psychological safety (Bowlby, 1988; Holmes, 2001) with a native impulse to explore themselves and the world. A child raised in this environment would have an implicit ground in the myriad rhythms and patterns (Beebe et al., 2010, 2003; Beebe & Lachmann, 2014, 2002) of protest and response, engagement, and separation. But what about people who do not enjoy this gift of safety? As therapists, we take on the task of providing a nurturing framework for our clients to relearn how to be connected, safely, in collaborative relationships that are mutual and respectful.

Say that to a trauma survivor or a client with substantive attachment issues, and their eyes will lose focus as they sit in stunned silence. Or maybe they'll roll their eyes, responding with a reactive, "What, are you crazy?" Or as one of my clients would say, "Time to take off those rose-colored glasses. That wasn't how it was, and I strongly doubt it is how it will be." Those flippant remarks of our clients hide, not always successfully, the longing for an embodied reality connected to themselves and to others.

> *I watched Melissa look at the clock, know that it was time to leave, and still pause. Slowly she made her way to the door, pausing yet again. "I don't want to go," she said ever so softly. "This is where I feel safe. Out there I'll be on my own."**

Our clients leave our offices and are alone again. By themselves. Our offices, our relationships with them, provide the bridge connecting them to themselves. Then the moment comes when the session is over. This moment of being connected, to then being alone once again, can be heart-rending. You've seen this, I know. That moment when both you and the client know it's time to go. You watch the client wrap themselves up, put the pieces together in the only way they know how, so they can walk out the door without falling apart. Our task in therapy, and the practice for the client in almost every moment of life, is to recognize that underneath all the bravado no one has gotten off without suffering. Supporting our clients to connect to our common humanity (Neff, 2011) provides a way to ease the aloneness (Fosha, 2011, 2000).

Attachment theory helps us understand how difficult it is for even well-adjusted, healthy people to release the defenses that have kept them safe, and trust another person. Lacking the strong emotional bond of a secure attachment happens in as much as 40 percent of the population (Bakermans-Kranenburg & van IJzendoorn, 2009; Brown, Elliott, et al., 2016 Moullin, Waldfogel, & Washbrook, 2014). For our clients who have been chronically neglected, abandoned, betrayed, or traumatized, trust is hard to come by, yet it is the main threshold our clients must cross in order to heal their hearts, let alone their bodies and minds. It's in courageously stepping toward safety and trust that our clients co-create with us a new secure base from which they reorganize their attachment representations. In

---

* Ed. Note: all purportedly "client" names and case examples in this book have been fictionalized to honor confidentiality.

this explicitly integrative holding environment, our clients risk showing us their anger, contempt, judgment, disapproval, rejection, joy, vitality, and wisdom. As we welcome all aspects of their expression with appropriate boundaries, our clients develop internal safety, a trust in themselves that forms a self-structure allowing them to venture forth into the world from a new, more secure base.

> *"I've been alone my whole life. Even when I'm surrounded by others I feel separate. I'm constantly lost, scared, worried. I guess it has to do with feeling like no one will understand me. Sometimes I wish I had a broken arm or something physically wrong with me so I could say, 'That's why. That's why I'm this way.' But I don't have that, so no one knows why I'm so scared, shaky, anxious, depressed, you name it. I'm all those things. You talk about safety and being in the present, but I don't know what that is at all."*
>
> *"We've worked together for a while now," I say, "What's it like with me? In this moment with me, now?"*
>
> *Maddy looks up at me, shy and angry at the same time, "Yeah. Mostly I do. That scares me too. I wonder what you'll do to hurt me, or when you'll go away."*
>
> *I nod. "Of course you have those fears, those worries. That happens to everyone when they've been disappointed, hurt, or betrayed by other people. The past experiences cloud and influence this moment. It takes time to sort it out, and to trust. It's important to take the time we need. The more we build a solid foundation now, the easier it will be later on. I don't need you to trust me or feel safe with me if it's not right for you. Part of our work together is creating room for you to be with that distrust, and find new ways to interact with others where you feel cared about, understood, and safe."*

We all long to love and be loved—it's sort of the universal currency of being human. Yet, the pain our clients have endured habituates them to keep themselves "safe" by shutting off the natural longing for that kind of contact and connection. As Jean said:

> *"I could feel little droplets of compassion, but I don't know why I kept drifting back into the normal state of being separate from others, staying in my space even though it felt good to make eye contact and hear what people said. To feel connection for a second or two, but then something in my body would go back and it's almost like we've had a few drops, and that was all I could take."*

Everybody needs to feel safe, warm, connected. That longing to feel better, to be reassured, to not be alone, to feel cared about is native to our physiology, even before our psychology asks for it. When any human being suffers they want comfort. The body, perhaps not the wounded personality, seeks warmth, reassurance, closeness, wants to feel protected. Connection—when it is safe, respectful, and caring—eases suffering, letting us know we're not alone (Fosha, 2011, 2000). Our clients talk of wanting their suffering to end; they want out of pain. Understandably so. To accomplish this requires a multipronged approach in therapy, to go into the heart of that suffering while holding a larger field of possibility orienting to a repaired, earned secure experience of relationship to the world.

Healing comes as an inner landscape of ease, playfulness, and relaxation is practiced and cultivated, one in which warmth flows and self-compassion is cultivated. It becomes easier to be seen, without fear of being disappointed or crushed by negative blowback (Germer, 2009). This book provides theory and practices to encourage what Jean called a "few droplets of compassion" to flow in, retaining those droplets, remembering them, nourishing the inner field in which they fall. Our clients can thus meet their protector parts with kindness and care, something many parts of the system have always wanted. Given that we are working with attachment wounding, when the fear of the negative arises we invite the client to return to the practices, facilitating a new pathway while at the same time respecting the fear. Developing a safe base is possible, despite our clients' protests that since it didn't ever happen, they can't imagine it, therefore it can never be. Attachment theory, coupled with yogic psychology and practices, offers a way to give people a chance to build solid ground inside and between themselves and others.

Contemporary theoretical models for understanding the self and the self-in-relation, such as The Internal Family Systems Model (IFS) (Schwartz, 1994); the Accelerated Experiential Dynamic Psychotherapy (AEDP) model (Fosha, 2000); Mindful Self-Compassion (MSC) (Germer & Neff, 2013); Compassion-Focused Therapy (CFT) (Gilbert, 2010; Kolts 2016); and the Ideal Parent Figure Protocol (Brown, Elliot, et al., 2016) create bridges to understand and frame the psychological suffering and disorganization that comes from trauma and attachment wounding. The models offer maps to use in therapy, each addressing different fulcrums. These theoretical constructs linked to concrete practices of yoga and self-compassion (Germer & Neff, 2014) give clients methods to apply the theory in accessible, practical, concrete ways.

The Internal Family Systems Model has a well-thought-out frame for Self, the larger presence of compassion, clarity, curiosity, connection; it features both "protector/manager parts" that dynamically interact in a fluid self-system, and "exiled parts" that hold the trauma and the disowned joys, love, and positive energies. The emphasis is on unburdening parts in order to free them from roles that no longer serve them or the whole system. CFT, in drawing on evolutionary psychology and neuroscience, provides a contemporary multi-modal approach to cultivate compassionate mind training. To deal with emotional dysregulation, distress tolerance, and all difficulties of life, CFT emphasizes affiliation, safeness, and motivation. The Ideal Parent Figure model (Brown, Elliott, et al., 2016) was devised to help remap the client's representations of attachment, moving them from insecure status to secure status. The orientation comes from positive psychology, emphasizing the fostering of inherent, nascent secure characteristics. AEDP uses the dyadic relationship of therapy to support the felt experience of being whole despite experiences of being broken. MSC explores developing self-compassion to encourage our common humanity in being with suffering. Yoga provides a wide-ranging model of transformation (Feuerstein, 2013; Singer, 2015, 2007; Stapleton, 2004; Weintraub, 2004) grounded in the reality of the present moment, framing life circumstances and experiences as life energy (*prana*) that is insistently moving us back to connection with Self. By providing a map for the body's physical, psychological, and energy fluctuations, yoga provides step-by-step instructions for engaging with the inner world while making sense of the outer world.

Underneath the stories and reasons our clients give us for being in therapy is the deeper, abiding, inchoate connection they are longing for—to return to their Self, their soul, their heart, while gently holding the many threads of their life so they feel put back together in a more satisfying way. Our clients require us to be skilled at entering the dark lacunae of their lives (through psychotherapy), guiding them across the chasm of trauma to repair attachment maps (via attachment theory), while helping them remember who they are underneath that pain (utilizing yoga). Doing this helps clients make sense of their lives, supporting them to know when the past is invading the present moment, and helping them set aside traumatic schemas in order to reorient to where they want to go. We support our clients between sessions, not necessarily by scheduling more sessions or with more phone calls or emails, but by providing developmental steps formulated into effective life skills that they can practice on their own between sessions.

CHAPTER I

An Integrative Approach to Healing Trauma

MOST CLIENTS ARRIVE at our door wanting out of the pain. Naturally we want to help. On the surface this looks like easing the symptoms from which they are suffering. This is the first phase of trauma treatment (Chu, 1998; Fisher, in press; Herman, 1992; van der Hart, Nijenhuis, & Steele, 2006; van der Kolk, McFarlane, & Weisaeth, 1996). Even as the trauma symptoms are eased, the greater issue is to ease the fractured sense of belonging, helping the person to remember who they are.

Contemporary attachment therapies remap historical representations by creating safety (Bowlby, 1988; Fosha, 2000; Holmes, 2009, 2001), easing the pain, reassuring, calming, soothing, validating, and fostering courage, to enter into the dark morass of a client's psychology that is embedded in internalized nonnarrative patterns. If trust develops that the other will be there when seeking safety and reassurance, a sense of belonging is created. This connection to self and others is what Bowlby and Ainsworth called the "secure base" (Ainsworth, Blehar, Waters, & Wall, 1978; Bowlby, 1988; Holmes, 2001).

Three dynamic tasks are at play for the therapeutic relationship to help the client. The first is to assist the client in organizing their inner world, making sense of their intrapsychic configurations, lessening identification with distress, so they can begin to experience themselves as whole. The second task is to help the person organize themselves interpersonally, understanding themselves in relationship to others and the world. The third task is a cosmological function, to aid the person in developing a meaningful map for the pain and suffering of life, one that contextualizes the immensely confusing world of suffering in which they find themselves.

Performing these three tasks together requires the therapist to help the client build internal relationships with divergent and conflicting parts of the self. Some parts of the self don't want integration into a larger, containing Self. That has to be factored in, while at the same time building trust between the client, and you, as a safe other. Successfully integrating these various components in a therapy hour contributes to a client's internal and relational healing: it isomorphically assists the client in managing their own inner life while supporting them to move out into the world with confidence, clarity, and generosity of spirit. Attachment-focused therapy provides a map for people to be known and understood, reconnected to themselves. The contribution of yogic psychology offers a model of transformation in which suffering has a natural place, encouraging security not just in relationships, but in the experience of life. Combined, these give the person ways to ride the painful process of healing and help in integrating their histories to expand into living the life they had always wanted to live.

The Present Moment

The primary lens through this intersection of theory and practice is the "present moment." Most people, especially those with attachment wounding, are unknowingly flooded by the past, precluding an alive experience of the present moment. The constant filtering of the present, while lost in the suffering of the intruding past (which feels like it is happening now), makes it hard to parse out this present moment enough to shift within the subtle mind-moments that rapidly build into larger segments of time. From an attachment perspective we look at how the past invades the present. Psychoanalysis points us to enactments (Bromberg, 2011). Internal Family Systems explores how our exiled parts are holding burdens from the past that haven't yet been able to be integrated. Hakomi Therapy (Kurtz, 2015) and Sensorimotor Psychotherapy (Ogden, Minton, & Pain, 2006) teach us about character strategies. Sensorimotor Psychotherapy and Somatic Experiencing (Levin, 1997) guide us to resolve trauma through the body. Neuroscience tells us that we are evolutionarily oriented toward danger, that the Default Mode Network operates in the background, preparing us for the possibility of danger, cautioning us to not get overly relaxed. Yogic philosophy details how the fluctuations of the mind make it hard to experience our true nature. Integrative psychotherapy mines the best of all these to provide skillful tools creatively and collaboratively designed to meet each person uniquely in each present moment. Developing mindfulness helps with this, giving people tools to slow down and enter the present moment. Becoming aware of the many layers in one moment, we more easily clear the mists that fog that moment.

We need tools to help our clients inch toward trusting us, to reassure them that we are safe and won't hurt them, physically, sexually, or emotionally. This is hard for our clients, especially those with trauma and attachment histories, as they are fluidly besieged with memories and associations, often unbeknownst to them. On one level they know they are with us in our office. At the very same time they live Parallel Lives (Fay, 1997) with different parts living in different metaphorical time zones. This moment "feels" so real to our clients, yet what they feel is the layering of memories, habits, beliefs, and patterns that instead veil the present moment: the past invading the present. Maddy came to terms with this in a session we had recently. Afterwards she wrote:

> "I can't believe how stuck I am in the past. I guess I shouldn't be surprised. But I'm a visual person, and found it amazing that even seeing your timeline, in black and white, I had to concentrate so hard on comprehending that it's 2016. I've decided I need to keep reminding myself and my parts throughout the day that it's 2016, so we can hopefully have more experiences of 2016 to draw from and be grounded in, as the part tries to pull me back into the past."

The more we coach our client to live in the present moment, the more possible it is to choose how we want to live (Germer, 2009). Dropping the stories, concepts, or conditioning, and learning to perceive life without the many interpretations and associations layered onto the pure facts, gives a glimpse of freedom. For our clients, it means putting a wedge into traumatic schemas to find they are not *just* their pain and suffering. This requires learning to slow down the quickly moving moments, unpacking the charged residue of history.

Clinically, Stern (2004) has a finger on the contemplative approaches to therapy, as he points out the present moment in psychotherapy as the components of specific, tiny moments of consciousness, full of raw data that is first lived on a felt sensate level and only later expressed through language. These moments unfold organically, without shape or agenda about the course or outcome, entering the subjective world fresh and unexpected. In Stern's poetic words, ". . . the present moment carries an implicit intention to assimilate or accommodate the novelty or resolve the problem" (p. 34). When we tend to the present moment in therapy, we focus on how everything unfolds without interpretation or association, creating space instead of exploring past memories or future fears. Being with the client in a nonlinear way allows the client's unconscious to express itself while holding the meta-perspective of patterns and conditioning they are remapping.

Belinda, who like all of us was used to her perceptions of reality, first looked skeptically at me when I wanted to explore how her perceptions clouded and shaped her experience, keeping her feeling stuck in hopelessness and despair. Having a long history of dissociation, living in a family culture of dissociation, prone to psychotic-like hallucinations, Belinda found it frightening to entertain the thought of witness consciousness. For her, the thoughts in her head were real. The thought of quiet in her head was actually scary. Who would she be? What would happen? To help her untangle this new way of being, we played with her felt experience of the present moment, inquiring into bare noticing, to be with experience without altering it in any way. As we sat together I wondered with her what would happen if she heard the sounds in the room and outside the room—listening, without reflecting or creating stories about them. We started with listening to the arc of sound the bus made as it drove by. Belinda looked at me perplexed. Huh? I suggested she only listen to one of the sounds outside, in this case the bus driving by. Nothing more than that. She was able to isolate the sound of the bus from the other sounds outside the window. Then she practiced listening to the bus as it drove up to the stop, settled, then started up again. "My body quiets down as we do that," Belinda told me, rather surprised. Subsequent sessions involved practicing this in many small ways, simplifying the senses, listening, seeing, hearing, tasting—feeling, without adding to it. (A simple practice for this will be found at the end of this chapter, and will be elaborated on through other practices in the succeeding chapters.)

DEVELOPMENTAL AND THERAPEUTIC TASKS

Everyone on a healing path at some point faces the painful realization that the solution isn't going to come "from out there." Every client deals with this. There eventually comes a moment when the client angrily protests, "It isn't fair! I shouldn't have to be dealing with this now!" or "Why is it always me that has to do all the work?" This is a fundamental pivot point in healing. As much as anyone pushes away at possibility ("It wasn't there! Why should I believe it's possible now?"), reframing this as protest normalizes the inchoate longings for someone to come fix them and make it all better. As these are confronted and normalized, resistance eases. Yes, they should have had "it" (secure attachment, love and nurturing, an entire matrix of being welcomed, known, cared about, respect, delighted in) when they were young. That's what should have happened. The developmental task of a child is to get "it" from "out there." If they had received "it," they would more likely have grown up securely attached. Their family *should* have provided that kind of experience.

The developmental task as an adult is different. Instead of "it" coming from outside, in order to have a better inside, the task of an adult is to build a secure self in order to safely and comfortably explore and interact with the world. As Jeremy Holmes says, "The aims of therapy are to provide an environment that fosters attunement, is secure enough to cope with relevant protest and, therefore, where new meanings and secure-autonomous narratives can arise." (2001, p. 49) If as a child the client did not have an attuned environment in which emotions were safe, they had to filter their experiences, morphing their emotions into active or passive protest behaviors. In therapy, the more we are able to safely encounter our clients' emotional variations with compassion, and even play, the easier it is for the client to know they can be real without losing us (Fosha, 2000), thereby gaining the integration that was missing for them so early on.

In the language of IFS, not only do our clients exile pain and distress, but they also exile the good, vibrant innocence and purity to keep those qualities safe. Yet, as sometimes happens when we put something away for safekeeping, we often can't find our way back to it. In therapy, we enter the painful cauldron of our client's lives, not only to excavate but to help them find the precious links back to their Self, which is where the healing path emerges (Fosha, 2000). This process can only be sensed opaquely by piecing together the micro-momentary world of implicit happenings, as Daniel Stern describes in his book *The Present Moment in Psychotherapy and Everyday Life* (2004). Yogic psychology suggests the way back is through the body, translating the inchoate messages into understanding, remembering the heart's longing for more, and providing the psychological structure to reclaim their native truth about themselves, the good, the bad, and everything in between (Feuerstein, 2013; Stapleton, 2004).

This cannot be done alone. The self-sufficiency model of our Western culture is often replicated in our therapy offices. There is no escape from connection, attachment therapy reminds us. What was broken in connection needs to be repaired in connection (Fosha, 2000). Instead of instructing our clients to go into their bodies by themselves, we need to venture in there with them, with empathy and care for the intersubjective matrix (Stern, 2004) we are creating together as well as with all the therapeutic skills we are trained in. Our task as therapists is to understand the level of disconnection our trauma clients live in; to support them in piecing together the jigsaw puzzle that is their inner life. Our relationship with our clients is an integral shaping as together we put their inner world together in a new, much more adaptive, and nourishing way.

Clients who turn to meditation or yoga to deal with their distress often do so out of the hope of managing it by themselves. In the late 1990s, I interviewed many long-term meditators whose trauma histories emerged during the course of many years of practice. Every one of them talked about how much they tried to use their meditation and yoga practices to deal with their trauma. At first, and with persistent, committed effort, they were able to use their practices to deal with the distress. At some point, however, their histories would no longer be contained by the meditative cocoon. Inevitably they entered some form of structure-building psychotherapy, to anchor and sort through the cauldron that meditation cracked open.

There are times when people are drawn to spiritual practices in hopes of immersing themselves in warmth, kindness, and gentleness as a way to find refuge from the dark sides of their undigested histories, by fleeing from the impulses of rage, contempt, judgment, disgust, or hatred. During the time I lived at Kripalu Center, we would notice this tendency to "prematurely transcend" the more disturbing aspects of being human. Gilbert's research (2014) on compassion indicates a similar phenomenon of people to "ascend away from," rather than developing the "courage to descend into," their experience.

Karlen Lyons-Ruth (1999) describes a model of "collaborative communication" for mothers and child that we can adapt for adults, as they venture into a safely connected world: inclusiveness, willingness to repair, scaffolding, and support in struggling. This model allows people to develop security, flexibility, and coherent working models of attachment, through inclusiveness (responding to the entire range of their experience, and staying curious about internal needs, wants, desires, and beliefs, which fosters a relaxed approach to psychological exploration); a willingness to repair disruptions (as we as therapists take ownership of our own parts, while being appropriately transparent, which allows the client to learn and expect that disruption doesn't disrupt the underlying solid therapeutic connection); scaffolding (helping the client to find the necessary baby steps in accessing their inner world, translating that into words, linking what's going on inside their self-system with the intersubjective presence of the therapist); and support the client in a willingness to struggle (actively engaging, setting limits, making room for protest, all while staying connected through the conflict).

Trauma survivors need to build internal structure to contain the vast spaciousness of good experiences, as well as the dark, foreboding, destructive tendencies that lurk within. Jack Engler (1993) famously advocated how necessary it is to have a self before letting go of a self through meditation practices. The Ideal Parenting Figure (Brown, Elliott, et al., 2016) remaps attachment from insecure status to secure status by valuing the distress while simultaneously reorienting the person to the positive possibilities. Instead of being caught in the attachment style, the therapist keeps revectoring the client toward the possibility of secure attachment through imagining a more ideal parent and more ideal family system. The Self-Awakening Yoga that Don Stapleton encourages has the same premise as scaffolding, finding incremental movement inquiry as the person enters the body in graduated sequences (2004). The Becoming Safely Embodied™ Skills (Fay, 2007) does this by distinguishing the basic building blocks of present moment awareness that allow a person to psychologically reorganize their internal experience.

The models used in this book map out developmental steps, to move from distressing past experiences to a life that is freshly created through possibilities arising in the present. As will be discussed in the next section, yogic psychology frames the crucible of distress as a pointer toward our deepest longings.

The Embodied Present Moment: Yogic Psychology with Trauma Treatment

Atha yoga anushanasam, "Now the teachings of yoga . . ." are Patanjali's open-ing words to the Yoga Sutras, the compendium compiled around 400 CE, pulling various threads together into what we now call yoga. Patanjali's first word is "Now." This present moment, Patanjali says, now, is the very moment in which we can find connection with our Self. Michael Stone, a contemporary yoga teacher, writes that "The only place to investigate . . . is the present moment, because *this* is all that is actually occurring. . . Begin paying attention . . . within this very experience as it unfolds right now, right here." (2008, p. 8) To do this simple task on a consistent basis takes many of us a lifetime of training our bodies, hearts, and minds. We need to navigate despite what's been imprinted (known in yoga as *samskaras*); not getting unnecessarily caught by the flood of beliefs, feel-ings, sensations, and memories (our *vrttis*), held captive in what yoga describes as the many layers of the body (the *koshas*).

Entering the embodied present moment via yoga gives entrée to a dynamic flow of healing. The Sanskrit word *yoga* is often translated "to join" or "union" (Bryant, 2009; Feuerstein, 2013; Singer, 2007; Stapleton, 2004; Taimni, 1961; Weintraub, 2004), wherein we are connected back to who we really are, whether we call that source of our connection the "soul," "true nature," "consciousness," "God," "core self," or an "essential energy," or in the terms of Internal Family Systems, "Self energy." Don Stapleton, the founder of Nosara Yoga Institute, encourages us to define yoga as a sacred relationship with Self, where everything we perceive engages a dynamic relationship expanding and including all parts of the Self (2015). It's through yoga, states Amy Weintraub, founder of LifeForce Yoga, that we get a sense of belongingness and connection to something larger than our small self, healing the disconnect of our early wounds. These contempo-rary approaches have us welcome whatever arises—the good, the bad, and every-thing in between—embraced in the whole, where nothing is separate and everything is connected (Miller, 2014, 2010).

The yogic path to connection is much more elaborate than the singular prac-tice of *asana* (postures) that have become so popular in the West. Patanjali describes the eight "limbs" of yoga. Hatha yoga is built on the ethical and character foundations of the *yamas* (integrity) and *niyama* (character and spiritual support), combined then with *asana* (postures, to balance the physical body); harnessing breath to integrate life-force energies (*pranayama*) and clear the energy body; *pratyahara* (developing an internal locus, through withdrawing the senses); as well as *dharana* (concentration), *dhyana* (meditation), and *samadhi* (the dissolving of separation). These practices aim to return the yogi to pure Awareness, that vast, spacious, presence which sees, observes, and radiates through all, without agenda or intentionality (Bryant, 2009; Miller, 2010; Singer, 2007; Stapleton, 2004). Yogic psychology, as in IFS, holds a framework for the Self as well as for that which obscures the Self. Patanjali, in his most famous sutra, "*Yogas citta vrtti nirodhah*" (Bryant, 2009; Taimni, 1961), tells us to inhibit these clouding patterns of mind, heart, and body. Simply said, to reach the sacred connection with ourselves (Stapleton, 2015), we need to release all that veils and clutters our true nature.

The Yogic Model of Transformation

There's a wonderful story in the Upanishads (a collection of philosophical yogic texts) of how we know of ourselves as separate. In the ocean of nonseparation, the fetus floating in the warm embrace of the womb is given its "instructions" by its own soul about who it is meant to be in this lifetime. The pain of birth blocks out this knowledge. The rest of life is about remembering this early knowing, navigating the pain and imprints that cloud our remembering, and block out memories of pleasure, contentment, and satisfaction. Yogic psychology tells us this is the purpose of our life: to remember and return to this native, natural connection.

The propellant fuel for this is the life-force energy known in yoga as *prana*, that flows consistently and persistently through everything, everyone, all the time, effortlessly, unimpeded, and without separation or distinction of self/other, and that is not located anywhere but everywhere at the same time. The great yogi, Muktananda (1992), points out that we experience *prana* as a tension in the body, vibrating, pushing, urging, nudging us always to remember and to return to this pure state of nonseparation; it is there from the moment we're born, until when we die. Always moving in one direction, the force of *prana* pushes us to return to our true nature. It's like the water rushing down from the mountains to the sea; it cannot be stopped. It moves around, moves through, and moves over whatever is in its way. Its singular agenda is to remove obstacles that keep us from Oneness, a connection with the luminous Awareness. This torrent of energy is always pouring through us, making it difficult to concentrate and draw inwards. The developmental task of being human is to harness this energy, learning to contain it, so that we can use it and direct it. If we don't have the distinction of *prana* as "life force," we confuse it with emotional states, because of the very power and potency of the energetic flow.

The free flow of energy at some point gets impeded. Inevitably something happens, interrupting union with all, and creating separation. The interruption could be something positive and pleasurable that we want more of, or it could be negative or painful and something we want to get away from. Whatever the case might be, these effects are imprinted (*samskara*) in consciousness. Let's say someone says something to you, causing you to feel hurt. You notice a constriction in your heart. The Gestalt of that moment is imprinted in sensory awareness. If the hurt gets repaired, the constriction eases, but the imprint lasts, lessening its strength the less it is activated. Over time, as life continues to ping, ricocheting on these imprints, larger knots are developed in the consciousness, creating even more separation, erecting physical armoring and psychological defenses to keep any further hurt away, and to compartmentalize whatever hurt and pain is already imprinted. The free flow of energy, this *prana*, hasn't stopped moving though. It's still there, moving through, urging, pushing, shoving, cajoling for that return to the vast spaciousness of Awareness.

As *prana* pushes up against *samskaras*, something else occurs. The imprint holds knots of painful thoughts, feelings, and body sensations, called *vrttis* in yoga. The *samskara* holds the Gestalt, and the *vrttis* are the fluctuations trapped within the *samskara*; we get identified with these clusters of traumatic schemas and attendant experiences. Think of *vrttis* as a beehive, with bees wildly buzzing around, or hummingbirds ducking and dashing around the sugar spigot. This swarm of *vrttis* become our focal point, clouding the senses, making it hard to know where to go. Identification is caught in the *vrttis*, instead of expanded in Awareness. With no map of how to deal with this, we think this is all there is to existence, becoming hopeless and despairing.

Yogic psychology says there's more. Encountering these stuck and painful knots *is* the path. This perspective teaches us that we aren't stuck, we're only identifying with less satisfying "things." One remedy, Patanjali tells us, is to look for the opposite (II:33). I think of it as the Nourishing Opposite (Fay, 2010) not just any opposite, but something that will actually invite more nourishment into our experience. Pain, then, is a process of pointing out the way to remember and return ourselves to our true nature. In integrating opposites, holding these opposites simultaneously (Bryant, 2009; Miller, 2014), a third higher synthesis occurs (Patanjali 2.48), in which suffering is eased. This model will get unpacked in later chapters; here I want to present the overview, and how it connects to attachment theory.

Integrative Perspective of Yoga and Attachment

Our clients long for more in life than the pain they are in. Yoga and attachment theory offer a frame in which that longing is harnessed and used for motivational change. Attachment needs, of connection, warmth, soothing, and care, are biologically embedded in each of us, along with the neurological underpinning to protect against danger. Instead of squashing this native longing (as our clients have been prone to do), an integrated approach opens up the mammalian need for attachment safety and security, while embracing the innate yearning for something larger, something bigger. The beauty of life is that there is no one prescription for all of us. The approach that one client needs is not an easy prescription for any other client. An integrative perspective understands the evolving nature of consciousness, allowing people and therapists to fluidly combine models with ease, creating their own cosmology, in a way that is collaborative and immensely creative.

Being a trauma and attachment therapist means we train in gently holding our client's everyday suffering, as well as seeing the patterns and condition that organize a habitual pattern of the pain in which they live. Even as attachment patterns are set early on, the great relief for therapist and client is that those patterns and styles can indeed be changed over time. Yoga supports developing these healing patterns with energetic and embodied experiences, accessing that inner world. In Patanjali's Second Sutra, "*Yogas citta vrtti nirodha*," we learn that yoga is the stilling of the states of the mind (Bryant, 2009). This is an interesting interplay with the work of those in early childhood development, like Beatrice Beebe and Daniel Stern. Both Patanjali and contemporary neuroscientists like Panksepp and Biven (2012) explore how early life experiences are imprinted into sensory imprints, and into sequences of action tendencies, thoughts, images, memories, beliefs, and feelings. Yoga suggests that we can intervene and effect the stream of our own imprinting: we have in our hands the reins of our experience, to steer this as we choose. To help, we need our developed consciousness. This is what therapy encourages, within the person and through the therapeutic container of a conscious and curious observer, informed, interested in, and exploring the options to help. This is likewise the stance of a securely attached parent, caregiver, or therapist who remains interested in the other person, encouraging baby steps to help the other scaffold their emerging explorations without agenda, fascinated only with how the person will shift, change, and become who they fully are.

These patterns flow in combinations of energies known in yoga as the three *gunas*, interacting on a fundamental, essential level, to evolve into physical form, present in every moment, in everything, everywhere. Together, the energy of fire (*rajas*), solidity (*tamas*), and serenity and lucidity (*sattva*) shift and move through all interactions, emotional expressions, and attachment patterns. Learning to be curious about these energies, one of my clients, Bill explored how to engage the *gunas*, to balance what he had, and nourish what wasn't as fully cultivated in him. Since he struggled with depression, Bill began working with *rajas*, to introduce more fire into his bodily experience. Using Sensorimotor Psychology provided Bill with ways to experiment with pushing energy in a safe and contained way. Simultaneously, we repaired attachment wounds by reaching for and attuning to the felt experience of serene (*sattvic*) energy. Bill practiced slowing down, through breath work, meditation, and using LifeForce Yoga cooling and energizing sounds (Weintraub, 2012), to notice the effect this slowing down had on his nervous system.

Jean Klein, the great non-dual yogi, writes in *Transmission of the Flame* (1990) that a relaxed body and mind opens a person to welcome and receive Awareness. Klein taught that the spacious body-mind was a near expression of true nature. It is almost impossible to be receptive to grace, when our body/mind is peppered with conditioning. Learning to unpack the loaded or charged elements of the present moment means introducing our clients to where they are caught in "time capsules" of memories (Fay, 2007) which are not always connected, integrated or consolidated in the present moment. These fragments of body feelings, narrative memories, and physical sensations that happened in the past are packed in "time capsules" of experience, or what the Internal Family Systems calls "parts" of the larger system. "Staying in the here and now helps identify filters placed on the moment.

Activation does not relate to the present but to triggers held in memory banks." (Corrigan, Wilson, & Fay, 2014a, p. 199). These fragments, or conditioning, Jean Klein taught us, are undone not by pushing them away, but by first seeing them clearly (1990). Even as the client is beginning to trust that they can be safe with you, their psychic configuration tends to hold very different perspectives or parts (Schwartz, 1994). As therapists we need to be aware that this matrix of inner complexity is always operating invisibly, yet influencing present moment experience.

The overarching perspective of yoga and contemporary psychotherapies hold the client in a larger context, one in which our clients are more than their pain, distress, and disorganization, caused by whatever traumatic experiences have happened. Combining attachment theory, contemporary psychological approaches, and yogic psychology, we are as Richard Schwartz says "Hope Merchants," peddling the reality that our clients can change and that life can be different. All this assumes a safety, both physical and psychological, that many of our clients do not feel. As trained clinicians we are aware of the need to provide a contained environment in which the client can explore their own world. Most of our clients, as we well know, are caught in a crucible of relational pain. They have been hurt, deeply and often repeatedly, in relationships. Just coming into our offices is an act of courage. To then share the extreme disorganization of their inner world requires even more. It means thoughtfully, intentionally, and repeatedly engaging the tripwire that activates that past trauma, and doing so within a safe holding environment.

ATTACHMENT

Attachment theory is a linchpin of this integrative approach, part of an interwoven systems of behavior including fear, exploratory, sociability, and caregiving systems (Cassidy & Shaver, 1999), of which Bowlby highlighted fear and exploratory systems as the most relevant to attachment systems. Mutually connected, fear increases the need for proximity to an attachment figure, whereas exploratory behaviors reduce attachment activation, as a child (or adult) ventures out to explore beyond the dyad. These two systems combine to give children a secure base from which to explore (Ainsworth, Blehar, Waters, & Wall, 1978). In a securely attached relationship, most infants balance flexibly assessing environmental hazards while predicting a caregiver's responses. Affiliative needs (Murray, 2008) to belong and be emotionally connected come online later in the child; they are broader and distinct from attachment needs (Bowlby, 1969).

Physical and emotional security and self-worth are interconnected. We need to know we belong, that we are connected to others, that we're wanted just as we are. Safe connection to others provides an intangible felt sense that everything will be okay. It alleviates the painful distress of being alone, not knowing what to do, of relying completely on oneself with no internal guidance on what to do, where to go, who to be. Without support of others, our appraisal mechanisms rely on faulty assumptions, being prone to negative conclusions, especially if we've had weak attachment bonds. Rather than moving toward a secure base ". . . minor setbacks may come to look like disasters; the world becomes threatening; the mental pain associated with loss of status, rather than acting as a spur to the formation of new bonds, may gain a life of its own and feel overwhelming." (Holmes, 2001, p. 2)

Attachment theory describes not only physical safety, but the connective tissue that joins us to particular others, providing emotional safety to evolve. Having this secure base helps contain the longing we all have to belong, to be a part of something, to feel safe physically and emotionally, building the foundation for the affiliative and caregiving systems of being cared about, heard, understood, reassured, and validated. Without this, it's hard to ground in the body or open the heart.

Nancy is a physically beautiful, accomplished professional, who despite great intelligence, feels insecure and less than most of the people she comes in contact with. Being seen as competent is critical, forming the essence of her identity. Yet in my office, the confidence melts, her body loses its erect stance. She reports an internal trembling that rattles her. No longer furious at me for bringing this out of her, she has become more open to the guidance I suggest, harnessing her intelligence to deal with the conflicting, tumultuous emotions that undermine her identity. Cracked open at fifty by a broken marriage, on the outside Nancy ferociously clings to an eroding presentation that all is well. She's successfully been able to push aside doubt, despair, and insecurity—until now. The fault line blown open by the marital woes exposed the falsity of the polished exterior she's cultivated for years, highlighting the broken self-structure inside. No longer able to hide from herself, she collapsed into drinking, drugging, and sexual acting-out in order to numb the intrusive memories of being verbally dismissed by her father as not good enough, not smart enough, not entertaining enough. Putting the pieces of her life together, Nancy came to realize that she hadn't wanted to belong to the child she saw reflected in her dad's eyes and words. She wanted to belong to someone who was delighted in her, saw the best in her, cared about her, and reassured her when she was scared or uncertain.

Before I understood the relevance of attachment theory in healing trauma, I had a conversation with the poet David Whyte, about the importance of belonging. In describing my work with trauma survivors the conversation inevitably led to the suffering that is a natural byproduct of trauma. David brought up the notion of *belonging*. I wondered aloud about belongingness with respect to those who often don't think they belong anywhere. After listening in quiet silence, David pointed out that they *do* belong; that everyone belongs somewhere. He reflected that some of my clients might feel they belong to the hospitals they'd been in or belonged to the suffering they'd lived through. He suggested I find a way to orient them to other forms of belonging. Sitting with that in mind over the years, I realized how critical it is to nurture a sense of belongingness—to ourselves, to others around us, to the small, overlooked experiences that connect us to the world. The inquiry of "belongingness" became an integral part of the Becoming Safely Embodied™ Skills, exploring how to offset the deep, abiding loneliness of attachment loss that is so corrosive to the heart and soul. To do so we need to feel ourselves belonging, connected—compassionately including all parts of ourselves, while spaciously open to the suffering in which we find ourselves. Held in this nourishing bond, suffering is the ground out of which wisdom arises.

Fostering the main conditions of secure attachment, of safety, attunement, soothing, expressed delight, and fostering self-development (Brown, Elliott, et al., 2016), therapy provides a safe base for the client to depend on. Emotional and psychological attunement, offering reassurance, delighting in who the client is, and collaborating with them in taking steps toward a more nourishing life, gives a steady structure for our clients to repair their histories. In addition to the therapeutic relationship, the client needs our help in remapping their internal representations to integrate new ways of being, aligned with their new external possibilities. This is the work Nancy and I are engaged in. Before the fault line cracked open, she belonged to her competence and beauty and all her external symbols of success. With that challenged, Nancy at first rejected belonging to the feelings of insecurity, self-criticism, self-contempt contained inside of her. It was in grappling with how rejected she felt in the past that she was able to clean the filters of mirage she'd worked so hard to erect. Even as she fought with herself, Nancy began to trust her native signals, that she was good, kind, responsible, and a caring person. She began to belong to herself, not just the despicable parts that she had left behind so long ago, in remembering the qualities and essence that resides natively within her.

DEFINITIONS OF ATTACHMENT

Ideally, belongingness is the natural byproduct of secure attachment, which Mary Ainsworth defined as the affectional tie formed between one person and another specific one. This tie connects and binds them together in space, and endures over time (Ainsworth, Blehar, Waters, & Wall, 1978), providing protection, and the security that is biologically rooted in the function of any protection from danger. This enduring emotional connection between people produces a desire for continual contact, as well as feelings of distress that can arise during separation.

Daniel Brown (2005–2015) distinguished instrumental love from emotional connections, making sense of the dissonance that comes with developmental trauma. "I had everything I needed," the clients say, "I didn't have any big trauma happen." Yet they suffer, and feel crazy in the suffering. The emotional neglect and rejection they've experienced makes developmental trauma more insidious. Cal puzzled about this. "I knew my parents loved me, I guess. I mean, they took care of me and put me through school. It's crazy though. I didn't feel loved or safe. I knew I had to be who they wanted me to be. There were certainly expectations on me. They didn't want to know why I did what I did." As long as he was being who his parents expected him to be, the relationship more or less worked. Trouble began when Cal was anxious or insecure, and when his mom wanted him to be confident. What Cal wanted, and needed, was for either one of his parents to be with him, curious about his inner experience, to help him make sense of what was happening. Instead, he developed survival strategies to navigate family, social, and educational environments, splitting himself off from his fears and insecurities. Years later, when his bosses wanted him to perform at a significantly higher level, he courageously dealt with the troublesome aspects of his history. He had the outward signs of care (schooling, clothing, food, housing). What he didn't have was the psychological conditions of attachment that provide an internal secure base.

Secure Base

Ideally, if a child has older, wiser people in her life who are attuned to her inner world, who are curious about how she is different and similar to them—where she can be physically safe when she needs to be, supported in harnessing, containing, and structuring the energy pouring through her nervous system, and held within appropriate boundaries—then she finds it easy to express herself and safely explore the world.

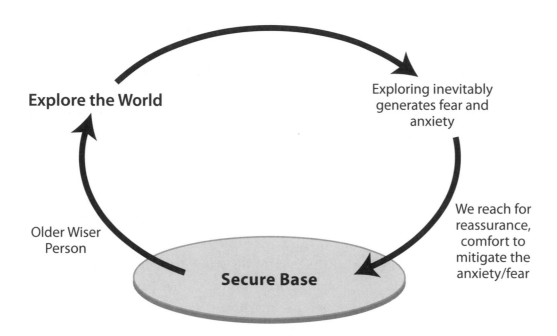

FIG 1.1   SECURE BASE

Ideally, this child would have the courage to step outside the comfort zone of her known world, knowing there would be safe people to provide reassurance as she inevitably encountered turbulence when encountering something new (Agazarian, 1997).

This encounter with turbulence is the natural result of such explorations. An older, wiser, caring person, the Transformation Other that Diana Fosha talks about, provides reassurance to help contain and digest the anxiety of something new and unknown, providing comfort and ease. As Bowlby tell us, "For not only young children . . . but human beings of all ages are found to be at their happiest and to be able to deploy their talents to best advantage when they are confident that, standing behind them, there are one or more trusted persons who will come to their aid should difficulties arise. The person trusted provides a secure base from which his companion can operate." (Bowlby, 1973, p. 359). When we traverse the edges of our comfort zone and find safe others there to mitigate the anxiety of exploration, we are relieved. We consolidate there, finding it easier and easier to take steps into the unknown, confident we will be able to navigate it, or have others to help us, if needed. This provides the felt experience of a secure base.

Internal Working Model

Knowing that our clients feel isolated and alone even when involved in community or held in a family structure gives a perspective into our clients' Internal Working Model (Bowlby, 1969). This representational structure gives us clues of the attachment map each person has: who is there, how they had responded back then, what roles were played. We are also given holographic models of what kinds of representational frames are being set up for the future.

"In the working model of the world that anyone builds a key feature is his notion of who his attachment figures are, where they may be found, and how they may be expected to respond. Similarly, in the working model of the self that anyone builds a key feature is his notion of how acceptable or unacceptable he himself is in the eyes of his attachment figures. On the structure of these complementary models are based that person's forecasts of how accessible and responsive his attachment figures are likely to be should he turn to them for support. And, in terms of the theory now advanced, it is on the structure of those models that depends, also, whether he feels confident that his attachment figures are in general readily available or whether he is more or less afraid that they will not be available—occasionally, frequently or most of the time" (Bowlby, 1973, p. 203).

Attuning to how the client perceives, organizes, and experiences the world helps us, their companion on the journey, help them find more satisfying ways to live. They come to us feeling alone and lost, fearing that they are doomed and life won't get any better. Like Hansel and Gretel, in the Brothers Grimm fairytale, we enter the dark forest of their Internal Working Model, dropping breadcrumbs to find our way out, together—together providing the essential connective tissue of attachment. We join with our clients, offering a subjective hand, integrating their past into a more whole and satisfying world.

Contemporary Applications of Attachment Theory

It's critical to understand the historical imprinting of early attachment representations and how those imprints influence the present moment. More importantly though, for those with trauma wounding, is to understand and organize the internal representations that have become concretized into current relational interactions. The Internal Family Systems Model takes pains to build, for any given person, internal attachment between the person's Self and the parts that are needing attention, by first inviting witness consciousness: the inquiry is, "How do you feel toward that part?" This orients and activates attachment qualities of connection, warmth, compassion, and interest. Once there is even a slight activation of attachment, the therapist might then ask, "How close does that part of you let you come?" Proximity is one of the cornerstones of attachment; when we feel safe, we move closer, and physical separation is decreased. IFS emphasizes the subjective connection between Self and internal parts, in forming greater attachment.

Many people first need to feel connected to a safe external "real" person, before, or so that, an internal self-to-parts relationship can be formed. AEDP does this within the therapeutic container. Belinda resisted "going inside" or separating into parts. "I want to have a relationship with someone . . . not be all alone inside myself." Over time as she felt our connection grow, she was also able to feel connected to herself inside. Contemporary and contemplative approaches to attachment psychotherapy place greater emphasis on the emotional connections between intrapsychic parts of self than on the interpersonal connection between one person and the other. This relational intersection integrates subjective experience within an intersubjective matrix (Stern, 2004).

The approach of this book is to explore attachment as a movement toward a greater felt sense of belonging to oneself and to the world, while incorporating a secure base of safe exploration internally and externally, where one is curious about life, the motivations of self and others, and oriented toward a positive perspective in which one feels safe and comfortable to be seen, known, valued, and respected. Characteristics of this orientation include: feeling safe; seeking and receiving support from others; being confident in psychological and physical proximity to self and other; being emotionally balanced without becoming caught in the dramas of life; understanding and making space for the emotional reality of self and others; being sensitively attuned to others, without losing oneself; becoming comfortable with conflict, and able to reduce that conflict without needing to retaliate, punish, or injure self or others; having the ability to comfort, soothe, and reassure; be self- and other-reflective; taking responsibility for how one affects others, while not taking on the sole responsibility; having high levels of relational satisfaction, commitment, and trust; and feeling safe enough to be playful.

Attachment theory helps us to understand how relationships form attachment styles that have been extensively researched since the 1970s with Mary Ainsworth's "Strange Situation" paradigm. Secure Attachment happens when the child is able to play and explore freely, returning to the "safe base" of the responsive and attuned caregiver. When secure, a child engages with others, even strangers, when the caregiver is there. The main conditions are safety, attunement, soothing, expressed delight, and fostering the best self-development (Brown, Elliott, et al., 2016). Since trauma inevitably sits on a ruptured attachment base (Brown, Elliott, et al., 2016), insecure attachment styles were developed. Parents who are sensitive, available, and responsive tend to have children who have secure attachment styles. When parents are inconsistently responsive, their children tend toward anxious attachment. Those parents who are distant, rigid, and unresponsive tend to have children with avoidant styles.

A fourth category was described by Main and Solomon (1986) as they researched behavior in infants that didn't easily fit into the above categories. This fourth category of infant attachment, unresolved/disorganized, describes the spectrum of push-pull combinations of preoccupied-dismissive behaviors that happen either alternatively or simultaneously. Disorganized attachment produces multiple and contradictory internal working models for attachment. (Brown, Elliott, et al., 2016). Over the years, many have put out explanations for the genesis of disorganized attachment (Main & Soloman, 1986; Solomon & George, 1999). Caregivers who are both frightening (loud, disruptive, aggressive), and/or have frightened behavior (such as being confused, disoriented for periods of time, fearful, tentative), seem to disorganize the child (Lyons-Ruth, et al., 1991). "Fright without solution" is what Main and Hesse called it (Cassidy & Shaver, 1999. p. 549). The parent or caregiver doesn't do anything to help the child deal with these hyperactivated attachment behaviors (Solomon & George, 1999, p. 24). Other predictors were maternal dissociated behavior (Schuengel, Bakermans-Kranenburg, & van Ijzendoorn, 1999), and depression and alcoholism (Solomon & George, 1999).

With the help of Carol George and Nancy Kaplan, Mary Main developed the semistructured Adult Attachment Interview (AAI) to study adult representations of attachment, exploring how each person organizes these attachment representations. Once we know how the person's relational world is laid out, new options can be explored that can help rearrange their internal world. The potential for this reorganizing happens in each present moment of the therapy hour. As therapists, we hold the distress with the possibility of change in the present moment to create space where small and large transformations can happen. In the Gestalt of the therapy hour, we contain the client's multiple realities and perspectives, validating their subjective reality while also encouraging, motivating, and inspiring the client to release traumatic schemas and embrace a more satisfying life. Both therapist and client deal with these multiple layers, at times confronting the old procedural habits to pierce through "stories" and interpretations of life experience, supporting, reorganizing, and reorienting toward this longed-for life that is as yet not articulated. For most clients it is more terrifying to articulate what's new and longed for, than the stories and events of the trauma itself (Fosha, 2011, 2000). "Without frustration there is no need, no reason to mobilize your resources, to discover that you might be able to do something on your own, and in order not to be frustrated, which is a pretty painful experience, the child [the adult here] learns to manipulate the environment." (Perls, 1969/1992. p 32). Shifting nonnarrative patterns means inhibiting previous ways of being, to begin to explore new ways (Polatin, 2013). Trauma and neglect inhibit the client's SEEKING (Panksepp & Biven, 2012) behavior, making it difficult for the client to explore beyond a constricted safe zone.

Whatever the origins of insecure attachment, we see the effects in our clients who live with intense, chronic states of high fear arousal, negative emotions, and a poor capacity for affect regulation (Brown, Elliott, et al., 2016; Cassidy & Shaver, 1999). Their attachment patterns run the gamut of being controlling, punitive, aggressive, or overly caretaking. A collaborative stance of the attachment therapist with clients who have dysregulated states is to be steady and reassuring, reducing negativity and fear, and to be actively engaged, without involving the client in our own internal states, or being a source of fear. This also means we need to be in an active relationship with any negative projections and transference that the client has with us, which of course is harder to do when we're in the thick of it. What makes it easier, is remembering how the subjective force of the past is thus launched into the present, filtering and obscuring the present moment. In the midst of it, both client and therapist are generally unaware that the incomplete patterns from the past are being projected onto their current experience, making it difficult to interact with that present moment. When the projective apparatus is in place, we are caught in reenactments (Bromberg, 2011), making reality fungible. Digesting and integrating the past organically builds, as our clients are responded to, attuned to, and learn about their emotional world, and how to create an internal secure base. Exploring the subtle inner world, our clients can become mired in confusion.

Each moment can be fraught with multiple and conflicting "voices." The Internal Family Systems Model provides a helpful way for most clients to make internal distinctions, by training the client to "unblend" each distressing "part," thereby creating internal organization; also by consistently orienting to the qualities of Self energy, which are: calm, confident, content, compassionate, curious, clear. Even small amounts of these qualities can pierce the cacophony that overwhelms or shuts them down. With clients, I describe the Parallel Lives (see Chapter 4) they are living, because it's easy to get lost when those discordant realities are contained within the very same moment. Our task with our clients is to help them then tease those moments apart.

One quick "Cliff Note" for clients is to learn that "if it's too much, then it's likely from the past." I often tell clients that, if it's too much for you to hold and integrate in this moment, it must have been impossible when you were younger, when your brain wasn't developed, when you didn't have the capacity to understand what was happening, or why it was happening. If it's too much for them now, then it's safe to assume the client is having a feeling or body memory that's exploding into the present moment.

Sam and I explored this, when he fought with his longing to spend more time with his son. He realized that he felt too humiliated to want contact; it was even worse when he realized he also wanted his son's love. Anytime we got close to the longing, he had he shut down, finally realizing this was a way to protect himself. Over time, he realized that he kept making an implicit decision not to show his truer heart to his son. The only problem was that he was confused, and ended up feeling stuck. Because of all the confusing feelings he embodied, he never did anything with his son, passively pushing the son away and communicating through these behaviors that his son wasn't important to him—when in reality, the complete opposite was true. We spent time making room for Sam's feelings, normalizing the importance of love, of wanting and needing connection, until Sam sorted out the difference between his internal experience and these external behaviors. With time he has been able to create situations with his son that are mutually satisfying, and slowly repaired the pain engendered by pushing his son away.

Holding onto the truth of these multiple worlds acknowledges the truth the client is afraid of, while at the same time interrupting the schema with direct moment-to-moment experience: "In this moment, nothing bad is happening. Check and see: Is that true?" The client "confronts" the discordant primary and secondary realities opening into this present moment. Once realizing how the past

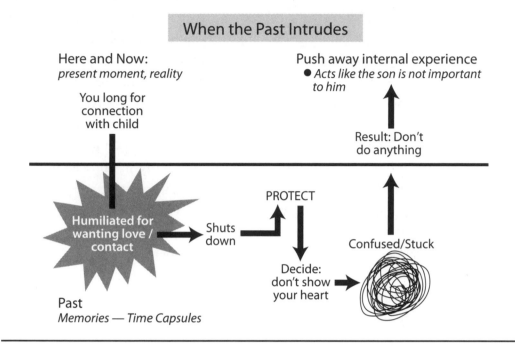

When the Past Intrudes

Here and Now:
present moment, reality

You long for
connection
with child

Push away internal experience
● *Acts like the son is not important
to him*

Result: Don't
do anything

Humiliated for
wanting love /
contact

Shuts
down

PROTECT

Confused/Stuck

Decide:
don't show
your heart

Past
Memories — Time Capsules

FIG 1.2   WHEN THE PAST INTRUDES

schema is intruding into this moment, we have a "choice point" (Fay, 2007) to deal with—a chance to stand right here, in the present moment, and nudge ourselves toward a more satisfying future.

Activating the attachment systems, in safe, clinically appropriate ways, allows the client to practice nurturing a longing for connection and contact. Practices that activate attachment while cultivating embodied safety include the five developmental infant patterns of movement: pushing down, reaching out, grasping, pulling, and yielding (Aposhyan, 2014, 2007; Bainbridge-Cohen, 1994). Most people with attachment issues have deactivated these developmental patterns, or have counterphobically engaged them as defense. This is what Sam did, pushing his feelings down, pushing away his son and others. He had to learn that even though reaching out for what he wanted felt excruciating at times (which it does, if the person is expecting humiliation, disappointment, or rejection), he could learn to ride the felt experience in his body, and shift his experience of it (the subject of Chapter 2). This wasn't in Sam's experience, but if a person has been trained to be a good child, they tend to fear grabbing and pulling. Yet those who are anxiously attached need to learn to release their grip, soften the impulse to cling, learn instead to yield and to let go. Those with a more dismissive attachment style are generally better at pushing away, yet in turn, have difficulty with reaching, grasping, pulling, and yielding.

These fundamental body movements (of yielding, reaching, pushing, grabbing, pulling) can be practiced while dropping the storyline, to help the body activate native embodied attachment movements. Most of us are restricted in one or more of these five patterns because we didn't get the responsive attunement, reinforcing how normal it is to reach, grab, pull, push away, or let go. A child who is secure will naturally reach for the safe other. Their body has procedural learning, that someone will respond more often than not. Without that safe experience, a child stops reaching, deactivating the attachment system, over time going into protest—or despair—detachment phases (Bowlby, 1979).

These developmental patterns are embodied, whether activated or deactivated (Aposhyan, 2007; Bainbridge-Cohen, 1994; Beckes, IJzerman, & Tops, 2015). A person who comes to our office might not know how much they have deactivated their attachment response, yet under their resistance and rejection often lies the embodied impulse to reach for someone, the longing to know that someone is there, and who will respond. Everyone longs to be seen, known, to feel safe to open, to pull what they want toward them, and to yield into that safe holding. The last one is the tricky one—receiving; yielding, receiving, then taking in, tends to be the most complicated movement or psychological stance of all these essential tendencies.

For example, when someone says something nice to you, notice your internal response. Do you say, "Oh! That's great. I've wanted to hear that for the longest time, it means so much to me" or do you shrug, sidestep, or dismiss the compliment? With clients, I have them pause and receive it into their bodies, and explore taking that in. Asking them to be with what it is like to open up to the positive, activating the longing, receiving it into the body, into the heart. In groups, people will talk about how they've learned to deflect, and push away. We remind our clients that repairing attachment wounding creates a new center of gravity, one in which they are grounded and securely held in the heart. In the words of one client, after practicing receiving, "This is happiness-making."

Engaging her longing for more, Anita played with the developmental movements of reaching out, noticing that it brought a positive return to being a child, "When I do this, I start it with just give me, give me, just like a baby. I love this. Give me, give me, give me. Loved being demanding, and knowing I would get what I wanted. I choose love and kindness as the quality, because that's what I want. Love and kindness. I liked it. I especially liked holding the view that I could get what I want. I don't often do that."

Or, as Saralee describes, "The exercises that involve the body and the mind and feelings and all that, all at once, are really good for me, Multisensory, kinesthetic, whatever it is, and so what I was wishing for and hoping for, I'm trying to pull these qualities in to my body and view myself with equanimity, because I started out being numb to the activity but then I decided to try to turn it in a positive way, and just the act of pausing long enough to not be reactive to things that make me react, is really good. I have to remember these exercises. Maybe, if I'm in an argument with someone (laughs), I'll say, "Pardon me I need to go do this; and do the exercise. It would be very useful and helpful to me."

Activating embodied attachment is difficult for people; that's to be expected. Some will find it impossible to explore movement, in which case simply imagining the movement can be just as fruitful, especially in finding places where movement is restricted. Others, like Alison, will first find the movement mechanical, having to separate from the experience to do it, "It took me a minute to figure out how to do it. Then it felt really good. It felt really right. The only thing is, I don't feel like I, like I was just kind of touching the outer surface, like I don't feel that connected. I felt like I couldn't go so much deeper. It felt mechanical in some strange way, like my body was doing it without me there. I got confused. Then when you suggested slowing down and meeting that confusion or the mechanicalness I hung out there. Didn't get very far." Yoga, as I reminded her, isn't about "getting very far." Yoga is about meeting the moment, being with what is there, curious about what is unfolding, without agenda. Sometimes you do one small movement and hold it, sometimes you go in and out of the same movement or posture, twelve or fifteen times, because you're reworking the pathways. Again, it's not right or wrong, it's about exploring what's happening, with nowhere to go and nothing to do with it. This "being-with" is the cornerstone of attachment healing.

Intersubjective Contact: The Present Moment in Therapy

Since attachment wounding occurs inherently in the context of relationship and our clients are coming to us within a therapeutic relationship, we need to explore the special kind of intersubjective contact that helps repair connections, involving the "mutual interpenetration of minds that permits us to say, 'I know that you know that I know' or 'I feel that you feel that I feel.' There is a reading of the contents of the other's mind" (Stern, 2004, p. 75). This knowing of the mind and heart of the other is the essential container for psychotherapy (Fosha, 2000).

We are endowed with an inherent intersubjective motivational system turning us toward connection, requesting regulation from others. This is where the bulk of attachment repair happens. Stern (2004) writes in *The Present Moment in Psychotherapy and Everyday Life* that we engage with our clients on a spectrum of " psychological belonging versus psychological aloneness" which has "at one end cosmic loneliness, and at the other, mental transparency, fusion, and disappearance of the self . . . the intersubjective motivational system regulates the zone of intersubjective comfort somewhere between the two poles. The exact point of comfort depends on one's role in the group, whom one is with, and the personal history of the relationship leading up to that moment. The point on the continuum must be negotiated continually with second-to-second fine-tuning. Too much is at stake for it not to be" (p. 100).

We can take for granted our interest in collaborating and creating a safe holding environment with our clients. Yet despite our best intentions, our own attachment styles get activated when our client's wounded attachment patterns emerge, when they want to cling and hold on, or when they push us away, dismissing our best efforts. It's in this sometimes very messy space that attachment healing takes place, holding the frame for trauma to be eased.

Having a willingness to engage in all aspects of the client's interpersonal world produces a rhythm of exploration within the secure base, which over time opens up a greater zone of comfort in the world. Beebe and Lachmann (2014) point us to how valuable this is with infants, identifying the rhythm of nodding that happens between infant and caregiver. This bobbing head phenomenon indicates a physiological mutual resonance, where the head automatically nods in agreement, "Yes. You understand. You got it." Jaffe et al (1970) researched the speech rhythms of adults that communicate mood, empathy, and effective dialogue. Beatrice Beebe (2003, 2010), Daniel Stern (1985, 2004) and Ed Tronick (2007) joined in the wider exploration of communication, studying mother-infant interactions, including gaze, vocal quality, touching, head movements, posture, and facial expression. Zlochower and Cohn (1996) found depressed mothers had longer, more variable, and less consistent switching pauses with their four-month-old infants than did nondepressed mothers. Operating largely out of consciousness, these forms of communication impact the substrata of interactions.

A secure child has someone who looks with a softly fixed gaze, is responsive, and calmly attuned to minute moment-to-moment fluctuations. These caregivers have a dynamic rhythmic communication (looking at the infant, turning away to give space, touching the child), with facial gestures that are attuned to the infant's internal and external expression (Jaffe, Beebe, et al. 2001). In contrast, caregivers that are insecurely attached have a confusing or incongruous affect, not noticing the subtle shifts and changes in the other's expression. Eye contact might be minimal or appear to "loom" intrusively (Beebe, 2010, 2003). Mother–infant synchrony of switching and pausing is interrupted. We see this with insecurely attached clients, when a communication rhythm of "turn taking" is difficult to maintain, resulting in a speaker cutting off another, not pausing and waiting.

Noticing this communication with our clients, we "intrude" into the nonconscious pattern of our client. Remembering that our clients want to be known, underneath their protective strategies, helps us be with our clients as they get confused when we "interrupt" their procedural pattern. What we together encounter at that point is a tenderness and vulnerability of their longing to be heard, known, and understood in a way that was previously impossible. Daniel Stern (2004) writes that "our nervous systems are constructed to be captured by the nervous systems of others, so that we can experience others as if from within their skin, as well as from within our own. A sort of direct feeling route into the other person is potentially open and we resonate with and participate in their experience and they in ours" (p. 76).

Evie's household was dominated by a father who filled the emotional and psychological space, allowing very little interaction or turn taking with him. When Evie was first referred to me for therapy, at age twenty-one, her mode was to talk without pausing. If I attempted any form of verbal interaction, she would talk over me, continuing with what she was saying, oblivious to any input I might have. Over the many years of her "growing up" in therapy, she began to realize that I actually was interested in her, wanting to know about her. My questions and explorations were to understand how Evie was organized inside. This helped her gain a greater sense of her inner world, distinct from others. Now we have a rhythm and pace that allows Evie to let me collaborate with her, responding and giving her a sense of not being alone in her internal process.

Our clients with trauma and attachment come to us for this precise attunement, a second-to-second fine-tuning of their inner states. They want to belong; they want the connection. Their plea to us, as therapists, is for us to reach an intersubjective hand to them so they can reel themselves out of the past wounded schemas onto the solid ground of connection. Yet they can't move faster than their internal development will allow. "Scaffolding" (Lyons-Ruth, 1999) happens when the caregiver challenges and titrates experience so the child can take the small, incremental steps to the larger goal. The research of Elizabeth Meins (1997) illustrates this with adult-child ball playing, in which the adult never pushes the child to do more than is developmentally possible. Step-by-step the child has a sense of success: waiting for the child to initiate, the adult then finds the next developmental step for the child.

Encouraging exploration while waiting to hear what our clients are wanting to express, we then enhance and support them by finding developmental steps for them to explore. Paying close attention to the multiple modes of communication, our client engages with us as we develop a subjective understanding of their internal reality. We both apprehend what's happening in their body, as well as comprehend how they are making meaning. Responding with a subjective appreciation validates the client's communication, acknowledging them and helping them elaborate on their experience as they learn to negotiate the similarities and differences that naturally happen between people, especially when navigating conflict and repairing disruptions. We both listen to what the client is telling us while also looking for a small developmental step—walking them, gently and kindly, toward a more secure world, one in which we are suggesting possibilities that they long for and are hardwired to have. This nascent, unformed possibility is the core of the longing for which they need us, the therapist, to affirm, validate, and normalize, before they are ready to more comfortably sit with it and then more confidently and securely move out into the world on their own.

Practicalities in Dealing with Resistance to Meeting in the Present Moment

Many of us have been well trained to take a history when we first meet with clients. Most of our trauma- and attachment-wounded clients will comply and report their histories while dissociating and disconnecting as they're doing so. Or they might shut down and freeze, visibly or internally, erecting stronger defenses to protect. Diving in too deeply in the first session (or even with some clients, for a protracted period) sets up a dynamic of uncertain insecurity. By not being aware of the possible effects, we signal to the clients that we are not attuned to their inner worlds of chronic and pervasive distress, thereby setting up from the start the stage for reenactments. If, instead, we slow down the moment, tending to the small micro-moments our clients aren't aware of, we signal an entirely different frame for therapy, one in which we are attuned and interested in what is happening on a moment-to-moment basis. Our attunement and metaunderstanding of what happens in the body, mind, and heart of those suffering with trauma can allow us to trust the natural arising of the contents of life history, without needing to push essential defensive boundaries.

Dealing with resistance is an important part of every therapy hour: doing something new (and that happens frequently, as clients practice the skills in this book) you can count on the client having some kind of resistance. Turbulence will arise. It might not be an obvious resistance, like saying, "No, I won't do that." More likely it will show up in small ways. Each person has a different variation. Some blank out, some get numb, some get contemptuous of the exercise, or say they've already done something like that and it didn't work. There are endless variations. Over and over, we need to hold the stance with clients that there is no right way. There's also no wrong way. There is only exploration. Curiosity. Wondering. Welcoming. Experimenting. This is the perspective of attachment theory, AEDP (Fosha, 2000), iRest Yoga Nidra (Miller, 2015), Gestalt Therapy (Perls, 1969/1992), MSC (Germer & Neff, 2014), CFT (Gilbert, 2010), Sensorimotor Psychotherapy (Ogden, Minton, & Pain, 2006), and of Internal Family Systems (Schwartz, 1994).

No matter how secure a person is or how much support they have from someone older or wiser guiding them, any step outside the normal comfort zone, to explore the world alone, can inevitably bring some form of fear or anxiety. Those who were lucky enough to have a good attachment figure had someone to come to for reassurance, guidance, advice, or physical comfort, to mitigate the normal anxiety and fear. Our clients, for the most part, didn't have that. If they did, we can almost guarantee that they wouldn't be in our offices, showing these symptoms. They're here with us precisely because they didn't get that kind of care or understanding. Ultimately, in the therapeutic relationship, we encounter the internal threshold that our clients aren't sure they want to cross. Yes, they want to get better, they will tell us. But they'll wonder with us: "Do I really want to touch this yuck inside? Do I have to?" That exploration on the threshold of being present is an important one. As my client Bill reports, "Vegging out, slipping away psychically, is something that I do so easily and naturally. I want to be present, but sometimes it's just so hard. It's easier to do what I can do so easily—slip away."

In IFS, protector parts (Schwartz, 1994) are always engaged and have an important role in keeping a person insulated from being too affected, either positively or negatively. Protector parts fear that being present will reduce the capacity to contain the distress they know will automatically arise. In a group I led, Mary put it this way, "I was appreciative of what others were saying, all the good things. It was like they were giving me a cookie or a piece of chocolate. I wanted it, and at the same time I could feel myself worried about what it would be like when I opened all that up, and had to be alone with it again."

Along the way, people will necessarily encounter resistance. That's normal, and needs to be validated and included in the practice. Playing with resistance, while exploring his developmental patterns, Elliott described his experience of listening to a guided yoga *nidra* of mine that we had recorded together in a session. "I liked what you said, which allowed me to do the movement. Your words resonated with something inside me. And then I felt some shame come up and then I was like, I don't really like that one. And then these different feelings came. First I went to a shamed child place and felt like I was beginning to go down a horrible shame route, but I hung on to your words and took it really slow. Stopping. And then I kind of went to a different child place—a good child place—and it felt more natural, like, oh, yeah, I could feel like this is a normal thing. It feels good. This is what I would want any kid to feel. Somehow that opened things up for me. I realized, wow! This is good. This is what I want. Like I could open up to it and receive it. Crazy."

LETTING GO TO EXPERIENCE THE PRESENT MOMENT

Letting go of agenda is hard for most of us to do; we're so tied to achieving or making meaning of something. Dan described his experience, "It's just not a way that I'm used to reaching out. Sure, it felt like a good stretch, and different, but I didn't. I sort of thought of something that I wanted and then got, you know, like can't have it, won't happen, forget about it. Why do you think you could get that?" We practiced the simple movement, letting go of what the movement objective was. He explored reaching for the sake of the movement, not to reach for something. In learning to discover movement without agenda, Dan was able to feel the pleasure of being in his body. He began to enjoy the way his hand and arm moved through space. "It's funny, this simple movement is so relaxing. My back feels better now." Effortless movements encourage integration as time is slowed down, giving the mind more details to explore.

Inviting people to be surprised by their experience gives them a chance to normalize what is naturally going on without having to do "it" right. Many will automatically have resistance, fearing a positive outcome that will ultimately disappoint them. "It's not going to happen, so why am I bothering." Reminding them to "sit and have tea with" their expectations of right or wrong invites the possibility to be with what shows up; a reminder to welcome and explore what it's like to be surprised by something coming in, even as they wait with open space.

Despite making the practice as slow or safe as possible, others, like Annie, will encounter difficulty. "I was clearly dissociating. I started thinking I'm, I can't reach out, I can't do this." When there has been a pattern of separating from the body, connecting back into it feels awkward. Annie continues, "It felt very inauthentic. It felt like I was pulling away. It just felt like I was watching it, not doing it." Encountering moments like this are doorways into attachment repair, by introducing positive imagery that can remap possibilities (Brown, Elliott, et al., 2016) Annie had deactivated her attachment need of reaching out ("I can't"), describing pulling away even in the reaching toward. That contradictory movement pattern is perfect to explore: what images, thoughts, feelings, body sensations, and memories are there when she reaches? When she pulls back? When she's doing both? Is the retreat there when it's something positive she's reaching for, as well as when it's something negative? Is there anything that she enjoys reaching for? If she drops the background commentary and focuses only on the movement, what is she aware of?

Others, like Sinclair, talked about how ". . . It was more like being in a yoga class, and they're telling me to put my arms out and do this. You know, I couldn't do it. I don't know why I couldn't do it, so I stop. It's that resistance, like the whole thing about reaching out and like, why bother? I mean, I didn't think 'why bother,' but I don't know how to explain it. I just didn't feel…you know I just felt like I was doing it. I was trying to be with it. I tried to just say love, you know. Reach for love, you know you want to have love, but I didn't really feel it. So why bother." So we started where she was, working with not wanting to do this, making space for her judgment of the practice, finding out what thoughts, feelings, and body sensations were there at each tiny moment of time, welcoming the disdain and contempt for me for suggesting it. Each time, we made it okay to have all these parts, welcoming resistance, being with it fully, enjoying it, making all experience okay. Other times, we stayed with what happened in her heart, in her spine, feeling the difference in her back, solid and strong, noticing how her back was different than her front, which felt like it needed protection.

To move away from old patterns, it helped to heed Patanjali's advice, and explore the Nourishing Opposite; what did she want? What wasn't there that she would want to be there? What impact would that have? Activating a positive body experience encouraged her, "If I had someone there in real life, wanting to guide me, like you're doing now, well, that would be easier." "If someone encouraged me when it got bumpy that would be nice. You do it, but you're not always there." We explored what happened in her body, when I was there, training her to take somatic impressions of that experience so that her body could help her remember when she was alone. Inviting in these positive opposite movements allowed Annie to shift her pattern of meeting new experiences with negativity and resistance over time. "It was kind of like . . . oftentimes it's hard to receive or reach out. So it was good practice, to put them all together. Yeah. It was good practice, and it was very good, especially, to be with all the resistance that is so automatic. It was just good to notice it and like, what you had to say about repeating things so. It was kind of working through that. I've learned to wave to things instead of being caught in their web."

WORKING WITH VULNERABILITY TO FIND BELONGING

One of the great subsets of resistance is feeling vulnerable, the fear being it opens us to something horrible happening. Those with attachment wounding weren't seen with kindness and gentle goodness, but rather with variations of neglect and contempt. Our clients, as you well know, are terrified of exposing themselves to anything that will repeat this deeply engrained schema. They've been shamed or humiliated for trying things or doing something imperfectly. Knowing this fundamental reality of our clients informs us and teaches us to go slowly into these tender inner worlds as we initiate change processes. This kind of statement from our clients is typical: "I *felt* my fear. I couldn't experience what was going on. I guess I blanked out. It's really hard for me to open up. I don't even know what the fears are. I so freaked out. I could say words but I don't know what I was feeling when I said that. It was even scary for me when you demonstrated it for me. I felt like I was going to cry and that was too much. I had to shut down."

As awful as those moments feel for the client, both client and therapist need to recognize those moments as a doorway into possible healing, knowing the beliefs that are encrusted in the fear (i.e., "People will hurt me"), and to explore ways to shift that in the present moment. It's only in these felt present moment experiences that transformation can occur. Sensorimotor Psychotherapy, Somatic Experiencing, and Accelerated Experiential Dynamic Psychotherapy models suggest moment-to-moment processing of experience as a way to unpack the experience. Being able to be in something, while at the same time observing and reflecting on it, cultivates the basis of a secure internal structure.

The other vulnerability we need to be cognizant of is the fear of empathy or compassion for oneself, parts of self, or for others, especially when vulnerability is high (Gilbert, 2010). Having had to protect against vulnerability for years, the person automatically disconnects the good parts as well as the scary, distressing parts. Guiding them to notice what is nourishing helps the client orient in that direction, stepping them toward the natural longing and yearning for safe connection, remembering how the body can feel good, activating the instinctive movement toward proximity and connection. Affiliative needs are met by turning toward others for comfort, support, warmth, enjoyment, and interest (Corrigan, Wilson, & Fay, 2014a). Over time, the client learns to trust that those nourishing experiences will reliably be there.

The psychologist Daniel Brown uses a form of subjective scale, asking "how present are you now on a scale of zero to ten," to have people develop metacognition. Yvonne Agazarian, in her Systems Centered Therapy approach, asks, "Are you more here, less here, or about the same?" I playfully ask my clients to explore their Subjective Unit of Presence (SUP): "On a scale of zero to 100 percent, how present are you in this moment?" It opens the door to wondering with our client, if they're here 30 percent, where's the other 70 percent? With individuals and groups, I suggest making a Belongingness Box, compiling bits and pieces of things that remind the person of who or what helps them feel connected. For example, Kathy, who spent years in a group with me, had been isolated and depressed, with very few friends, for many years. Her pain enveloped her like a cocoon. It buffered her from the pain of connections that didn't work, that hurt and caused her pain. Using the Subjective Unit of Presence, Kathy was willing to look at how often she separates herself in social situations of any kind, acknowledging that she was a pro at it. She described how she always wants to say the right words, or be the right way, but the protective parts take over and keep her from being who she really is inside.

To antidote this, Kathy created a Belongingness Box, as part of one of the exercises to help her orient to being present and belong to this world, her body, and her life. She filled her box with reminders of things that made her feel more connected, among them a picture of her dog, the old lady who sat outside the house and smiled at her, a small stone, crayons to draw with. Over the weeks of being together the group members and I watched her shift, slowly taking time to learn to connect with others in the group, who patiently sat with her week after week. One day she came in and told us she had decided to go to church, deliberately choosing a church that had young people in it so that she wouldn't be the only single person there. Again, we watched as she unfolded. Week after week, she would tell us about connections she was forming, people who liked her, who listened to her, called her, who liked when she called them. Her face softened, her body relaxed. Her language changed, her edges whittled away. She belonged.

Over the years, others have contributed many things to their Belongingness Box—like the rock Harriet found on a trip to Fenway Park, to watch the Red Sox. Being there in the stands with other fans, she feels connected and part of a larger community in which she can relax, even if the Sox lose. Carrying the rock around in her pocket reminds her of an important connection, that there are people like her, who belong to the same team. This rock represents an opportunity for Harriet to connect with others, and certainly is one of many doorways to a more productive therapeutic experience. Caroline wears a locket with a wee picture of herself as a child, innocent and joyful; Natalie sings songs that help her heart to open; Sam brought in a drum that he plays in a small group. Many people have brought in pictures of children and animals to whom they feel they belong. People have also brought in pictures and stories, where someone reached out, saw something, kindled a connection. The inquiry of belongingness is vast enough that all can find a place in it.

Amalie lived at a domestic violence shelter after living in an abusive relationship. Inspired by her experience, she became a therapist at the same shelter she had found refuge in. She introduced the idea of the Belongingness Box at holiday times, which are especially hard at shelters. Safety at the shelter often comes at a cost of having to sever connections. Belongingness has been ruptured. People are there because there is nowhere else to go. Amalie felt the Belongingness Box gave a simple way for people to store precious memories, quotes, or phrases, to provide a source of comfort when life felt meaningless. "I wanted to help them shift their narrative. As you say in the Becoming Safely Embodied Skills™ Manual, our task is to remind ourselves that we really belong where we want to belong, rather than where we were fostered. We don't have to belong only to our pain or our history. I know I found this so important as I was trying to figure out who I was and where I was going. after I left the abusive relationship I was in."

Belongingness provides a form of self-compassion practice, a way to connect to our common humanity (Neff, 2011; Germer, 2009). The "Just Like Me" self-compassion practice (in the practice section below) is crafted for moments when a client feels isolated and alone. Together, we can wonder, "Might it be true that others (or other parts) might also be afraid? That just like me, they are vulnerable, or afraid, or protective?" This simple self-compassion practice connects us to everyone: Just like me, people suffer. And for our clients, it weaves in the incredible reality: they are not alone in their suffering. One of the things I love about this practice is that it can be done anywhere—taking a walk down the street, in line at the shopping center, doing laundry, anywhere. We're inviting in connection, focusing attention on what joins, instead of what separates. For example, one of my clients saw someone yell at someone else, and felt judgment. She caught herself as the judgmental thoughts cascaded, deciding instead to try the practice, "Just like me, this person doesn't always know what to do with their feelings." The judgment eased, and she felt some opening for the other person's humanity. "It's really helpful to talk about," Maddie said one day in a session, "Some of these things never occur to me 'til we talk about them, like realizing I'm not alone, that other people are just like me, worried, scared, insecure."

When I've led this with groups, members have worried that they're making assumptions about other people, saying, "After all, we don't really know what that other person is wanting." It's a great question. This exercise, though, is less about assuming what's going on in the other person and more about changing our perceptual experience of that person. Judgment or criticism arises, but that separates us from the other. "Just like me" assumes a human connection, assuming that we are more similar than separate. It's in finishing the sentence that we find that connection. "Just like me, this person is trying to control how things are happening." Or "Just like me, this person is learning to deal with difficulties." Or "Just like me, this person has had things happen that I don't even know about." This "Just Like Me" practice can create a more loving and open space inside, bringing connection to oneself and to others, without getting overwhelmed by intense feelings or body sensations. It also supports finding a different way to motivate or mobilize oneself that includes kindness and compassion, instead of harsh judgment or rejection.

ORIENTING TO A MORE SATISFYING WAY OF LIVING

Our clients come to us for healing. They want to get better. They want a way out of suffering. They want the pain they are in to mean something. These existential questions are everyday realities for them. Attachment theory and yoga can offer our clients answers. For many with complicated internal lives, one of the most difficult things to do is to respectfully interact with adaptive strategies that have previously formed powerful defenses against any kind of feeling—understandably so. Learning to make contact with these defense structures invites a return to the true spirit of yoga, return to one's True Nature, grounded in knowing of Self, listening to the guidance of how to find their way back to themselves in a way that is most meaningful for them. The practices of yoga, self-compassion, and attachment therapy teach us a lot about the present moment, about the individual sensate moments that happen, and how we can organize all that raw data into an understandable, meaningful whole. This gives our clients access to the healing state of being.

From an attachment perspective, the way we interact, make mistakes, and repair ruptures with our clients is important. This turning of the wheel of therapy happens over and over again. It's in the relational cauldron that we offer a motivational possibility for a different future. Essential to this is our own self-reflection, training, and consultation as therapists, paving the way forward to guide our clients through the dark and often treacherous paths. We become the older, wiser person our clients need, through the work we have done on ourselves. That authentic presence, more than the techniques we learn, is what makes the biggest difference to our clients, as we model boundaries and ways of being safe in our bodies, minds, and hearts, both tangibly and intangibly.

Integrating yoga into trauma treatment includes holding a positive attachment perspective, orienting the client toward self-connection, self-compassion, and belonging to the world; reversing the isolation and sense of not-belonging has to be fostered and encouraged through multiple practices. Although addressing trauma symptoms is an important part of therapy, yoga, compassion, and attachment theory invite a different orientation, one in which the suffering occurs within a larger frame of belonging, union, and connection. To nudge open stuck schemas endemic to trauma, I might suggest using a yoga posture modified to encourage physical and psychological integration. Using the metaphor of the archer raising her bow, targeting something in the distance, taking aim, and releasing the arrow, can develop concentration and focus. In addition, as in the Modified Half Archer posture, it encourages taking a quality into the body. For example, I have my client, sitting or standing, bowing and acknowledging the suffering they are in, while orienting toward someplace they want to go. When Maddie did this in my office, sitting down, she found she was able to make more contact with a future possibility: ". . . actually pointing felt like I could get closer to it. I always find it scary to put out what I want. This wasn't any different, still scary, but I found myself wanting more than I didn't want to." Agnes's experience also described grappling with wanting more than she allowed herself to usually want, "I found myself wanting something impossible, trying to picture ways in my mind to make it happen. I started to get frustrated and stopped thinking of ways to get there. Then remembered being at the grocery story today, and there was a moment that I became aware of. I was really out of it and something about the experience really pierced me. There was this older guy singing and making jokes and one of the staff was relaxed and open. His demeanor and his kindness came off him. I watched the two of them joking and laughing and then more people smiling because their enjoyment was infectious. I thought this is what I like, this is what I want. That's part of my wish—my intent. It seems so impossible and yet wanting it brings tears to my eyes. It feels so simple and right. I don't know how to do it but having that thought as I was pointing to what I wanted. I thought I should take this in even though it wasn't really happening to me it was happening around me. Maybe it's not having to know how to do it exactly but taking it in. Somehow being moved by it makes a difference."

Foundational Practices

YOGA PRANAYAMA: UJJAYI BREATH

Objective: *This soft, soothing pranayama practice is often called "ocean sounding breath." There is some thought that the back-of-the-throat vibrations in the larynx stimulate the vagal nerve, inducing a calming effect (Brown & Gerbarg, 2012). The balancing effects of ujjayi removes heat in the system and in the words of Swami Sivananda "the practitioner becomes very beautiful." (2008, p. 62). How's that for inspiration!*

Instructions: With a soft, open jaw, take a breath in and exhale long and slow making an audible "ha" sound. Do that a few times noticing the effect it has on your body. When that's familiar gently close the mouth, the tongue relaxed at the back of the mouth, continue to make the "ha" sound breathing out through your nose. After a few rounds of that let go of the "ha" sound breathing in and out allowing the ocean sounding breath to move in and out.

PRACTICE: BARE NOTICING

Objective: *Training the client to use their senses without embellishment. To see simply develops mindfulness; seeing without judging.*

Instructions: You might want to join your client in this exercise, as it helps to do this with another person. Delineate an area of space for you and your client to explore. It could be everything within view against the far wall, or perhaps noticing what is outside a certain window. It's best to not have too crowded a field of view, however.

In silence, both of you should occupy yourselves in independently noticing all that is in that area and listing each item on your respective sheets. When done, compare and contrast the differences and similarities.

PRACTICE: REACHING OUT, OPENING UP, DRAWING IN

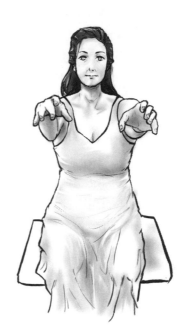

Objective: *Using developmental movements to activate attachment needs.*

Instructions: This exercise can be done seated or standing. Begin by placing the feet flat on the ground, in line with the hips, the toes pointed forward. Take a few minutes to ground in your heart.

Imagine there's something wonderful out in front of you, something that you want. Notice what happens in your body as you see something there that you are drawn to. Can you feel the muscles engaging, wanting to move toward it? Where does that movement happen in you?

FIG 1.3A   REACH OUT

When it feels right, begin reaching, feeling the muscles that get stimulated, to move toward something. You might feel a twitching in your fingers, the arms pushing, or an area of the back moving. Let the movement take its course. Perhaps you feel happy that this wonderful thing is there, knowing full well that it is given freely and without agenda. As you reach,

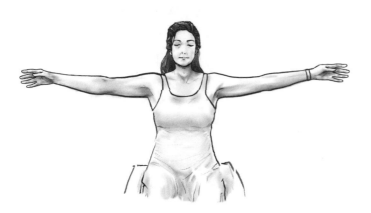

FIG 1.3B   REACH OUT

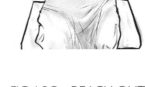

FIG 1.3C   REACH OUT

notice exactly how your body reaches too, playing with the simple movements and enjoying them.

Open up to this wonderful thing or person. Letting your arms expand out to either side, feel the stretch that occurs along the front of your neck and shoulders, the muscles in the back pulling together, to allow you to open fully. Open as much as you can to let your body experience how good this feels. It is wonderful to open without fear.

Grab hold of this wonderful thing/person with your arms, reaching around this bounty, and drawing it toward you. Take all the time you want, to experience what this feels like. Bring it closer, and see what it's like to receive that goodness into your heart and belly.

As you learn to do this, you'll probably find different kinds of resistance—either in your thoughts, in your body, or in the energy of holding and moving. Even as you notice the resistance, accept it. Of course you're scared, worried, or uncertain. All of that is normal as we do something new and different. It's okay to reach, what you're reaching for is there, if you can let your arms reach out, and open wide. Open to it and receive it, and bring it in close to you.

What's it like to receive, to take this in?

Reach out again, doing it over and over. Become familiar with the movement, reaching out toward it, opening yourself toward it, training your heart, body, and mind to receive this goodness. Open wide, then bring it in.

Reach out again, This time, visualize something specific, say, a quality of being that you really want. Maybe it's light-heartedness. Maybe it's graciousness. Maybe it's kindness or goodness, or relaxation, or wonderment? What calls to you?

This time, as you reach toward this quality, it's right there, waiting for you. Reach toward it, open toward it. And then draw it in, expecting it. Allow it to come in, and be surprised by it. Feel your body yield to it.

Then, once more, reach out, reaching for that exact, specific quality. Open toward it, knowing it's there. There's no doubt in your mind it is there. And then imagine that you're receiving it.

PRACTICE: MODIFIED HALF ARCHER YOGA POSTURE

Objective: *Since the body is so much more concrete than just thoughts and feelings it's good to find ways to shift body experience. This posture integrates top-down (setting an intention) and bottom-up (moving in and through a yoga posture), to integrate what the client is wanting to bring into possibility. Doing so will naturally engage some resistance. Meeting the resistance without needing to change it suggests ways to break the posture down into smaller and smaller pieces, which might be to first lengthen the spine; notice what happens.*

The posture is also designed to encourage positive attachment movements of reaching and pulling. Many clients have had their developmental movements truncated because there wasn't an adequate nurturing environment to encourage the movements. By stretching out, reaching, and pulling toward we are stimulating the development of attachment needs. With that, of course, might come the deeper, nonverbal resistances. If the client grew up in an environment where she wanted and that need was not met, then reaching out for something might have an affective charge attached to it. Being sensitive to that we can keep encouraging our clients to stretch, reminding them that we are there with them, willing to process whatever comes up as they do this.

Instructions: Take a moment to contemplate *why* you want healing, integration, and soothing. What's your intention in learning these new experiences and ways of being in your body—what do you want to get out of doing this? Where would you like to be at the end? As you consider these questions, allow the answers to arise inside you.

Instructions: Modified Half Archer Yoga Posture

Start by standing or sitting, with the spine erect, but still relaxed.

Place one hand on the belly, and the other hand on the heart. Notice what happens inside. Is there turbulence? If so, what form does it take? Are there thoughts, feelings, body sensations?

Feel the warmth of the contact between your hands and your torso. Does the warmth from your hands reach into your skin? Into your torso? If so, what happens inside? Do any of your muscles change or tighten? Something happens. What might that be? Without expressing it as being either right or wrong, what is it that happens?

The posture is a variation on the traditional Archer Yoga Posture. I'm adapting it here to make it more accessible for those with trauma and attachment issues. As we know, anytime we experience even a light touch on the body, there can be a sense of vulnerability and the fear of being exposed. For many, there are places inside that feel victimized, small, and afraid. This particular posture can be very empowering.

With this exercise, we're going to aim the "arrow" of our mind and body toward the intention ("target") we're setting for ourselves. We're training the mind

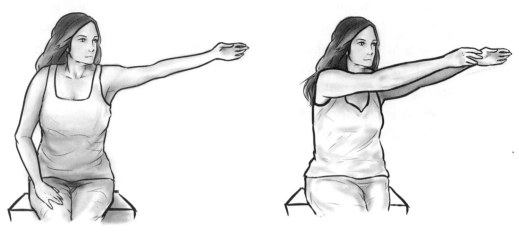

FIG 1.4A   ½ Archer   FIG 1.4B   ½ Archer

to go where we want it to, rather than getting caught in old states of mind that might feel more comfortable. The more we train the mind to go in the desired direction, the more the body can shift and change with it. Conversely, the more we let go of our ideas about posture, the more the body takes on this new state, and makes it more concrete, shedding old ways of thinking along with it.

This posture teaches us patience and strength of focus, through imagining being an archer. An archer has to see ahead into the distance, and take aim at a specific spot. The archer aims her arrow directly at this spot, focusing her mind, while at the same time engaging her body, bringing this into a position to follow the intention of her mind's focus. With practice, the steadiness of mental focus and posture will become native. Our eyes can relax, even as they orient toward the target. Settle into the breath, letting go in the present moment.

Benefits from this posture are strengthening of arms and shoulders, increased hip mobility, and the softening and opening up of the heart and chest muscles. If you have shoulder/lumbar/disk injuries or are pregnant, take it slower; in any case, never stretch beyond what is actually comfortable for you. Make the posture work for you, rather than working too hard to achieve a specific posture. Does the sensation inside feel good, or is your body telling you to stop and not go there?

Softly close your eyes and turn your attention inward—or soften your gaze, if closing your eyes seems too much.

Internally explore your intention. What are you wanting? What motivates you

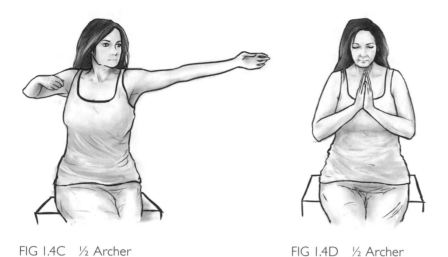

FIG 1.4C   ½ Archer   FIG 1.4D   ½ Archer

to shift something on this day, or in this moment? Where do you want to go? Looking ahead, what do you long for; wish for? What is right outside you that you want to draw in closer? You might have a name, or it might just be a longing, a felt sense of something that you want. Become aware of whatever is just out of your reach that you're longing for. What is your intention for this moment?

Sitting or standing, feel your spine roll; if you're against a chair, move your spine against the chair back. Is there tightness, is there a way for your neck to be more at ease? Search for movements that feel good and linger over them, enjoying them. Noticing as you do so what sensations and movements bring pleasure. You might find your body sharing colors or internal sensations that are pleasurable.

When you are ready, begin by lifting your arms to shoulder height. Softly swinging your upper torso, rotate your arms, shoulders, and spine, enjoying the movement. Stretching one arm out in front of you, and then the other, feel the changes as they move fluidly through you. Stretch your arm and hips too, as you move around. Decide what feels good, and follow that sensation.

Leaning your body to the right, keep your hips facing forward, and not moving. Stretch your left arm toward this intention you have, this hope or wish that you've identified. What is this that you want to move toward? Let your left arm move toward it, feeling it rotate in your shoulder socket as it points to this intention. Reach for it, focus on it, feel it; it's right there. Delight in it.

Bring your right arm over to the left arm, with both pointing forward, keeping your spine straight and strong. Your right arm tastes this longing. Then slowly pull your right arm back, as if it's pulling your intention along the parallel left arm, and right across your heart, bringing this intention into and through your heart. Pulling your right arm back, pull the intention into your body, keeping your head steady and your left arm still pointing to the future, while your right arm brings the intention into and through your body, pausing at the torso, and cocking the right elbow up and behind you. Moving your body slowly, capture every tiny movement you feel, reveling in these movements that come with any safe exploration of the body.

Bring your right hand back to the left, then bring both hands together, moving them toward your heart in a prayer position, as you also notice what happens inside of you.

Be open to all feelings, thoughts, and sensations. Be aware of any confidence that you might feel, in doing this, in your body or your mind.

JUST LIKE ME: A SIMPLE PRACTICE OF SELF-COMPASSION

Objective: *Develop the awareness that we are all in this life together, all wanting similar things: to be at ease, to be happy, to release suffering. Practicing this opens us to our common humanity.*

Instructions: Imagine someone you love and care about. Hold them for a moment, in your mind's eye and in your heart. Then imagine saying to them, "Just like me, . . ." finishing this sentence in whatever way feels comfortable to you.

Then imagine someone you barely know, someone who is at the periphery of your world. Again, hold them in your mind's eye, and imagine saying to them, "Just like me, . . ." and finish the sentence.

Then if you feel up to it, think of someone you're having some difficulty with, and do the same with them.

Do this a few times, and see what happens in your heart, to your thoughts, and with your feelings.

PRACTICE: RIDING THE BREATH

Objective: *This simple practice is about getting used to riding sensations in the body, by being with the breath. Effortless breathing allows the parasympathetic nervous system to calm.*

Research indicates that breathing in and out at a rate of five or six breaths per minute is the most efficacious pattern (Brown & Gerbarg, 2012). For some clients, counting breaths is very important, and can be soothing. Others get trapped into trying to do it "right." I offer them the option to experiment, starting with a simple noticing of how the breath is happening now, and then expanding it in whatever ways work best for them.

Instructions: Breathe in. Breathe out. (pause) Let your breathing be simple and easy, without effort in any way.

Breathing in; imagine the breath softly leaving your body.

Whenever it's comfortable, take another breath in, holding it to a count of two. At the top of the inhalation notice how the breath turns over into an exhalation. Exhaling to a count of two.

Breath flowing easily in, this time to a count of three, then exhaling to a count of three.

If it feels comfortable, simply breathe in and out to a count of four.

Expanding it to counts of five or six if your body is at ease with that.

Then, starting again with an easy breath, breathing in, breathing out.

Again breathing in and out to two (then three, four, five, even six if comfortable)

Take a moment to notice what it's like being in your body after doing this.

Try it again for a few more rounds, moving at your pace, staying curious about your own experience.

BELONGINGNESS BOX

Objective: *The practices in this book are about reconnecting with what connects you to this moment, to this life experience—including the pain and the goodness with this breath, this beating heart. It is also about remembering the things that connect us to others, to places, events, and objects. When the suffering is there it is hard to remember those little moments when things are easy or restful, or even fun. This practice is about having a portable remembrance box.*

Instructions: It may be hard at first to think of ways that you are connected, ways that you belong. That's normal. You might have an internal working model where you didn't feel that you belonged; you may have many memories of not belonging, not being included or valued. It may take some time to reflect on what does help you feel connected. For example, a young woman, Juliet, remembered living down the road from an organic farm. Juliet started hanging around after school until the owners invited her to come and do some chores with them. It was the only place she felt safe. The herbs were planted all over the farm, mingling together. It was the lavender, though, that stood out for Juliet. That smell, all those years later, would instantly transport her back to the safety of that secure connection to the family and the earth. After having this memory, Juliet brought in a spray of herbs loaded with lavender. Is it any surprise that years later, when I heard from Juliet she had moved with her husband to a cooperative farm?

Take a small tin, something easily portable like an Altoids tin. If you like, use paint or nail color or sparkles or dime store bling to decorate the tin. When you're done, admire your handiwork. It doesn't have to appeal to anyone but you!

The goal is to fill the tin with small objects that help you connect to yourself. These are things that help you remember that you belong. This reminds me of the Buddhist monks who painted *thangkas* (portable paintings of the Buddha or the spiritual path that could be rolled up and carried with them on their travels). This way they could always create a sacred environment around them. Your tin need not have any spiritual significance. What's important is to find items, words, and pictures, that help you feel good. Things that help you feel good are sure fire access routes to belonging.

Here are some examples to help you get started:

Pictures from magazines.
Sentences you've read in books.
Photos of pets, small enough to fit in the tin.
Quotes that make you feel good.
Thoughts you've had that brightened your day.
Small figures of animals, spiritual objects.

Make them small enough to fit into the tin so they are easily accessible. Some people like to have folded, paper-based items so it's more of a mystery when they open them.

CHAPTER 2

Foster Self-Compassion to Ease Shame

"Aggh!" My heart captured Karen's cry as she writhed on the chair in my office. Her hands covered her eyes and ears at the same time, her mouth opening with the agonized cries. Holding her anguish, grounding myself in compassion, I spoke to her to bridge into her aloneness and reach her, cocooned in shame. "I'm here, Karen. I'm here, right here with you. You're safe. You're here with me in my office. These are old feelings churning through. I'm here with you."

It takes enormous courage for our clients to show us how vulnerable and out of control they feel when caught in these shame cycles. As therapists we open to the intersubjective space that allows our nervous systems to mingle while staying solid in our embodied experience. "I'm here with you, Karen." My voice seems to reach through the distress as we meet in the space between. Karen's body both tightens and eases at the same time. "These are wretched moments we all have," I say. "You're not alone. I'm right here with you." Moment-to-moment tracking of her felt experience reminds Karen of our connection, grounding her in the present moment. I let Karen know that whatever she is experiencing is welcome and digestible between us.

These godawful moments of shame take over in a nanosecond. Anyone who has had the experience of shame can recall the acute experience, the physiological horror of wanting to die, hide, numb, disappear—or as one of my clients says, "zeroing out." Definitions of shame miss the actual experience that can come on so instantaneously, the whole body submerging into molten lava wanting to do anything to get away from plunging into psychological chaos and horror. The body knows the experience first. Within a moment defensive responses come roaring online with the demand to hide, disappear, shut down. In the tightly packaged aftermath, the frontal lobe shuts down, information processing gets cut off. People often describe themselves at this point as blank, numb, or confused (Corrigan, 2014; Gilbert, 1998). The tsunami of shame sets off every alarm in the body igniting a cauldron of intensity, filling the person with seething self-criticism, self-hatred, and every other dastardly self-attack.

None of us arrives into adulthood without being scarred, some deeply. To be alive is to want all kinds of things, while not always getting what you want. Despite that, the longing for more continues, and is a motivational force. To be in a body, to have a heart, is to explore beyond, reaching for life, wanting contact, to engage with life (Holmes, 1996). That innate need coupled with being chronically misattuned fosters an inevitable belief that "there must be something wrong with me." This is what distinguishes shame from guilt (Tangney & Dearing, 2002). Physiologically, this torrent of shame pours forth, teaching us to not reach, not to engage. The extraordinary pain of wanting something and not getting it grinds into our psyche, shaping hearts and bodies in gruesome ways. People with trauma and attachment issues fall into deep wells of shame. The crushing experience collapses the heart, soul, and body, as the person is sucked under by the powerful undertow, into an utter cacophony of pain. Scrambling to escape any vestige of shame, people narrow their attention, pull into themselves, and recoil from connecting with any possible triggers.

Under Shame is Developmental Trauma

When we take a step back from the physiological anguish that occurs, we uncover the underpinnings of attachment: the need for safety, and the longing to be seen, to be known, to fit in, to be heard and understood. When unprovided for, these longings launch shame attacks, spiraling people into shutting down, acting out, and various self-destructive behaviors. Without a secure base of connection or a network of support to rely on when triggered, people are catapulted into shame spirals that can last days or even weeks, which for some stretch into long-term self-destructive patterns.

Combined with an inner dialogue of self-criticism, hostility toward oneself can verge on self-persecution. Whether criticism comes externally or internally (or both) the force field of shame is overwhelmingly setting up the self to fragment with a need to shut down immediately. Consequently, people feel there is no safe place inside their own skin, or outside with anyone else. In these moments there can seem no way to soothe or calm the resulting torrential distress except to compartmentalize the shame (Fisher, 2015). In the aftermath of such "shame attacks," metacognitive beliefs are formed of the person not deserving love, compassion, goodness, (Gilbert, 2010), or of being a "loser for needing those very things," as many people tell me.

Over time, protective strategies form to guard the wounded parts that are exiled (using the language of Internal Family Systems) from consciousness, yet carved deeply into the psyche. With the entrenched beliefs embedded in nonnarrative schemas, it can be hard to deal with the shame head on. As therapists, we know how threatening it is for our clients to ease the schemas that keep them feeling small, worthless, and undeserving of love, attention, kindness, and care. For many, the thought of being positive or feeling good raises fears that they recoil from, horrified of becoming narcissistic or self-aggrandizing ("I'll be too big, too important, too seen."). On the other side of the nihilistic pole can be fears of "It's not worth it," "It's hopeless," "Nothing good ever happens anyway." Across this continuum, the client believes they don't deserve the simple forms of compassion, kindness, and goodness.

Teaching skills to increase self-reassurance/warmth and self-soothing to antidote the intensity of threat that arises poses its own set of complications, as painful, neglected childhoods make it difficult to access soothing internal processes (Brewin, Gregory, Lipton, & Burgess, 2010; Brewin, Lanius, Novac, Schnyder, & Galea, 2009). Gilbert (2009c) has repeatedly found that self-criticism exacerbates the evolutionary, physiologically based threat system, making it hard to defuse the enflamed nervous system. Those who haven't had a secure attachment while growing up lack the implicit navigational beliefs and tendencies to turn toward support or connection during turbulent moments. Given that lack of support, they are in dire need of developing new internal templates for those times when life goes awry, to mitigate their faulty evaluations of what is happening. Without that, Jeremy Holmes writes, "Then minor setbacks may come to look like disasters; the world becomes threatening; the mental pain associated with loss of status, rather than acting as a spur to the formation of new bonds, may gain a life of its own and feel overwhelming" (2001, p. 2).

Those with any kind of trauma need to walk gently into the practice of positive psychology, or training in compassion. As Paul Gilbert's (et al) research tells us (Gilbert, McEwan, Matos, Rivis, 2011; Gilbert, McEwan, Catarino, Baiao, Palmeira, 2014), sometimes cultivating compassion exacerbates the negative self-criticism or hatred. Anyone who has been on long-term retreats will know the experience of offering *metta* (loving kindness) or *karuna* (compassion) to themselves and being caught in what Chris Germer calls "backdraft" (2009) describing the type of explosion firefighters can be confronted with when fresh air arrives into a fire deprived of oxygen. "A similar effect can occur when we practice loving-kindness. If our hearts are hot with suffering—self-hatred, self-doubt—when we begin to practice, sympathetic words can open the door of our hearts, causing an explosion of difficult feelings" (2009; p. 150).

What our clients, what we, long for is often just what we are terrified of. Our clients come to us wanting to be guided back to their own internal secure base, or what the IFS model calls "Self-energy" (Schwartz, 1994) and what yoga calls our true nature. At the same time, we need to be aware that our clients' protective parts/strategies are often furiously determined to protect and defend against old wounds reoccurring (Schwartz, 1994). Complicating this is our clients' histories of fear or neglect, producing approach-avoidance conflicts (Liotti and Gumley, 2008).

USING YOGA AND ATTACHMENT TO BUFFER AND COOL THE INTENSITY OF SHAME

Reminding our clients that being cared for safely, respectfully, and compassionately is a natural, normal need that all human beings have is a gift we can offer them over and over again. It's exactly here that the contribution of yoga and attachment theory provide ground for healing. The common ground of our human suffering is one of the tenets of self-compassion (Neff, 2011). And shame, certainly, is a painful form of suffering. It's in that cauldron of suffering, yogic philosophy teaches us, that our longing arises to return to our true nature. It comes disguised as protest, anger, and resistance, vocalized and/or buried in the body.

Safe attachment normalizes the need to be safe from harm, of returning to a haven, belonging, instead of being and feeling alone. The evolutionary model of attachment theory proposes that life's difficulties are made manageable when held in physical security, the root of which lives in the attachment bond (Bowlby, 1988). Mammals in the wild, when threatened, move closer in proximity to larger mammals. Humans have a similar response when threatened (Cassidy & Shaver, 1999; Gilbert & Choden, 2014; Levine, 1997; Ogden, Minton, & Pain, 2006). With a secure attachment we move toward a safe person or space when distressed, to contain and help with any anguish that occurs (Bowlby, 1988; Brown, Elliott, et al., 2016; Cassidy & Shaver, 1996; Holmes, 2001). To become secure inside, or classified with an "earned secure" status in the Adult Attachment Interview, our clients need to construct a secure base, which is essentially why our clients turn to us for psychotherapy. Our stance of being reliable, warm, caring, consistent, responsive, with thoughtful boundaries and skillful knowledge, helps facilitate our clients' development of an internal foothold.

In the 1990s I led a workshop in South Africa, soon after the Truth and Reconciliation Commission had started. After the workshop, someone (I wish I could find that person again, to acknowledge how meaningful this story has been for me) opened up about their experience working with one of the country's tribes, and how the tribe dealt with shame. When someone did something wrong the entire tribe would all gather, circling around this person. Perhaps you're like me, starting to imagine a crowd of people gathering, circling around someone who has done something "wrong," this someone getting hyperaroused preparing for hostility and aggression. But no, that's not what would happen in this tribe. Instead, people would stand around the individual who had "done wrong," telling them over and over again all the things they've done right, all the wonderful qualities about them, all the good things that they are. The tribe would provide a counterpoint to the inner shame of doing something wrong, by holding up a mirror of who that person "really" is. Not implying that they hadn't done wrong, but rather mirroring back their true nature.

What would that be like, for any of us?

What this story brilliantly describes is how shame activates the affiliative need to belong, highlighting what we wanted, but might not have had. Even as shame activates fears of not being wanted, cared about, respected, or valued, shame also activates our attachment longing to be seen, known, and loved. Research mimics intuition, showing us that we need balance to contain and absorb the painful negative effects of shame on our psyche and body. Despite the scarring that shame inflicts, it is possible to alter its insidious course and dissolve the toxicity of shame attacks. It's possible to understand what's happening and why our clients are filled with shame, but that by itself almost never shifts the dreadful felt experience.

The remedy for shame is to create a larger field of consciousness in which shame can be absorbed. To do that the client needs to befriend their body's disruptive splatter. For those who have come from neglectful or abusive environments, this doesn't come naturally, even though under protective barriers their heart longs for reassurance, warmth, kindness, and validation. These attachment mechanisms are broken in such people, both with others and with themselves. The therapeutic task of attachment repair is to fearlessly hold the suffering, while inviting ourselves and others to walk with us through this distress together.

Cultivating secure attachment (Brown, Elliott, et al., 2016) guides our clients as they learn to titrate emotional distress, allowing them to peer at distress from some "distance," without falling in. With this, our clients gain a perspective to deal with the unaddressed, unfulfilled longings for connection. In therapy, we support the client by seeing the patterns of distress and training the client how to be with their body's physiological states without being caught in the quagmire, even as we are with their fear of being stuck in the shame.

This is generally the hardest part for our clients. Having trained themselves not to know what they need, they are confident that they will be disappointed, or shamed for their needs. Doing this, they turn the valve of their hearts' longing off so tight they no longer know what they need. For them, having a need is shameful. Needing comfort is horrifying. Wanting reassurance is a desire set up to be ridiculed and humiliated. With this backdrop, we begin the repair, inviting our clients to slowly open to what they might need. It might simply be to face the truth of the suffering, while at the same time offering a safe haven for them to explore this pain with you.

What then might the antidote be? What helps someone be with the undercurrent of need that is arising? In response to the inquiry, clients throw out big answers, "Someone to love me," or "A job that will cover all my bills and a boss that doesn't humiliate me." All those are true but we, and they, can't meet that need in this moment. To pick up on the importance of the present moment discussed in the last chapter, what does this person need, right in this moment? Right now, when they are sitting with us, grappling with this distress? The need might be as simple as safe touch, with one's own hand on the heart, a soft breath as Mindful Self-Compassion practices do (Neff & Germer, 2014) or letting you see how bad it is inside their heart and body. Addressing the need in the moment has no rote answer. Needs arise fresh, raw, and threatening. To inoculate shame, we learn to metabolize it. The practices of self-compassion guide us in creating a buffer zone to antidote shame (Germer, 2009; Gilbert & Choden, 2014; Neff, 2011). Meridith used the Mindful Self-Compassion practices I taught her to be with her "old friends." As she said, "You know, after all this good stuff happening to me, I found myself at home, my husband and kids downstairs, I was getting ready for bed, and I heard my thoughts: I'm ugly, nobody loves me, I'm fat, I'm never going to amount to anything. I heard those thoughts and was startled. They were almost reassuring. Crazy, right? Here they were, saying all these negative things to me, but somehow they were kind of comforting. I sat with that and realized they were like my old friends; friends I had outgrown a long time ago, but didn't really leave behind."

THE LITERATURE ON SHAME

Of late, there is a wealth of study on shame (Fisher, 2015; Gilbert& Miles, 2002; Kaufman, 1989; Nathanson, 1992; Tangney & Dearing, 2002): exploring how shame exists in a world of parental humiliation and rejection (Stuewig and McCloskey, 2005); shame in dealing with sexual abuse (Feiring & Taska, 2005), and dissociation (Fisher, 2015, in press); shame resulting in obsessive rumination, especially in depression (Cheung, Gilbert, & Irons, 2004); and how shame and criticism from others can result in cortisol stress responses (Dickerson & Kemeny, 2004). Benau (2013), Fisher (2015), and Gilbert & Irons (2005) are all exploring clinical applications to shame.) There are studies defining the phenomenology of shame and guilt (Tangney & Dearing, 2002), specifying the underlying motivational systems (Gilbert & Choden, 2014), the organization of cognitive and emotional processing distinctions between them, as well as internal and external shame.

Parsing out the conceptual understandings of shame, Paul Gilbert's Compassion Focused Therapy (CFT, 1997, 1998, 2003) model describes the aggressive defense to shame that triggers dominating behaviors, while a submissive response to shame would be to hide, avoid, curl up the body, lower the eyes in response to external situations. External shame occurs when we fear, worry, believe or have had actual experiences of others viewing the self in a negative fashion or with feelings of anger and contempt, leaving a felt experience of being unwanted, unattractive, reject-able, or in some way open to attack by others. With those experiences the world feels unsafe and unwelcoming. Internal shame (Gilbert, 2003; Lewis, 1992) comes as we evaluate ourselves as flawed, broken, or bad in one or many ways, resulting in high self-criticism. And of course, there is always the option to fuse external and internal shame together, into what Lewis calls the "exposed self."

There is a difference between shame and guilt (Tangney & Dearing, 2002; Gilbert, 2010) and even what Benau (2013) calls "self-righting shame." Guilt produces feelings of remorse and sorrow while shame generates anxiety and anger. This can be explained by describing what happens when one apologizes "out of" guilt versus shame. Perhaps because shame is more physiologically destabilizing, when someone apologizes from an internalized shame, the apology might not come across as remorseful, but rather as an attempt to get the other person to feel better about the one who did wrong, thus allaying the desperate disintegration of self that comes. As one of my clients says, "It doesn't feel 'clean.' It feels like there's an ulterior motive." With guilt, however, there tends to be more mentalization, when apologizing, sometimes producing genuine remorse, while maintaining a relational connection between the ones involved.

Shame is one of the biggest blocks to affiliative emotions (Gilbert, 2009b, 2010), even as healing shame happens best when in connection with safe others who offer kindness, understanding, support, and validation. Benau (2013) claims that the paradox of shame is that one connects to the shaming other (internal or external) and disconnects from one's core self. From his point of view, it helps to distinguish the active and passive shaming that occurs: active shaming coming from either an introject or from an external person ("You little piece of . . .") and passive shaming from the failure to be seen, recognized, or responded to when we are in our core self-state.

SAFE HAVEN. SECURE BASE.

Shame arises when the natural urge for connection is chronically rejected or dismissed. Bowlby (1969) articulated two main functions of the attachment system. Those provided with a "secure base" have a felt experience of protection and safety when vulnerability and tenderness arise. This engages the exploratory impulse to engage in the world with curiosity, seeing the world with fresh eyes. A "safe haven" gives us a respite to return to, when the inevitable turbulence of stepping beyond the comfort zone becomes disquieting. Batson (1991) suggests this evolves out of an empathic stance toward suffering, allowing perspective taking, and sensitivity to the inner world and the inner life of another. Having a larger perspective, that includes the heart and mind of oneself and awareness of others, reduces suffering and distress (Germer &Neff, 2014).

These attachment underpinnings imprinted in the very young form the body's understanding of how the world is constructed. Sue Gerhardt eloquently writes, in *Why Love Matters: How affection shapes a baby's brain* (2004), "We are not aware of our own assumptions, but they are there, based on earliest experiences. And the most crucial assumption of them all is that others will be emotionally available to help and process feelings, to provide comfort when it is needed . . . to help regulate feelings" (p. 24). Our present reality is often shadowed by the Internal Working Model in which we are unconsciously remembering "gist," if not historical truth, through body and emotional memories that point to particular experience, encoded at an earlier age (Beckes, IJzerman, Tops, 2015; Brown, Elliott, et al., 2016). The indelible imprinting can't be taken as historical fact, yet they provide a doorway into understanding. In IFS, this doorway becomes a "trailhead" to follow. In yoga, these are the fluctuations of the mind (*citta-vrttis*) that we are looking to ease.

Our early experiences influence our ways of being in relationship as we get older, and affect the wider context of social relationships shared between friends and groups in general (Cacioppo & Patrick, 2008; Mikulincer & Shaver, 2007). Developing a solid sense of self as an adult is a complex form of interrelating maturational tasks including: self-other distinctions; learning how to form alliances; belonging to groups; working in teams; developing sexual identity; relating to and caring for others as intimate partners or parents; and developing a sense of self-authority and self-worth. So much of this has to do with who we are in connection to others, how they perceive us and how we exist or imagine ourselves to exist in the minds of others, and balancing competitive urges with sorting and caring for oneself and others. This is almost impossible to do, authentically anyway, if we first haven't experienced the loving gaze and the body memories of affectionate care and being positively held in the mind of another (Schore, 1994; Trevarthen & Aitken, 2001). This longing, this "wanting to be chosen" (Barkow, 1989) continues throughout life (Hrdy, 2009), unless the protective strategies have successfully truncated the preemptive force of this connective tissue.

NOT GETTING AFFILIATIVE NEEDS MET

Attachment wounding, especially in the early years, negatively effects the infant's felt experience and affiliative memories (of warmth and emotional soothing), giving rise to anxiety and depression (Bowlby, 1969, 1973, 1980; Mikulincer and Shaver, 2010). Not getting what is needed brings forth a strong protest, which at first focuses attention on getting that one thing that is the focus of need. If there isn't any resolution the infant/child/adult becomes exhausted and psychologically lost, disconnected from self. In turn, that becomes unbearable. Turning off those distress signals becomes essential for new strategies to form, conserving resources and filtering out signaling, which in turn reduces the positive impulses to reach out, explore, and down-regulate positive affect (Aposhyan, 2004; Corrigan, 2014; Corrigan, Wilson, & Fay, 2014a; Gilbert, 2007).

Affiliative psychology (Depue & Morrone-Strupinsky, 2005; Gilbert & Choden, 2014) presents a neurobiological model based on several decades of psychological and neuroscience literature review, stressing that we are not "affiliative robots." Even as our first reflexes are automatic, we expand in complexity without simplistic cause and effect. Depue and Morrone-Strupinsky delineate two kinds of rewards: appetitive and consummatory. Appetitive rewards are associated with distal stimuli, such as smell, color, shape, or temperature. Consummatory rewards are unconditioned proximal stimuli, including light touch, grooming, mating, and so on. If we haven't been lucky enough to receive and be rewarded with kind touch, gentle humming, soothing sounds, or environments that cushion our developing bodies, minds, and hearts we may well tend toward threat-based protection strategies, protecting even as those very strategies keep out just that for which we so desperately long. We effectively learn to mute and numb out the basic longing for connection.

Those who come to us for therapy generally haven't had this kind of caring, or kind physical, emotional, or psychological attention and can be negatively activated by kindness. Their attachment systems, not grounded in affiliation, will activate aversive emotional memories of trauma and neglect (Bowlby, 1973, 1980). This erodes the natural body movements of yielding, reaching, grasping (Aposhyan, 2004, 2007, 2014; Bainbridge-Cohen, 1984) and provides the structure for less desirable metacognitive beliefs to form (Gilbert, 2010), those of not being worth connection, not deserving kindness, compassion, goodness, and perceiving oneself as a "loser" or a "failure," or not needing the normal, natural body-heart-mind warmth.

Gilbert describes three Affect Regulation Systems in the Compassion Focused Therapy (2009b, 2009c, 2010) model that help clients orient to their emotional world:

- *Threat- and self-protection-focused system:* evolutionarily we have a system to detect threat and enable self-protection, giving capacity to attend to, process, and respond to threats. These threat-based emotions include anger, anxiety, and disgust. Defensive behaviors include fight, flight, submission, and freeze.
- *Drive, seeking-, and acquisition-focused system:* we also have built-in systems that enable us to orient to and pay attention to advantageous resources as well as tendencies to activate experiences of pleasure in pursuing and securing those resources.
- *Contentment-, soothing-, and affiliative-focused system:* especially important for those with trauma and attachment wounding is the system that enables states of peacefulness and openness when not threat focused or seeking resources, allowing the body/mind/heart to be satisfied and experience positive well-being. This system is linked to soothing, safeness and affiliative behavior, allowing parasympathetic responses, calm mind, and coming into balance.

Affiliative connections down-regulate the threat system (Gilbert and Irons, 2005), allowing safeness to be established enough that people can engage in exploratory behaviors, mentalize, reflect, and change (Allen & Fonagy, 2008; Liotti & Gilbert, 2011; Wallin, 2007). Kristin Neff and Chris Germer's Mindful Self-Compassion training provides a step-by-step process of developing safe compassionate connection to oneself (Germer & Neff, 2014). Compassion Focused Therapy (Gilbert, 2010) cultivates a compassionate self; Internal Family Systems (Schwartz, 1994) connects the client with their Self-energy; Accelerated Experiential Dynamic Psychotherapy (Fosha, 2000) works through safe connection to a therapist.

DISCOMFORT WITH AND FEARS OF DEVELOPING COMPASSION

Why then do we not all flock to developing this counterpoint to shame, becoming more compassionate, more respectful of others, more open and loving and kind to people, including ourselves? It's sort of a conundrum, isn't it? I recently posed this question to a group I was leading over the course of many weeks. Confronted with the question, honestly exploring the inquiry, people spoke of fearing that what they long for couldn't be. They spoke of the reality that they never had this safety, this sense of connection, this kind of body ease. Never having it, they asked, why would there be a different outcome now? These are the questions that Paul Gilbert and his colleagues (Gilbert, McEwan, Catarino, Baião, & Palmeira, 2014; Gilbert, McEwan, Matos, & Rivis, 2011) have explored over the years, developing measures to sort out fears of compassion from others, for others, and for the self. I'm sure it comes as no surprise that the fear of compassion for oneself is highly correlated with not having received compassion from others. This is linked to experiencing self-coldness, self-criticism, and depression (Gilbert, et al., 2011). Even the thought of warmth and care coming toward our clients can trigger beliefs of not deserving these very qualities (or any other positive quality for that matter). Held with a compassionate stance, someone's nervous system might activate a grief response for all that hasn't been there or for their own disconnection from how important this is for them. There's also the fear of "Who will I be?" without this protective layer of self-critical or shame-based schemas. Yet underneath the fear, attachment theory, Compassion Focused Therapy, Accelerated Experiential Dynamic Psychotherapy, and yoga psychology each urge us to remember the inherent longing for connection, for the warmth that folds us into security and reassurance, letting us know that even in the midst of the world falling apart, our urge is toward proximity and contact with others.

THE THERAPEUTIC TASK OF HEALING SHAME

Clinically, healing shame happens as a person develops a larger container than the one they had to constrict into. Held in a larger force field of real and imagined compassion (not dissimilar to the African tribe described above) a person can find ways, internally and externally, to antidote shame and the suffering that goes with it. The attachment mechanisms that are broken in our clients affect how they think and feel about themselves, tending toward the negative impulses of feeling worthless, unwanted, or thrown away. The therapeutic task is to fearlessly hold our client's suffering, while inviting them to walk with us through this distress together. Imagination can play an enormous helping hand, as we encourage, motivate, and facilitate our clients to turn toward more positive images (Brown, 2013; Brown, Elliott, et al., 2016; Falconer, Rovira, King, et al., 2016; Falconer, Slater, Rovira, King, Gilbert, et al., 2014). As someone develops new, more nourishing internal working models that activate secure attachment, shame is buffered, becoming less invasive, and therefore more able to be explored and unburdened. Self-compassion, and the compassion of safe others, helps inoculate the shame of our clients. The more our clients open to the possible reservoir of self-compassion, the more they reduce the crushing moments, collapsing completely, being sucked away by the powerful undertow of shame. Self-compassion provides a wedge, allowing our clients to unfreeze enough to have a tiny sip of breath, keeping them from getting swept into the utter cacophony of pain. Self-compassion then is not a conceptual understanding, but a practice to ease the suffering of the heart, right now, inside all of us, in the present moment.

YOGA AND SELF-COMPASSION

As a person builds a bigger, better, stronger internal and external self-container of connection, belongingness, and self-compassion, the toxicity of shame is remedied. At first, connections and attachments to the therapist buffer the shame, so that it can be therapeutically shifted. Over time that psychological buffer expands, creating a force field of compassion and kindness that eases and then softly releases the toxic grip of shame. As a client understands that their body is not just one singular seething cauldron of distress, they develop psychological distinctions that help untangle the horrid felt experience of shame. Children brought up in a psychologically secure environment generally have these foundational principles cultivated in the family system through repetition of implicit and explicit guidance. This builds character over time, forming a container for the self to develop, creating safe boundaries for the heart to open and be nourished. As a child learns that she can make mistakes and still be loved she is enveloped in a secure base. These character traits can be cultivated (Brooks, 2015; Brown, 2013; Peterson & Seligman, 2004). Doing so allows self-compassion to more easily arise. For trauma survivors, this waters their arid inner world, countering the self-hatred that's constantly fulminating on the sidelines.

THE YAMAS AND NIYAMAS

For those with difficult histories, entering the internal world stimulates awareness of needs, activates longing for native attachment urges, and opens the door to backdraft (Germer, 2009). Therapy can unburden the alarm, but the painful reality is that our clients generally need time to adjust, to buffer the shame from not having had these needs met, and to learn to live in a different world, one in which their needs matter. Their nervous system is invaded by shame, day in and day out. Learning practices of cushioning the heart, filling their inner and outer environment with the *sattvic* energy of compassion and kindness, eases the intense vulnerability of suffering alone.

This kind of lifelong practice is addressed in yoga as one develops protective riverbanks of ethical and characterological orientations called *yamas* (nonviolence, truthfulness, nonstealing, energy management, trusting) and *niyamas* (purity, contentment, self-discipline, self-study, surrender). These form the first two limbs of Patanjali's Eight Limbs of Yoga, providing internal and external "restraints" that build a container for the self and safe boundaries for the heart to open and be nourished. In this training of the mind and heart, to embrace suffering, turning toward kindness, self-compassion arises as a byproduct of practice watering an arid inner world, countering the self-hatred and traumatic pain that for many constantly threatens to invade every moment. The *yamas* and *niyamas* create a buffer zone, a force field to contain physiological distress, so the shame doesn't have to cripple a person.

In the traditional teacher-student relationships of yoga, the *yamas* and *niyamas* are part of the everyday relationship developing character before moving into later forms of practice. Anyone having watched *The Karate Kid* will remember the teacher telling the student, "wax on, wax off" (Adele, 2009). Repeating that over and over, the young student's character is formed. This is true with any practice; it takes repetition to carve out a new neural pathway.

The *yamas* provide skills for positively restraining the full force of *prana*, organizing and training the mind, heart, and body into a balanced way of living in the world.

Ahimsa is the practice of nonviolence or nonharming. Within the obvious ways of practicing nonviolence are small baby steps to develop courage, balance, vulnerability, and self-love (Adele, 2009). This moment-to-moment practice encourages us to be with the background noise of our being. What is the automatic response when good things happen, or when we do or say things that we're not happy with? How are we with our neighbors, or the bus driver, or the client who raged at us, or wants special considerations, or didn't pay their bill? When our parts are active and unyielding, how can we engage and hold them nonviolently? *Ahimsa* challenges us to find the least harmful ways to move through the day. In the excruciatingly painful experience of shame, what would be a simple, kind, internal, or external expression to help inch away from shame? For trauma survivors, *ahimsa* helps a kinder, less harsh, more *sattvic* energy emerge, so that courage and strength can develop without fear of being humiliated, submissive, or dominated. The self-compassion break described at the end of the chapter helps build and strengthen a nonviolent field.

Satya is the practice of truthfulness, and can be seen as authentic self-expression going hand in hand with the practice of nonviolence. When shame takes hold we only listen to the physiological pain of *samskaras* opening. At those times it's impossible (in the beginning) to not get identified with and caught in the cyclone of painful schemas. *Satya* asks us to hold onto the underlying truth that exists under the shame: we are whole and unbroken, despite the barrage of physiological distress that floods our system. As therapists, we provide *satya* to our clients as we remind them, over and over again a thousand different ways, of small acts of kindness, thoughtfulness, or consideration they make to themselves or others.

Asteya refers to nonstealing, that is, not taking what hasn't been freely given. From a psychological viewpoint, it inquires how we steal from our own inner storehouse of goodness. When we think badly of ourselves, putting ourselves down, we're stealing from the reservoir of our true nature. Instead of directing love and kindness back to ourselves we're stealing it.

Brahmacharya, though narrowly defined as celibacy, has a broader definition of energy management. Managing the nervous system to not be swept under a shame tsunami is a vital skill. The inquiry with *brahmacharya* is to be with our body when there is an explosion of energy churning through every system of body, mind, and heart. *Brahmacharaya* coaxes us to learn sensate language, shifting away from huge explanations or experiences of shame into smaller, more bite-sized components. This allows us to learn to trust the burning instead of roiling in memories of humiliation of some previous time or projecting nightmarish scenarios into the future. When there's a wide-open firehose of energy, which happens with shame, we are asked to reach, often feebly at first, toward trust that life can be more nourishing, even as shame roars unendingly through the heart and body.

Aparigraha is the practice that releases the grab at life, people, and situations. This *yama* is about developing trust that *prana* is moving us steadfastly toward a more nourishing and sustaining life. *Aparigraha* encourages those parts of us that cling to people, places, and things, asking us to loosen the fearful grip, to explore the subtle nature of breath, bones, muscles, and heart. This *yama* trains us to come home to the heart, building an internal locus of control from which we then learn to more deeply trust the unfolding of the healing process.

Character and spiritual support come from the *niyamas*, which are the practices that build wise character:

Sauca is the purity and clarity of how we can be with ourselves and with others. It builds on the foundation of the *yamas*, requiring trust that we are more than our wounds. *Sauca* is the faith that there's more, even when our patterns tell us there isn't. It's about turning toward the simple, small things that nourish, instead of grabbing onto old, familiar, no longer satisfying ways of being. To hold ourselves with *sauca*, we develop perspective, repeatedly asking the parts of us that muddy clarity to give us room to remember who is underneath the distress.

Santosha is the contentment that comes when we're with life as it is. The inquiry here is to tenderly hold vulnerabilities, making it safe to live from and in the heart. Contentment then is an experiment with self-valuing instead of striving to be someone else or squeeze ourselves into a someone we think we should be. With contentment comes an easing of the viscera making the body an easier home to live in.

Tapas is the burning heat of self-discipline to stay focused as inner ground is cleared. Healing is an Olympian task, requiring enormous discipline, focus, and dedication to find the way through. Developing *tapas* helps deal with the many parts that try to convince us that change is not worth it. *Tapas* is the discipline of holding *prana* as it moves through *samskaras*, cleansing and clearing.

Svadhyaya is the practice of self-reflection, growing and developing beyond any wounded identity. It requires a capacity to steer the heart and mind toward where you want to go, instead of being caught up in the stories we have. Reading, writing, contemplating the wisdom in spiritual texts, workshops and trainings, or self-help books encourages reflection, and exploring how these truths map onto our own experience.

Ishvarapranidhana is the contemplation of the sacred nature of life, surrendering to what is. This is the cultivation of compassion in everyday life. A contemporary, and recent, expression of this was the grace shown in Charleston, South Carolina, when nine church members and their pastor were gunned down. Teaching the nation about redemption happened as the community of faith was able to forgive the killer. I say this with a caveat that for many of our clients being with the sacred nature of life isn't necessarily always about forgiveness, but rather to be fully with ourselves even when we're not ready to forgive. This *niyama* is to hold our hearts, surrendering to whatever life circumstance we are in with grace, love, and compassion.

These interwoven qualities and ways of being are practices for a lifetime, building an internal structure to hold and develop an earned secure attachment for the heart to open into tenderness and vulnerability. Discipline, *tapas*, helps keep us focused on healing, and is instrumental in steering the mind and the heart, regulating the felt experience. Along the way, the *niyama* of *svadhyaya* studies the felt experience of the body, untangling thoughts, feelings, and body sensations. *Svadhyaya* helps clients use therapy and helpful reading and courses to shift the painful stories that continue to replicate patterns of pain. This takes a commitment and dedication to cultivating their Self/Higher Power/Wise Being/true nature or sacred source. Over time these practices benefit the client, bringing a greater percentage of *sattvic* (serene and balanced energy) into the body and heart. As the inner garden is weeded of self-critical thoughts, envy of others, and reality distortions, a more beneficial felt experience is cultivated inside, which is also mirrored in the outside reality. Shifting the automatic negativity bias provides protective riverbanks for *prana* to flow more smoothly, watering the seeds of *sattvic* energy, making room for compassion to naturally take root.

I learned this the hard way. In the intensity of my own trauma history erupting I found *metta* (loving kindness) retreats a necessary antidote. With an activated nervous system, I would sit at the Insight Meditation Society in Barre, Maine. I had a difficult time slowing down into Patanjali's four positive attitudes (1:33) and what Theravada Buddhism calls the *Brahma Viharas* (heavenly abodes of the mind). May I be happy. May I be at peace. May I live with ease. May I be free from suffering. The phrases provoked the "reality" that I was not doing well. Metta practice, however, is to cultivate the qualities of loving kindness despite what is being activated. I needed the *niyama* of *tapas* (discipline) to orient consistently and persistently toward what I wanted: to be at peace even while realizing I wasn't. *Ahimsa,* nonviolence, gave me a foothold. Rather than trying to force myself to have an experience that I wasn't having, which would have felt more difficult and create resistance, the *yama* of nonviolence guided the practice.

CULTIVATING SELF-COMPASSION

The best counterpoint to the levels of reactivity and toxicity that shame engenders is the cultivation of compassion and self-compassion (Germer, 2009; Gilbert & Choden, 2014, Neff, 2011). Science has been developing a wealth of research on the benefits of these principles, yet what is it? "Compassion can be defined as behavior that aims to nurture, look after, teach, guide, mentor, soothe, protect, offer feelings of acceptance and belonging in order to benefit another person" (Gilbert, 2010, p. 217). Differing from kindness or empathy, compassion includes the intention and motivation to alleviate suffering (Germer, 2009; Gilbert, 2010 Keltner, 2009; Neff, 2011), not by fixing, changing, or giving advice, but rather by being mindfully with the suffering. When someone is suffering—and shame is one of the most excruciating forms of psychological suffering—we need to first befriend the intensity of suffering before we can even entertain anything else.

Self-compassion is one of the first steps in forging a life worth living, especially for those whose lives have been caught in the wounds of distress. People start to find ways to move toward a more satisfying life as they shift from an isolated life, caught in the swirl of the past, and begin to practice and cultivate an alternative path. Rather than being stopped by an encrusted fearful attitude toward life, compassionate practices and perspectives motivate and are linked to well-being (Gilbert, McEwan, Catarino, Baiao, & Palmeira, 2014). Practicing self-compassion shifts a passively oriented perspective, to deliberately orient to the inner and outer worlds in new ways, forming habits to soften defenses and befriend aversive feelings.

This more psychologically active stance promotes a foundation for what the AAI calls an "earned secure" style (Brown, Elliott, et al., 2016) where curiosity and exploration are native traits, knowing there will be reassurance and support even if life goes amok. Contrary to fears people can have, compassion is not about becoming passive and becoming stuck in negative loops, but rather fosters positive emotions by embracing the negative. In having a compassionate connection to other people who are suffering, we feel less alone, giving room to welcome suffering, allowing a percolating sense of enjoyment, finding meaning, optimism, and wisdom rather than merely surviving provides a renewed sense of hope for future steps in encountering the world (Heffernan, Quinn Griffin, McNulty, & Fitzpatrick, 2010; Hollis-Walker & Colosimo, 2011; Neff, Kirkpatrick, & Rude, 2007). In fact, despite people's fears that they would become passive and decrease any motivation to change, Gilbert, McEwan, Matos, & Rivis (2011) and Neff (2004) found that self-compassion reduced maladaptive perfectionism, making failure less risky (Neff, Hsieh, & Dejitterat, 2005). Remarkably, practicing self-compassion helped people try again even when they failed (Neely, et al., 2009) and to have greater motivation and willingness to shift mistakes into possibilities (Breines & Chen, 2010).

Kristin Neff, the self-compassion researcher at the University of Texas/Austin, describes three components to "self-compassion" (2011). The first is mindfulness: we need to know we're suffering. If we aren't aware we're suffering, there's nothing we can do about it. When we come to terms with the universality of suffering we encounter the second component, our common humanity: everyone suffers. The person next to you might not suffer in the same way, but they have known suffering in one form or another. The third component is meeting that suffering with kindness. Rather than responding with defensive strategies locked in by shame, self-compassion nudges us to develop warmth and understanding in the face of suffering, failing, or insecurity. The self-compassion break Germer and Neff (2013, 2014) developed, described in more detail in a subsequent section, has us move right toward the moment of suffering. This isn't an intellectual exercise, but a movement into the felt moment of suffering. Like Karen at the beginning of the chapter, the practice is to open to what is happening in the moment. Here it is. Here I am. I'm suffering. Right here in the body, in this moment. The practice is not to marinate in the suffering, stuck in that dreadful reality, but rather to soften into the fact of life: that all of us, humans, animals, all sentient beings—all of us suffer. In this place of suffering, we are connected. We are not alone. Holding these two realities, we can provide an antidote. Open to the suffering, feeling into it for the unmet need that has been shut down, there's room to respond in simple ways, to mitigate the suffering.

After practicing the Self-Compassion Break in therapy, Janice said, "Sometimes it [the self-hating part] listens and sometimes it doesn't. The instruction is so simple—to give ourselves the antidote, but really, it takes a really, really, long time to be able to acknowledge that I'm suffering—to catch myself in the moment when I'm dying inside. Usually I just fall apart. My practice now is to catch the moment, and hold it, building a dam against all the story of how worthless I am so that I can stop myself and know that right now, I'm suffering. Catch myself in that moment where suffering is being generated. I'm just off and running so quickly. I've slowly been able to catch it, more easily than ever before. Which is a huge relief."

At some point in therapy, after testing the waters to see if it's safe, our clients will humbly admit their vulnerable need to love and be loved. Confronting protective strategies is easier when the client feels held in the compassion and trust of the therapeutic relationship. The client comes to know that it's an innate need, this utterly normal and natural want to be loved. Automatic tendencies to protect are softened, and the person's nervous system eases.

CLINICAL APPLICATIONS FOR HEALING SHAME

In the therapy hour, confronted with the acuteness of suffering, we find ourselves needing to reduce the pain on demand. Untangling the physiological horror unfortunately doesn't come quickly or easily. We can unburden some of the alarm in a session, but the painful reality is our clients need to develop a practice of opening cultivating compassion. Learning to buffer shame with positive qualities day in and day out cushions the heart, filling inner and outer environments with serenity, kindness, and compassion.

Ken Benau, a therapist in Kensington, California, and associate clinical professor at UC Berkeley's Graduate Program in Clinical Science, tells us the most important element of healing shame is being able to separate enough from the shame so that it's not overwhelming. If our clients can't witness the felt experience of shame nothing else can happen. As he says in a podcast (2013), "When we're in the shame, we feel it's me and there's nothing that isn't me." Benau's experience with adolescents and adults urges us to develop a relationship with shame which is not about getting rid of it but witnessing (as the IFS model also has us do) the shame that a part of us is holding, what happened to cause it, what the part is trying to accomplish, and what it's fears are. Ken's approach asks his clients to get in touch with their best self, and from that place, looking at the shame and developing a relationship with it.

It goes without saying that any practice is easier when one is not in acute pain. In a therapy session I ask clients to think of a difficult time, though not the worst moment they've ever been in. For the purposes of practicing, this could be a three, four, or a five on a Subjective Unit of Distress (SUDs) scale of zero to ten (ten being the worst). It doesn't help anyone to plummet down a shame hole when trying to learn something. Offer reminders to be gentle with the process and to reel in the understandable desire to "make it all better right now." Dealing with something in the three to five out of ten range allows there to be breathing room, so that "learner parts" can stay on board instead of being hijacked by the pain.

ANJALI MUDRA

Many clients struggle with giving themselves compassion. In groups with enough safety, they'll ask, "Why is it so hard to accept compassion from myself or others?" Rather than fight the resistance, I've found it helpful to work with one of Patanjali's ideas of cultivating the opposite (II:33). With attachment and trauma wounding we want to cultivate what is the nourishing opposite. When working with resistance, especially resistance to positive qualities like kindness, safe connection, or compassion, I invite the client to try an adapted version of Anjali mudra practice, putting the "resistant" part in one hand, while exploring a Nourishing Opposite to put in the other. This offers a way to explore the polarities that every situation offers, perhaps on one hand, a judging part, and on the other, a part that longs for kindness; or a part that is terrified and a part that longs for love. People generally swing between different poles, finding ease difficult. In this practice the inquiry brings polarities together while finding a new center of gravity in the heart.

I used this one day in a session with Andi, as she struggled internally. I asked her to get a felt sense of one of the struggling parts and to imagine holding that part in one hand. To help her sort this out, I offered her a menu of what that part might be like: was it a blob, a shape, a certain age? Or might it be a wise part, a part that knows about kindness and compassion. I encouraged her to feel that nourishing part in her hand, letting it come alive energetically. Then I had her imagine another part in her other hand, perhaps a hurting part, a wounded part, one that longs to be loved and reassured. Throughout the practice, I reassured her that there was no right way to do this, that this was an inquiry, a way to explore these different parts of her, to bring integration. Externalizing the parts in this way helped Andi to get a felt sense of their differences and similarities, taking the energy out of her body to give her some space. Letting her take her time, I then suggested that she bring her attention to her heart at the same time as she was holding these two parts in her hands. Holding that attentional triad (two hands and her heart) I also had her feel the strength of her spine. Inviting her thoughtful attention, I guided her to feel the energy of all three points (hands and heart/

spine), while slowly bringing her hands together. I suggested that she pay attention to feeling what happened in her hands, her heart, and her spine; taking her time allowed her to notice the subtle energies there. When her hands came together at her heart, I wondered aloud with her if there was an offering she wanted to make to these parts.

Having fought the idea of compassion and kindness without being able to articulate why, I was curious to hear about her experience. Andi looked up, surprised. "I had a really good experience that I didn't expect. I have never done that before, taking two parts, one calm, sane, centered, which is the part I'd love to be more often, and the other part that gets triggered, not connected, not sure what it's saying, basically mouthing off. It's the part that causes me a lot of shame. I hate getting anywhere near that part. When that happens, I'm not aware, not tuned into what I'm saying or who I'm talking to. I so didn't want to do this, but when I started to bring them together—and it helped that you had me slow down—the weird thing is, they liked each other. If these two parts met they would like each other, and then I got this really good feeling, warm. I can't believe it."

Other people like Maddie have at times reported: "It was hard. I felt really resistant to giving in—having one part giving in to the other part. I didn't want to bring them together. I wanted to stay hurt." I asked her, "What makes it feel hard?" Maddie replied that those feelings made her feel out of control. I reminded her of what we had been reviewing the week before, that feelings have a cycle of rising, cresting, and falling. When we give space to feelings without clamping down they have room to complete their cycle. Trying it again, Maddie found, "Since there's no way to do it wrong. I had two wounded parts from different ages, and in this exercise they got introduced together, and became friends. They were like, 'Hey, me too!' I know my whole life across the whole continuum, but how did they not know each other? That sounds weird, but now they're friends."

It's in the mutual retooling of therapy that our client's nervous system, slowly reorients toward kindness, gentleness, and goodness. The past ruptures get repaired in the field of compassion. Their center of gravity shifts from protection against yet another moment of mean-spiritedness, instead opening the tender heart that was always there, buried under the pain. Melissa shared about how much she argued with herself, listing all the reasons why she shouldn't give herself compassion, why she wasn't worthy of it. She then surprised herself by arguing back with that part, fiercely defending her longing to be free of self-hatred. Melissa attributed this slight opening to the years of being with her therapist through thick and thin. The "safe haven" of therapy allowed her to explore new possibilities, opening to this crushing shame, knowing there was a safe other to return to if it all went bad.

To do this, though, our clients have to face the fear of vulnerability, something that was not allowed when growing up. As Annabelle said, "I know now that kindness makes me feel safer, but that old program is ingrained in me to hold onto my protection, just in case things get scary." Tony's version of this is, "I'm afraid I'll be caught unawares and not be ready. This person will hit me with meanness, and I'll die inside. Better to keep tough and not allow anyone in. It's too much, otherwise."

MINDFUL SELF-COMPASSION BREAK

Years ago, in the 1980s, I went to a talk that Steven and Ondrea Levine gave on compassion. I left that workshop completely distraught, realizing I had no idea what compassion was and no clue about how to be compassionate to myself. Rattled by this, I made the long trek home to Lenox, Massachusetts, where I was a resident at Kripalu Center. The drive on Interstate 95 was stressful even back then. The drive, combined with the residue left from the talk, hit me out of the blue. I found myself sobbing, pulling over into the breakdown lane, broken open by the lack of compassion I had for myself.

The Mindful Self-Compassion Break (Germer & Neff, 2014) gives a simple access route to learn self-compassion. There are three components to the MSC Break: first to acknowledge the pain, second to connect to the reality that we all suffer—recognizing that it's part of our common humanity—and third, to offer ourselves a simple moment of kindness. Encountering suffering, we notice what the underlying need is that isn't getting met. Perhaps it's kindness, or peace, or trusting that maybe this painful place will change. The practice invites us to look into our own suffering, responding with kindness and care to this place in us that suffers, held in an understanding that suffering is part of being human.

This practice was something that Gulia practiced in a variety of ways, to help her build a force field of compassion inside and around her. One day Gulia talked about being in a situation where she immediately felt some shame, noticing how an exiled part shut her down and cut off all her emotions, numbing her. Slowly, she externalized the part of her that shut her down by imagining separating from it, like taking off an old comfortable sweater and placing it in her lap. Having a sense of distance, we explored the IFS practice of asking how she felt toward that part, to activate positive attachment. At first she wasn't able to do that at all, but over time she could feel a sense of interest, curiosity, and even some compassion for it. Creating an internal intrapsychic connection, IFS explores if the exiled part can feel the interest or compassion. In Gulia's case, she could sometimes but not others. We found we had to slow the process down even more. The Self-Compassion Break helped her do that. Gulia acknowledged the first step: she was suffering. Then she would repeat, over and over, almost as if she was only now realizing the reality of her suffering, "Right now, I'm suffering. Right now, I'm suffering." Doing that helped her put a wedge in her tendency to run over the suffering, finding stories and explanations to move away from the felt experience.

Eddie used the Self-Compassion Break practice to realize, "I'm a very generous person, but I have a difficult time giving to myself. I'm loyal to others, understanding of their flaws, but have really high expectations of myself. As you suggested doing the Self -Compassion Break, I argued with myself about why I shouldn't give myself compassion. Then I had a part that argued back with that part! With that, I was able to find the antidote—I had to bring in that other, to give reasons why I deserved to be compassionate with myself. Gosh, it's so hard."

Learning to move away from protective mechanisms, to instead drop into the heart of self-compassion, is both hard and nourishing. Andi acknowledged this, "There's fear about changing into a person who is really vulnerable. I learned that growing up. When I try to be generous with myself, and try not to assume the worst about someone being with me, I end up feeling shamed and then angry with this person, for shaming me. I'm afraid I'll be caught unawares and not be ready, and this person will hit me with meanness and I'll be hurt. I would rather keep it tough. At the same time, I know now that kindness makes me feel safer. But there's still an old program that's ingrained, that I have to hold onto the protection; I need my old program in case things get scary."

CULTIVATING A FORCE FIELD OF COMPASSION

In addition to generating self-compassion, it's valuable to cultivate a felt experience of being surrounded by, and living in, a force field of compassion, to counteract the sense of isolation that comes with trauma. That isolation manifests in contraction, closing up, and in unconsciously pulling inwards, providing a protective pattern not necessarily needed in the present moment. With the focus in this book on the present moment, the orientation is to cultivate nascent mental, emotional, feeling states in the body that buffer the fierce swells of shame. The practice I use with clients uses visual representations to concretize new states externally, then to practice developing the felt experience that is associated with those images.

To help the client get started, I take a large piece of paper (poster size is best, or have them imagine a large piece of paper) and ask them to put themselves in the middle of it, either by drawing themselves or by bringing in a photo or another image that represents them. I then ask them to look for examples of compassion in their lives, of experiences they have had themselves, or through watching others, or even by listening to their longing of what compassion could be. As they gather these visual examples, they place the images around themselves on the poster board. People have drawn words and stick figures or used cut outs from magazines. They might have spiritual figures, many have used pets, some have used representations of music and songs that evoke certain qualities of compassion for them. Stretch yourself, I urge them. Focus on what it is you are looking for, find the small, sometimes insignificant moments, when you saw and felt compassion. What was that like to see or hear that outside of you? What does that feel like inside you when you see and hear that? The more examples, the more representations they gather, the more they then create this force field around them, buffering them.

Anne and I worked on this together. She had been struggling with the idea of compassion, pushing against it, claiming she didn't know what it was like. I led her in a guided meditation, which we taped (similar to the one below in the practice session), so that she could use this at home, especially since I was going to be away the following week. When I came back the next week, Anne brought in her patched-up, beautiful drawing, rolled, because she didn't want to have any folds in it. "This has become precious to me. I'm going to have it framed. I look at it, see those images, and practice taking that in. I want to stay in that place, to keep doing it, letting it grow bigger and bigger. There are times I find myself glowing from the inside," she says, as she starts to cry. "It was nice doing it with you, talking on the audio. It helped keep my mind focused."

SO HUM: MAKING ROOM FOR INTENSITY, RESISTANCE AND PAINFUL PARTS

Dissolving separation is an integral part of *advaita yoga*, the practice of nondualism (Klein, 1990; Miller, 2010, 2014, 2015; Maharshi, 1985; Nisargadatta, 1973;

Amelio, 1989/1994). The simple translation of the *So Hum* mantra, "I am" or "I am that" doesn't easily communicate the profound reality of nonseparation. One of my early *advaita* teachers, Thomas Amelio (*Shivanand*) describes the practice of *So Hum* as a "vast practice of spaciousness in which everything is included and there is no rejection or judgment or self-improvement. Repeating, 'I am . . . I am' over and over again can bring us into meditation of oneness, with no separation. We have the need to put an adjective to the end qualifying I am such as 'I am a mother, father, bookkeeper.' *So Hum* calls us to drop the need to identify with the quality and roles that we play. I am. We're called into the process of being instead of having to be someone (Amelio, 2015). To practice yoga, Don Stapleton, the Director of Nosara Yoga Institute, proposes that we be fully in the sacred relationship with our Self in which everything we perceive comes through this dynamic relationship (Stapleton, 2004, 2015). *So Hum* is that invitation to enter this dynamic relationship.

Dropping identity is difficult for all of us. When our body is full of distress and our mind is racked with mental constructs, prying identity from experience can feel like a big stretch. With clients who have shut down and closed themselves off to experiences and people, I offer this mantra as a way of integration, of reducing separation, of inviting in more spaciousness. "I am" or "I am that" proposes "that" is everything we encounter. This then is a practice of welcoming all parts of us and learning to be in relationship with all parts of others. Opening the arms is a gesture of welcoming. It encourages inclusion where we are part of the grand spaciousness, with no need of editing or censoring. Holding that perspective, *So Hum* includes: I am the irritation I feel. I am the protest I am having because of what you said. I am the terror that can engulf me. I am the hopelessness I feel. I am the incredible generosity that simple strangers offer to me. I am all of that.

The nice thing about this practice is that it's already something we're doing every day. The yogis say *So Hum* is the natural mantra occurring as the breath naturally inhales (*So*) and gently releases (*Hum*). When you sigh, you are making this sound effortlessly. In fact we often make this sound multiple times a day without knowing it's considered a mantra. To scaffold this practice and make it concrete, I invite clients to externalize an experience (for example, someone made me angry; there's something, some event I'm afraid of) or a quality that's triggering (fear, tenderness, care, compassion, worry, etc.), as described in the practice section below. Even when we want "it" to come from outside, we have layers of resistance keeping "it" out. This practice teaches a way to energetically, somatically concretize the quality, and bring it closer into experience.

CONCENTRATION PRACTICES

In the next section we'll delve into the whole arena of being in the body, using such practices to focus the mind, counteracting the extreme pull that shame exerts away from the present moment. The locus of shame buried in past schemas hijacks the person into the subjective experience of the past and blurs the boundary between past and present. This makes healing more complicated.

Concentration practices train the person to focus on one thing so closely that distractions fade into the periphery. There are times when trauma clients feel swallowed by the intensity of their symptoms, unable to separate from them. When the body is besieged with intensity a person needs a way to separate from the inner noise to get enough perspective to be with whatever tumult is occurring. This is a form of consciously and creatively using dissociation in a positive way. Training the mind to focus and concentrate is vital in getting enough perspective. Yoga describes two balancing energies of *citta* and *prana*. *Prana* is the flowing energy of life force, *citta* combines cognitive functions of intelligence, action, and the organizing function of the mind (Bryant, 2009). Concentration practices use *citta* to harness the incessant flow of *prana*. It is one of the many practices Sandy and I have been using to tackle the ferocity of her traumatic flashbacks. She has parts that hate everyone, including me. They live inside as seething, burning, energies that rail at the slightest intrusion. These parts hijack Sandy, in desperate attempts to get her to pay attention, to not let go of the "truth" as they see it.

Week after week, Sandy comes to therapy as these parts try to speak their fury through her. Her body wrenches in the chair, writhing with the pressure of coming into consciousness. Even as Sandy hangs onto her skilled and knowledgeable experience as an executive in the health field, her eyes lose focus, her body curling up into a ball, despite her best intentions. Repeatedly, we practice focusing her attention on the present, having her use her eyes to orient to external objects in the office and/or slowing down her breath, training her body to open up instead of shutting down, supporting her to make room for the burst of energy that turns her body into a rollercoaster. Focusing the mind on a small amount of information such as orienting to her breath in the moment, the books on the bookshelf, or the colors in the rug takes enormous effort. The result or narrowing attention over time is that the body/mind stabilizes into the present moment, pulled out of these past traumatic schemas. Once there is even a small amount of parasympathetic ease the body has a moment of rest. We're training the body to pause the cycle of traumatic activation. Pausing offers choice, building an internal platform to turn attention toward what is more nourishing, focusing on that, balancing intense body experiences. Sandy's next task will be to focus on one small thimbleful of the intense internal activation, drop the story, and ride only a tiny sliver of sensation on the bell curve to completion. That takes concentration and practice, to consistently slow down, focusing, not get distracted, and yield to the sensations rising inside.

Self-Compassion Practices

MEDITATION: SELF-COMPASSION BREAK*

Objective: *This meditation teaches clients to become aware of themselves when in a painful moment (mindfulness), then recognize that they are not alone, that everyone suffers. That there's a connection to a larger whole. In that moment of suffering lies an unmet need. The client explores what that is, and offers an antidote: "May I release this pain," or "May I be kinder to myself?"*

Kristin Neff developed the Self-Compassion Break, which can be used moment-to-moment to become aware of the suffering we are in and then practice ways to address the suffering in a new and nourishing way. There are three steps to the inquiry: Mindfulness, common humanity, and meeting one's need in the moment.

1. *Mindfulness:* The first step is to become aware that we're suffering. This develops the capacity for mindfulness. Prepare the client, before asking them to think of an interaction with someone that made them feel bad, though you don't want them to have an extreme situation. To practice the Self-Compassion Break, it's best to practice with a moderately activating memory, not one that will be overwhelming to bring to mind.

   Invite the client, "When you're ready, think of something that may have happened where you felt triggered, or felt badly about yourself, or when you were suffering, maybe a time when you were alone, lost, confused, disoriented, or said something, when you weren't received in the way you wanted to be. Feel into that moment. Have them visualize the situation until they are a little uncomfortable. Ask them to nod or speak of the event that is arising.

   When the client is ready, acknowledge to them, "Yes. This hurts. It's really hard. This was a moment of suffering." The client can use the words, "I'm suffering. Everybody suffers. This is a moment of suffering. We all have known what it's like to suffer."

---

* Used with permission. The Mindful Self-Compassion Training of Chris Germer and Kristin Neff

2. *Common Humanity:* Part of the antidote to suffering is knowing that you're not alone. Suffering, as painful as it is, connects us to each other. It can help to say: Suffering is a part of life. Other people know what it's like to suffer.

If you feel comfortable joining the client in this moment it can be immensely helpful to solidify the reality that we all suffer. Part of the antidote to suffering, for any of us, is knowing that you're not alone. Suffering, as painful as it is, connects us to each other. It can be helpful to acknowledge.

Once the quality is identified, it's important to feel it, imagine it, touch it with your heart. The antidote is not an intellectualization but a felt experience that we learn to receive. Many find it helpful to feel the physicality of presence by putting a hand on your heart—to feel the presence of your own self embodied. You might want to ask your client to put their hands on their heart, to feel the warmth of their hands and the gentle pressure of their chest rhythmically rising and falling beneath the hands. Model for your client by putting your hands over your heart and invite them to follow suit. Ask them to feel the warmth of their hands, the gentle pressure, and their chest rhythmically rising and falling beneath their hands.

3. *Inside, the suffering is a need for something, some quality.* What is the shame (or other feeling) needing? Wanting? Longing for? Part of the extreme difficulty of shame is feeling like we won't ever have that need met, or that there's something terribly wrong with us; we find ourselves fielding seemingly ample evidence of why we'll be disappointed or why we can't get that need met. Often, we hide that need from ourselves.

Your client might need some prompting or a menu of possibilities. Perhaps they need a certain kind of contact? Or some reassuring words, or to be validated in how hard this situation is.

I always invite the client to trust what arises. This practice might be different every time it's done. There isn't any right touch, phrase, or contact. It's more important to be authentically responding, with an open, caring heart, understanding the pain and suffering that's present. Half of the antidote to the suffering going on in the present moment is sensing that there is a need, even when we don't totally know what it is. The intention to be with ourselves with some quality of goodness, kindness, and compassion might be the most important element of all.

Feel into that moment, finding a way to respond to that suffering with some offering, some blessing, and some gesture of kindness. I always ask the client to take the time to let their body take in the kindness and care being bestowed. If you use parts language, ask the part that's been suffering if it can feel and sense this antidote.

Above all, it's important to remember that there's no right way to do this, no wrong way. Both of you are exploring what it's like for the client to be mindfully with their suffering, inviting in self-compassion. Phrases like, "I don't know how to do this, but I really want to try." Or "I'm learning, and I won't always get it right, but I'm going to keep trying." Or even simple phrases such as "May I be kind to myself (self-kindness)" or "May I accept myself just as I am." In the years of working with those with trauma and dissociative strategies for coping with life, people have come up with incredibly nuanced and profound blessings for themselves: "May I one day, perhaps someday, be able to feel peace in my body." Or "May I be free from self-harm." Or "May I find the way home to my own self."

ANJALI MUDRA

Objective: *The practice of bringing hands together at the heart is an expression of respect and an invitation to contemplation in many traditions. The instructions for this adapted posture for trauma survivors is to externalize conflicting feelings by placing them in either hand, while holding the expanded view of both at the same time. Consciously bringing opposite hands together integrates the polarity and naturally opens clients to compassion.*

Overview: This psychologically helpful posture brings two different parts (or felt experiences) into connection. In yoga the posture means "I bow to the Divine in you (or within all)." Bringing the praying hands together and moving them to the third eye is the posture of Anjali mudra. Anjali means "offering" and "mudra" means "to seal." Anjali mudra then is the sealing of an intention, an offering, in our body, mind, and heart. Since one of the definitions of yoga is union, with this posture we are inviting union between all parts of ourselves. I've adapted the traditional posture for those with trauma and attachment wounding, to connect and find ways to unify all parts.

For our purposes we'll be doing a posture of integration, bringing two polarities together. Everything in the universe can be seen in this aspect or the other.

For example, we have two sides of our brain. On a simplistic level, the left side of our brain holds the more logical, rational aspects while the right side holds the more creative, free-ranging natures. This posture we're doing is connecting two polarities, the left and right sides of the brain, in a yogic process of unification, yoking (which is what the word yoga also means) our rational and receptive natures.

Of course, there might be resistant parts that don't want to do this (which makes it a perfect candidate for the practice), while there might be other parts that want to heal the pain inside. This posture will be a simple exploration of any polarity, while bringing them together. Often clients will speak of the polarities they're struggling with, the judging part, the part that longs for kindness, a part that wants to be safe. Swinging between these poles, clients feel stuck. This practice is a way to bring the polarities together at a new center of gravity—the heart.

Script for clients: *You've probably noticed times when one part of you was saying one thing, another part saying something else. Sometimes we can clearly differentiate the polarities, sometimes those parts of us are separate, distinct, sometimes even unknown to each other. This adapted posture is a way I've found to integrate various polarities with our core self, our true nature.*

Traditionally in yoga, Anjali mudra is a grounding into the center of our being, our chest, the place where our energetic or spiritual heart lives. It's visualized as a lotus flower at the center of our chest.

One of the great yogis, Krishnamacharya, invites us to explore our potential in the posture, by bringing our hands together not quite flat against each other but where the knuckles at the base of the fingers are bent a little, creating space between the palms and fingers of the two hands, suggesting a flower yet to open, symbolizing the opening of our hearts.

For our purposes, in this posture we're looking at the polarities of life, the many different parts of ourselves that are integrated, as well as those that aren't necessarily in our awareness. We might find a fearful part, a judging part, a part that is longing for kindness, perhaps even a part that is angrily protecting another part that wants to be safe. Many of us find ourselves swinging between different parts of ourselves.

For this practice, rather than dealing with parts of ourselves intellectually, let's explore bringing these two parts together at the center of your chest, inviting them to live from a different center of gravity—your heart.

Intention: *Since Anjali mudra seals our intention, seals our offering to whatever we're doing, take a moment as we start to explore: What is your intention in doing this? What is it you're offering to yourself?*

Instructions:

- We're going to be externalizing different parts of you by placing them in your two hands.
- Chose a part, or feeling, or experience to place in your left hand. Get a sense of what that's like in your body. Can you feel the part there? It might not be anything fully formed, perhaps only a blob or a shape.
- What happens in your right hand, as your left hand holds this part? You might get a sense of this part being from a certain age. Perhaps it's a wise part, or maybe a triggered part, or a part of you that cares for others. Take the time to feel the part in your left hand, welcoming it, letting it come to life in your hand.
- Now bring your attention to your right hand, and imagine holding another part of you there. This could be a hurting part, a wounded part, a part that longs to be loved, to be reassured, to be wanted. There's no right way to find a feeling or a part of you. All we're doing is allowing these different aspects to separate from you so you can better listen and be with them. How does your left hand respond to the part in your right hand, if at all?
- Can you feel the different energies, the different parts in each hand? You don't have to feel it perfectly, you might only have a tiny sense of this quality, this aspect of yourself.

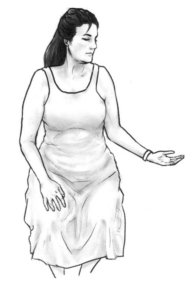

FIG 2.1A   Anjali

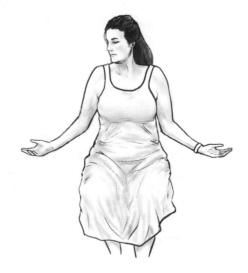

FIG 2.1B   Anjali

That's all right. It can help to take the energy out of your core body into your periphery. Sometimes that gives us more room, more space to breathe, to be with and listen to these parts of ourselves.

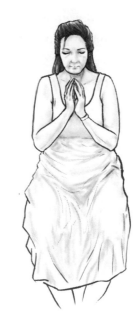

FIG 2.1C   Anjali

- Feel each hand, feeling the energy, not feeling it perfectly but holding the energy there, taking it out of your core body, externalizing the energy or feeling. Holding both energies, explore if one side feels heavier, lighter, thicker than the other. What's similar? What's different? Taking all the time you need so you can get a felt sense of each individual part. Find ways to play with the movements of your hands, perhaps slowly bringing the fingers and palms of both hands toward each other and noticing the effect it has on your heart, on the rest of your body. Notice especially the effect bringing these two parts together have on the opposite part.

- As you hold the two parts in your hands take some time to notice the rest of your body?

- What do you notice, if anything, in your spine and your heart? Ground there for a moment, while holding both parts in hands. Holding your attention on the two parts (hands) and the heart and spine at the same time, holding this triad together.

- Then bring your attention to your heart, even as you feel these two parts of you. Centered in your heart, notice how you feel toward these two parts?

- Feel what happens as you bring your attention to your heart, to your midline, letting yourself land in this center of your being. As you hold attention in your heart, slowly, with a lot of thoughtfulness, feel the energy of both hands, slowly bringing your hands together. Taking your time, feel the energy, the sensations of both hands at the same time. Bring your hands together at the center of your body. Continue playing with moving the fingertips together, with the palms slightly open and the base of the fingers holding space between them. What's it like to have this slight opening cradled in your hands? If it feels right, sense into this opening to see what qualities might be wanting to emerge. What do you hold sacred that you would like to offer to yourself, and possibly to the world?

• Feel what it's like to have the different parts separate and starting to meet at the same time. Feel the energy between them, as they meet, letting those two energies come together at your heart. What is it like to feel the different parts as they meet? Keep your attention on the simple body experience of these energies meeting together at your heart.

• When your hands meet at your midline, in front of your heart, notice if there's an offering you want to make. What would you like offer to these two parts? With respect, reverence, humility, and generosity, what is the offering or blessing?

• Then let your hands ease and relax.

• As your body lets go of the posture, what do you notice happening inside your body? Mind? Heart?

• Take a moment and write in your journal.

YOGA: SO HUM MAKING ROOM FOR INTENSITY, RESISTANCE, AND PAINFUL PARTS

Objective: *Slowing down and focusing on body experience, while compassionately making contact with intense emotion or sensation, fosters integration.*

Instructions:

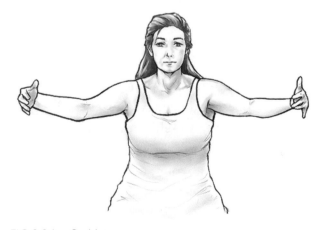

• Imagine the experience (or quality) in front of you about an extended arm's length away.

• What do you notice in your body with this experience, part, or quality in front of you? Are there places in the body that are protesting or resisting? Bring your attention to the center of that resistance. Invoke the mantra So Hum. Speaking it quietly, sounding it internally, or humming the mantra "I am" or "I

FIG 2.2A   So Hum

am that" or "So Hum," whatever is most comfortable for you. Make room, welcoming this protest or resistance

• Do you want to pull away? Move closer? Close your eyes? Does a feeling come up in you? What thoughts do you have? So Hum. Take all the time you need to be with this present moment, without changing, fixing, or making it nicer than it is. This really is the practice of So Hum.

• Feel yourself in your own skin, internally contacting your spine, feeling your back, not retreating into your back, but filling it, so you are held by your back. So Hum.

• Remind yourself "I am here." In this present moment, nothing bad is happening. Breathing quietly, grounding in this reality, saying "I am here, right here in this moment, and all is well." Repeat the mantra as you do this So Hum . . . So Hum . . .

• Bring your arms out in front of you, relaxed, palms facing you, encircling you. Quietly saying the mantra "I am" or "I am that" or So Hum—whatever is most comfortable.

• Pay attention to your body as you breathe in and out gently, arms extended. Again repeating the mantra, steady yourself in the breath, the sound, the sensations in the body, moving as slowly as you can, or need to, to stay present. So Hum

• Draw the person or quality that you envision toward your heart, pausing when you feel resistance. Hanging out there. Repeating the mantra, moving slowly, as you take in, incorporating the feelings, the sound, the breath.

• If this is as far as you get, that's fine. If it feels right to continue, draw the person or quality or part a bit further toward you, offering the mantra So Hum, feeling the breath, steadying yourself through the spine, grounding in your heart. Take all the time you need. Accept everything as it is, bringing in self-compassion.

• *Continue as it feels right.*

• Relaxing your arms down by your side, exhale, repeating the mantra.

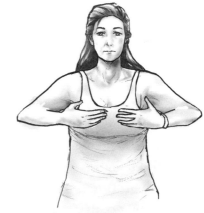

FIG 2.2B   So Hum 2

SO HUM VARIATION: INTEGRATING SECURE OTHER

Imagining the secure person or quality in front of you, slowly draw the image or felt experience toward your heart, pausing when you feel resistance, hanging out there. *So hum.* I am that too, opening to that possibility as it is.

While doing this, you're activating the attachment system and all its connected sensations. Moving slowly and with even a small amount of compassion invite in what you are wanting. Extending arms and hands in front of you, gather up the energy of this other to bring it toward you inch-by-inch, noticing any resistance, pausing as needed, connected with the resistance with both compassion and kindness.

Even when we want it to come from outside, we have layers of resistance keeping whatever it is we want out. It's important to find ways to hold both the resistance and the longing for more. Using the *So Hum* practice as well as Anjali mudra can help integrate resistance by identifying exactly where in the body the resistance is being held. Keeping attention on that place also evokes the desired quality. You then bring this longed-for quality into the exact place of resistance.

CULTIVATING A VISUAL FORCE FIELD OF COMPASSION

Objective: *This practice has the client create representations of compassion that he/she can observe. By focusing on positive visual representations the client alters previously internalized negative connections.*

Caveat for clients: If at any point the guided meditation becomes distressing and you don't feel comfortable with what is coming up, please stop. Your safety is important. It's never good to push too far past our own comfort zone. In order to heal, it can be important to engage, or lean into what feels "right" or comfortable. Over time we learn where that middle zone is. If we push too far past it, we can really trigger ourselves, which we'd like to avoid in this exercise.

Part 1 - Script for Guided Meditation

Bring to mind someone who to you symbolizes compassion. It could be a pet, a family member, a mythic figure, a spiritual figure, someone you know from TV.

Let go of any kind of right or wrong thought about "choosing" this person. Allow that person to come fully to mind. Drop any extraneous associations you have about the person, dropping the story you have about them and the story you have about what you need and want from them. At this point just allow the person to arise in your mind's eye. Allow them to be as real and full as you can.

As you have a good sense of this person, imagine them there in front of you, as if you are seeing the person in the room with you.

Be patient with yourself if you notice any resistance or turbulence inside. There's no need to force any of this. If the person only comes to you in small fragments, that's enough for now. This is the first fundamental aspect of any meditation—noticing, becoming aware.

Sometimes our minds will bring forward images of people, places, or objects that are not compassionate. If this happens, simply acknowledge whatever or whoever it is and allow it to pass like a cloud in the sky.

If the image doesn't shift, firmly let it know that you are looking for positive images and representations of compassion.

Take all the time you need for this.

Part 2: Journal Reflections

Open your journal and take some time as you respond to these questions:

Notice the effect this person has on your body, on your mind. What happens to your nervous system? What happens to your heart? This is where we practice the second important component of meditation: receiving the blessings that are being bestowed upon us.

Bring your attention back to this person. See this person looking at you, being with you. What are the qualities of their being? When they look at you, what is the energy that is being communicated to you?

Don't do anything to stress yourself out or scare yourself. We can sometimes become scared by love, by care of others. If you start noticing yourself getting a little frightened or upset, then either slow down the process or don't go any deeper into it. This is a very gentle process, meant only to surround yourself with compassion—to remind yourself that compassion is always there. This is a deeper level of receiving. Taking in the blessing of love and compassion.

Take some time and hang out here with this person, pet, or mythic object. There's nothing more important than this experience right now.

What is the experience like?

If you can, join with the person in beaming this love and support to you. Remember, our practice is also about receiving. Don't put yourself down if you can't receive for long. That's why this is a practice!! At this point, pause, while you take all the time you need to notice, allow, and receive.

Write and draw any kinds of images and words that come to you.

What were the feelings that came up in you?

What were the feelings and qualities of being that you experienced coming from the other?

How easy was it to take those in? How difficult? What got in the way? With no judgment or measuring stick in sight, take note of the length of time that you were present to this experience. This is only to provide some way for you to see yourself progressing on this path.

Part 3: Internalizing Compassion Meditation

Objective: *Using ancient practices from Tibetan Buddhism and the Sufi mystical traditions, in this meditation practice the client focuses first on externalizing qualities of compassion, feeling them with multiple senses, making the external expression as real as possible outside of themselves. Then the client imagines those qualities taking root in them, moving from the crown chakra down into their heart (akin to how a child learns to internalize positive qualities). It's one of my favorite practices, one which I use consistently to this day, and which helps people learn to receive and drink in the positive qualities. It's normal to have resistance and judgment come up during the practice. That's natural. If that happens, see, feel, and sense the positive qualities of compassion moving with and around and through the resistance, just as water flows easily around boulders in a river.*

Gather up the qualities of compassion. Bring them together into an area outside our body, close to you, so you can see the qualities, sparkling, shimmering, radiant in their fullness. Imagine those qualities merging into one glorious quality, merging joyfully into a ball of light.

Notice what responses happen inside as you bring your attention to this object.

Bring your attention inside, and notice your internal core from your crown to your heart.

Imagine that object at your crown.

Gently allow it to sink down into your crown.

If there's any resistance, just notice it. Let your object of compassion hang out with resistance.

Don't change anything—just hang out with compassion in that resistance.

When ready, continue to sink down until you reach your heart.

Let your heart soak it up, until it naturally opens to receive this quality.

When you're ready, let the petals of your heart fold around the qualities, leaving a kernel, a nut of it behind, then slowly lifting up, release this energy around you as well.

Variation: Compassion for parts we don't like

Now imagine this compassionate being with you. As you do so you might be in touch with parts of yourself that you don't like, that hold a lot of negativity or judgment of yourself. It might even be a part of you that you hate. Feel free to be as explicit as you can, in words and in images. *[The caveat to this is to not do anything that you find triggering, or too upsetting or scary. Use more than your best judgment! If you feel yourself getting too upset at any point, set down the work and go and do something nurturing.]*

Now notice what it's like to have that part there in front of you, feel your body, hear what words are reverberating in your mind.

Now, with the difficult part still in front of you, bring to mind the person, pet, or mythic object that holds the qualities of compassion for you. See, feel, and sense how the compassionate object interacts with this part of you that you are upset with.

Notice and watch and be with how the compassionate object is with the part of you that you don't like.

Write down the qualities, words, images, or the environment that the compassionate object extends to the part that you are not liking, maybe even hating.

Is there someone or a group of others that you feel safe with in your life? If so, I am going to invite you to take this drawing of the part that you are not liking to this safe person.

Ask them to write, draw, or tell you how they feel toward this part.

Obviously do this only if you feel the person is trustworthy and safe. If at any moment while you are doing this the other person says or does something that blocks your heart instead of opening it, simply thank the person (even if they're in mid-sentence), and take your drawing away.

When you are feeling vulnerable it's important to keep your heart safe, and not put yourself in emotionally painful situations.

After you have some feedback from inside yourself and from others around you, take a new look at this part that you were hating and see how you have shifted. There is often some shift.

If there isn't, notice that. Most likely you are dealing with an old relational strategy that kept you safe, keeping any nurturance out. You're up against your nourishment barrier. You don't want to push through this at this point. Noticing it and taking care with it will get you further in the long run.

Try making a practice of receiving kindness, love, gentleness, support, and care for others around you. Notice in your body where you keep that nourishment out. What thoughts do you use to push it away? What images or beliefs do you conjure up to keep this nourishment out?

Try noticing when others around you, even on TV/movies or in books and magazines, are gentle and kind with each other. How do you respond? See if it's the same internal pattern of thoughts, feelings, beliefs, and sensations that keeps nourishment out.

CHAPTER 3

Support Safe and Secure Body Access

The breakup crippled Madeline. Almost a year later she was still unable to breathe normally, living in constant panic, attempting to do her job even though she was spending a great deal of time in the bathroom crying. Her family and friends were worried. Madeline came to me for a consult on the suggestion of her own therapist. There were many things we tried that first session, the second session, and in sessions after, to interrupt the patterns that sped her into feeling so overwhelmed. Focusing on sensations, Madeline slowly got more solid, taking bite-size pieces of the grief, making cognitive links between the present and the past. As her body was able to be with the grief, she connected the despair to earlier pain. Her internal world began to organize. There were many things that helped, she told me. The biggest thing was knowing that she didn't have to be flooded with emotions. When she first heard me say that she could have control over her feelings, she was shocked. She thought they just happened to her, coming out of the blue, in big, frightful waves. Wanting a hand out of the tsunami, she learned not to feel every single feeling. She was terrified, gripped with fear that if she didn't, she'd be stuck. Not so, I assured her. Instead I offered her another choice: she would learn that she was more than her feelings, that they were there to inform her, not to define her. In time, Madeline came to integrate not only her feelings but the whole range of subtle internal experiences, to make her world a rich, dynamic place to live in instead of a cacophony of pain.

Entering the body means crossing a very new and different threshold, even learning a new language. Generally, people don't undertake that learning until life cracks them open and they find they can no longer cope. That was what happened to Madeline. She described her life as before the breakup and after it. Before, she could shut off her feelings, minimize stress by ignoring it, and pushing on. It was shocking to her to have those well-honed coping mechanisms seemingly evaporate when the breakup pulled the rug out from under her. She found herself unable to think, confused, flooded with feelings when she least expected it.

People with trauma or attachment wounding report feeling as if they are living with a terrifying internal fireworks display erupting in their mind, heart, and body, sometimes all at the same time. With huge amounts of sensate data coming in, it is difficult to parse out what information is useful and what isn't. On top of this sensate data are scripts from the past and worries about the future, combining with negative self-assessments and hopeful notions about that same future. The body is flooded with data that feels "real," especially if that body has been besieged by tsunamis for an entire lifetime. Learning to organize all this disorganized data is the chief task of anyone healing from trauma.

To slow down and titrate that incoming data to a manageable level requires keeping attention on the bare experience of life, without interpretation or alteration, something that is hard for any of us to do. For our clients, wounded by trauma and attachment neglect, information processing changes from a simple bell curve that rises, crests, and falls to shifting into an infinitely complicated pinball machine, ricocheting madly inside. It's disorganizing. Too much information flies around too quickly and on multiple levels. Organization comes as the person learns to sort out the vitality affects (Stern, 2004, 1985) or primal impulses (Stapleton, 2016/2015, 2004), with the various thoughts, feelings, and body sensations that occur in each moment. In developing sensate consciousness, the person learns to slow down, to observe the raw data of the moment to see what's behind the label(s) generally used to explain an experience. Dropping underneath the story and labels, it's possible to ride the swell of pulsing, tingling vibrations that form one's experience.

Yogic psychology details the workings of the body. One minuscule moment of experience activates any number of imprints, called *samskaras* in Sanskrit, which unleash the fluctuations (or *vrttis*) of the heart, sensations, feelings and thoughts with the potential to create massive internal disruption. When activated, and unable to stay with a pure sensation, any one piece of the internal puzzle pings chaotically in this way, activating thoughts, feelings, memories, sensations, and beliefs that create an internal, pulsing wave rushing toward what feels like sure annihilation. When trauma intrudes into a person's body, mind, and heart, the rich, complex array of sensations that move erratically and tumultuously through every moment are unleashed at disruptive paces. Uncertain of how to navigate this inner terrain, our clients shut down that which they often don't understand or know how to control. In this environment suggesting that they enter the body feels onerous to them, bringing anxiety, confusion, and distrust. It's not a simple task. Their feeling dial is preset to high activation, numbing or shutting them down.

Yet despite all the ways any of us try to get out of our physicality, we can't escape our body, our physical home. When we offer our clients a "map" of this territory, they often thrive. As they understand the moment-to-moment experiences that pepper their inner world, they begin to connect with their body. Many will only be aware of their physical self through the layers of negative cognitions, parts, schemas they have built up, making it difficult to perceive anything else. When they try to enter the body, they generally can't; many of them will say that it's impossible for them. They weren't given a "map" to distinguish the many components. Overwhelmed by every level of information processing, people close the door to their own body. This chapter offers a way to first knock on the door, to enter, and then reorganize what has been so confusing for them all this time.

Safe Embodiment

The fundamental evolutionary task for all living things is survival, allowing reproduction and continuation of the species. Central to this is the protection and nourishing of the young (Corrigan, Wilson, & Fay, 2014b). This protective environment becomes the bedrock of affiliative emotion and the biological basis of compassion (Corrigan, Wilson, & Fay, 2014b; Gilbert & Choden, 2014). Evolution primes all mammals for threat detection, then instinctively responding by initiating physiological, behavioral, and motivational reflexes (Lang & Bradley, 2010), Built into our physiology, this rapid-fire reflex occurs before any cortical appraisal system ever clicks in.

For those with traumatic imprints, the original trauma sets up conditioned responses that interfere with this normal processing, generating physiological patterns of anxiety and depression (Corrigan, Wilson, Fay, 2014b). Learning to activate the prefrontal areas can provide an important inhibitory effect on the threat system. Lazar, et al (2000) found meditation can decrease amygdala signaling. Cultivating compassion has also been shown to facilitate the ease in amygdala activation (Gilbert & Choden, 2014). The Becoming Safely Embodied™ skills do this by training people to slow down traumatic activation, so that the person can study the "mind moments" involved in each episode; slowing down time, to discriminate between thoughts, feelings, and/or sensations. Entering Body Time in this way breaks apart the traumatic schema, identifying the small building blocks of each moment and creating the possibility for new choices in the next moment. Having this kind of a map to the body's territory is helpful when a client is first starting on trauma recovery. Obviously, their main objective is to feel better, by decreasing reactivity and increasing organization of mind. For that, they need to know the terrain to be able to organize and disidentify with the cauldron of disruptions that is happening inside their skin.

One of the simplest maps is the Triune Brain (Cory & Gardner, 2002) developed by Paul MacLean, a researcher in the 1960s. He formulated a concept of how the brain evolved into three main parts. The oldest part, the reptilian complex, is common to all reptiles. These parts of the brain are involved with the basic necessities of life. Let's say you're thirsty. Being thirsty, you reach for a glass of water. You don't have to think, "I need to drink water." It's organic in your body. Then when you're full of water your body knows what to do to release that fluid. These functions happen in the reptilian brain. MacLean called the second part the limbic system. This major system of the brain is responsible for learning, memory, motivation and emotion, both positive and negative. The youngest part of the brain, called the neocortex or frontal lobe, is the part of the brain with the ability to process language, structure, abstraction, planning, and perception, and taking in and distilling information. Janina Fisher, PhD, the internationally known trauma psychologist based in Oakland, California, has found an ingenious way to teach the Triune Brain to clients through simple illustrations on a flipchart. Viewing the brain's mechanisms in this way reduces the abstraction, helping clients to disidentify with traumatic activation (Fisher, 2010).

The incredibly rich map of the body is not obvious for most of our clients. They deal in the concrete—wanting symptoms to abate. In their desperate state, clients want to ease the pain of their suffering. Who can blame them? The phase-oriented treatment model (Chu, 1998; Herman, 1992; Steele, van der Hart, & Nijenhuis, 2001; van der Kolk, McFarlane, & Weisaeth, 1996) is the gold standard for trauma treatment, generally agreed to be in three phases. The first phase of trauma treatment focuses on symptom reduction. Once the client is stabilized, the trauma can be processed in the second phase. In the third phase, the client is supported in moving out into a larger life. Subsumed by their symptoms, our clients want relief (phase one and two). They also want to know they are not just the package of symptoms that assault their bodies, minds, and hearts (phase three). A contemplative approach to the phase-oriented treatment model offers clients connection to their Self energy while guiding them through the phases.

People need ways to sort out what's so internally confusing for them. From an attachment perspective, affect regulation comes when a safe, caring person helps contain the affect while also being curious about what's happening inside. This requires the wiser person to have an active, noninvasive curiosity about what's happening in the other's mind. Doing so provides developmental scaffolding (Lyons-Ruth, 1999), disentangling a huge morass of disorganized experience into smaller, more bite-sized pieces. Breaking down these bits and pieces, clients can metabolize internal experience, bringing relief. The pieces of the puzzle can then be taken apart and looked at, as well as putting them back together in a format that works better for the client. Especially in the beginning and middle phases of treatment, this untangling process is revisited over and over again as the person learns to hold and contain highly charged feelings.

Let's explore the experience Elizabeth had. She had been in analytic treatment for decades. When she came to me, she had an extremely good understanding of her history, giving me well-thought-out explanations of why she was depressed. Her understanding was unhooked from her body experience. Understanding didn't shift the depression that had plagued her. Our work together involved separating out one feeling from the many happening at any one time and slowly helping her to sort out internal experience behind the words. She's learned to take a "thimble-full" of feelings out of the vast ocean of sadness in which she was lost. Elizabeth began to distinguish her body's feelings from the stories, memories, associations, and interpretations encoded in this "feeling." This kind of separation allowed Elizabeth to organize her internal work and gave her relief. With that, she began to feel less need to shut off her feelings. Then we were able to use the Internal Family Systems model to work with the part that was holding the sadness, helping it to unburden and live more in the present moment.

When our clients sort out the feelings from their broader tangled-up experience they are less defensively driven. They start to explore (one of the hallmarks of an earned secure attachment) their feelings as valuable clues about themselves, about life. They learn that feelings are messages, giving information about the here and now, or how the past is leaking (sometimes gushing) into their present moment. At that point, feelings become better messengers, directing us in Servan-Schreiber's words ". . . toward experiences we seek and the cognitive brain tries to help us get there as intelligently as possible" (2004 p. 26).

Understanding their psychological self better, our clients start to use their whole internal world more skillfully, resulting in a more satisfying life. Along the way, they are also informed about their likes, dislikes, fears, and hopes from a felt experience of themselves. This sensate knowing develops trust in navigating the internal shoals of experience, without being overwhelmed or shut down. No longer identified with pain, it is easier to explore sensations urging and directing the person into their own "developmental path" (Aposhyan, 2015). Linked to Self-energy, the person accesses motivational fuel to move in a nourishing direction, even while integrating fears and hesitations about the possibility of getting there.

ENTERING THE TRAUMATIZED BODY WITH A YOGIC PERSPECTIVE

Yoga provides a complex map, big enough to hold everyday experiences as well as immense suffering. Every starting point is in the present moment, no matter where we are on the journey. As mentioned earlier, Patanjali declares at the very beginning of the Yoga Sutras, "Now . . ." This ever-changing moment of now . . . "is the time of yoga." (I:II) Or, as Don Stapleton (2015/2016) says, "Now is the moment to inquire into yoga—which is to get interested in what you don't know that you don't even know you don't know." In defining what we inquire into, we give it shape and form. Amy Weintraub tells LifeForce practitioners, "It's important to keep in mind that so many people are living from the neck up and don't feel safe to be in the body. When we offer a sense of compassionate reentry we empower people to reclaim their bodies." (2013). When we attend to the body in this moment, we open the door to a new world, one in which language isn't the most efficient navigator. We suspend our intellectual understanding, to inquire into the felt nature underlying all the various fluctuations (*vrttis*) of thoughts, feelings, and sensations fluttering, cascading and obscuring the serenity of pure consciousness. When *vrttis* are activated, it is as if we are dealing with a startled hive of bees.

Inevitably, in the years of working with trauma and attachment wounding, especially with those who also had long-term meditation and yoga practices, people found their spiritual practices alone weren't enough to deal with their trauma symptoms. They needed trauma psychotherapy to integrate the past. Yoga and meditation practices are designed to open the person up. At some point doing spiritual practices, especially for those on long-term retreats, a fault line opens up, making them more permeable to previously compartmentalized information. For others, the fault line unexpectedly wipes out their capacity to hold onto former ways of being. In this process meditators realize their spiritual practices alone aren't working, and they need help of a different kind. Some abandon their spiritual practices, while most lighten the intensity of the practice. Those who continue with spiritual practices find it helps to create a larger field to hold the suffering, while giving it perspective. Augmenting their practices with psychotherapy builds a psychological construct to harness and contain the suffering. This necessitates learning different skills to reprocess and release the suffering they were carrying, while integrating the enormous benefits of spiritual practices.

In order to face the tragedies of their external lives, and the disorganization of their internal lives, those suffering from trauma and developmental wounding need to remember and cultivate the seeds of goodness, clarity, compassion, kindness, and who they were before the wounding occurred (even as their wounded parts protest that there isn't any part of them *not* wounded). Humanistic psychology orients us to this same truth. IFS tells us these are the inherent qualities of Self energy (Schwartz, 1994); positive psychology emphasizes the character strengths and virtues that are the innate qualities of being human (Brown, 2013; Peterson and Seligman, 2004).

How then to create safety out of chaos? Exploring what mindful embodiment of the Self would be. Corrigan, Wilson, and Fay (2014) found people generally define safety as the lack of something versus the flourishing of various states. Yoga and meditation practices invite us to consider that safety comes from being connected to true nature instead of being identified with the fluctuations of the mind. That requires decoding the inner working of body and mind. "The structural details of any yoga practice or spiritual system can be alluring; it is easy to mistake external technique for consciousness. But practice comes alive when you communicate with your body's sensations as you live in the question of what is unfolding from inside your physical world" (Stapleton, 2004, p. 38). In the yogic perspective, as with body-mind therapies, we explore what allows the client to be with what is happening while remaining grounded in their own body/self. Attention is held in a larger field of awareness, which includes pain and suffering, at the same time holding an attitude of welcoming whatever comes up (Aposhyan, 2004, 2007; Germer, 2009; Miller, 2014, 2015; Schwartz; 1994; Stapleton, 2004), embracing the distress while remembering, grounding, and being nourished in and by the larger consciousness of True Nature. In yogic cosmology, the metaphor for a person's true nature is the sun radiating warmth, even while the clouds filter and obscure (Bryant, 2009; Stapleton, 2004; Singer, 2007, 2015). Our task as people, and certainly as therapists, is to release the identification with suffering, so we can hold the woundedness in a different way, colluding less with fears. The poet Rumi says it well, "Don't turn your head. Keep looking at the bandaged place. That's where the light enters you." (Barks, 1995).

WITNESSING AND OBSERVING TO DIGEST EXPERIENCE

This is where yoga and psychology support the healing process. Not focusing exclusively on "putting Humpty Dumpty back together again," contemplative approaches to healing trauma incorporate the realization that we are more than painful distress (Germer, 2009). Yoga helps us break the dualistic imbalance of suffering. We are embodied. Our skin boundary encases our physical, emotional, and mental self. Yoga says we're more than that: we are infused with life force (*prana*) that radiates inside every part of our system, moves through us, and extends beyond into everything, everyone, everywhere. The yogic orientation proposes that our True Nature is, as Richard Miller writes, "simultaneously everywhere as it is omnipresent by nature" (iRest Level I Manual, p. 37). The IFS word for this is Self-energy (Schwartz, 1994).

Patanjali's second aphorism *Yogaś citta vrtti nirodhaḥ* is translated as stilling, restricting or modifying the patterns and fluctuations of consciousness (Bryant, 2009; Feuerstein, 2013; Stapleton, 2004; Taimni, 1961). To achieve yoga, we see these internal machinations without getting caught by them. We move from being identified with the story to being with what arises with less reactivity (Singer, 2007, 2015). Ah, the words make it sound so easy, yet the task requires courage, commitment, and dedication.

Yogic teachings invite us to experience the luminous clarity of our body, heart, and mind where *prana* flows in, through, and around us. These waves of energy infuse proto-sensate data that is pulsing, vibrating and shimmering at all times. Accessing these small sensate data points may be the route through which we touch *prana*, the life-force energy that animates all of life. Part of the healing path for those with PTSD and attachment wounding is to widen perspective, having a witness consciousness, holding a larger view, to be with the constantly shifting and unfolding flow of experience without being caught up in it.

Tabitha looked at me like I was cross-eyed when I told her we all had the capacity to witness our experience while being in it. "Wait. We've been working at slowing down dissociation and now you want me to actively dissociate?" I chuckled. She's right, in a way. It can be confusing. Those that have been identified with a disorganized inner world need to develop "witness capacity"—something that is different than dissociating. One way to create that kind of space is to explore pure experience by using the sense doors of seeing, touching, hearing, tasting, and/or sounding. Sitting in your office, you can have a person look at something in your office, seeing it, without getting overly engaged with thoughts about it, or listening to the sounds of the room or outside the room, hearing, without adding anything to it. Over time, Tabitha came to love doing this, "It feels like I get a break, but I'm there with it rather than not there." (The practice is outlined at the end of this chapter.)

Life experience gets digested when we're able to witness and observe what's happening, while experiencing it at the same time. Everything in life has a beginning, middle, and end. Imagine a temple or church bell sounding. Out of nothing, the sound emerges from the bell, building in intensity or vibration until it dissolves back into the space that it came from. Being with experience, mindfully observing, we learn to ride the unending currents, each moment rising, cresting, and falling away. Attention to what is happening opens a cycle of somatic change (small or large) to rise, reach a crest and then naturally fall, or in psychological terms, to integrate.

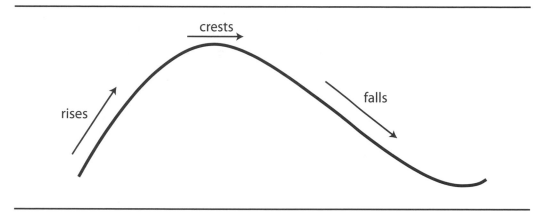

FIG 3.2   BELL CURVE OF SENSATION

This is true with feelings, as they rise up, crest, and pass through. It's also true with sensations rising up, cresting, and falling, and with thoughts as they come up, and pass without sticking to us. Experiences can move freely and effortlessly through our system without making a mess. Complications come when we're flooded by sensations or feelings, unable to digest the experience. When we can stay present inside our own skin and acknowledge that "x" experience is arising even when it's hard or even when it's astonishingly wonderful then integration occurs. At those moments we're not separate but completely alive in them and with them. This developed reflective function allows us to say, "I'm really triggered right now," rather than reacting. For those who use the language of parts, we talk about "a part of me is feeling like this," or "a part of me is having this experience," which is a form of reflection.

Being-with is the opposite of dissociating. It creates a wedge in experience, so that the frontal lobes can be present, exploring what's happening as it is happening (Corrigan, Wilson, Fay, 2014b). This being-with promotes a "dual consciousness" (Ogden, Minton, & Pain, 2006), describing when we can be in experience, while observing and naming it at the same time. Straddling a variety of moments allows integration, giving the body a chance to digest the vast amount of sensory data accumulating in every moment of time, and accessing this larger state of consciousness. The meditation traditions point to the analogy of the sun hidden by the clouds, making it difficult for us to experience the sun's bright, unobscured light and warmth. The healing path is about clearing the filters, the veils of confusion, doubt, insecurity, and fear that come between our knowing ourselves in the best possible way.

The Internal Family Systems model developed by Richard Schwartz (1994) speaks of this kind of witness consciousness in the form of "Self-energy." IFS holds that Self energy is the essential nature of every person having the qualities of calm, curiosity, clarity, compassion, confidence, creativity, courage and connection, despite all the trauma and personality traits. As a person differentiates their parts, they uncover what has always been there: Self energy. Different parts of the personality carry psychological burdens, as they adapted to life by playing various roles. This hopeful perspective of IFS allows therapists and clients to enter complicated psychological territory on firmer ground, where nothing and no part is wrong. "All parts are welcome" is the adage of IFS, creating room, igniting curiosity.

Richard Miller's iRest Yoga Nidra (2010, 2014, 2015) asks us to welcome whatever is arising while becoming sensitive to the array of feelings and emotions that occur. "Observe what passes in front of us as a neutral witness of all that arises, either internally as feelings, emotions, and thoughts, or externally as behavior of another or ourselves. Witnessing allows us to see the larger picture that so often escapes us when we fuse with and become embroiled in emotional reactions" (Miller, 2014, p. 78). The more we see, the more we observe everything, changing all the time. As Patanjali says, we begin to observe the *vrttis* (patterns and fluctuations of the mind), getting less and less caught up in living out the negative patterns.

Any person with trauma will acknowledge that being mindful isn't enough. Observing and welcoming is hard, when the body feels like it is being filled by a high-velocity firehose. The first step for safe entry is naming and identifying what is there, then welcoming it by helping the skin and muscles to open instead of habitually tightening against. We become sensitively attuned to whatever is arising without being hijacked by it.

Yogic texts present highly evolved distinctions, allowing us to encounter this infinite bell curve of experience (Bryant, 2009; Feuerstein, 2013; Singer, 2007). *Manas* is the function of consciousness that organizes sensory input and directs the senses (Bryant, 2009; Muni, 1994; Singer, 2007). *Manas* "imposes a conceptual structure on the chaotic field of raw *sensations*, recognizing and identifying sensual impetuses and categorizing them. It exhibits attraction to some sensory possibilities and aversion to others—in other words, the functions of feeling, emotion, and desiring. It is the bridge connecting the world of sense objects as accessed through the sense organs" (Bryant, 2009, p. 13). The sense organs "sense the world, convert the information, transmit the data through electrical nerve impulses, and then

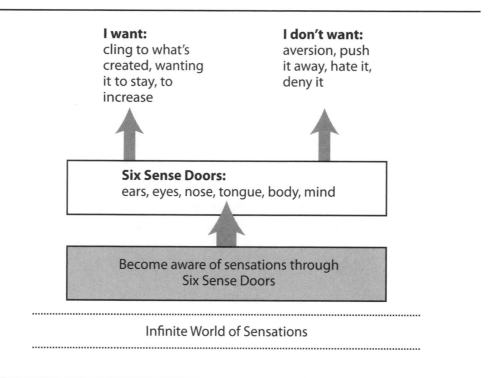

I want:
cling to what's
created, wanting
it to stay, to
increase

I don't want:
aversion, push
it away, hate it,
deny it

Six Sense Doors:
ears, eyes, nose, tongue, body, mind

Become aware of sensations through
Six Sense Doors

Infinite World of Sensations

FIG 3.3   SIX SENSE DOORS

the impressions get rendered in your mind. Your senses are, indeed, electronic sensing devices" (Singer, 2007, p. 51).

MINDFULNESS AND CONCENTRATION PRACTICES

To ride the bell curve of sensation requires skills from the meditation and yogic traditions in order to navigate the body's invisible terrain. In general, there are two kinds of meditation: mindfulness and concentration practices. Mindfulness practices help to develop an ability to watch and observe what happens, without judgment or being caught up in it. Mindfulness allows bare noticing, naming what's there simply and without embellishment. Mindfulness helps to enter into or witness and observe the painful or joyful experiences without getting caught by them. Concentration practices like self-compassion or loving kindness help focus the mind, orienting toward a point, moving to where you want to go instead of being caught up in various distractions along the way. Directing the mind lowers internal churning, creating ease.

Let's take a moment to be with how vital these two approaches to meditation are for trauma survivors. When triggered, everything becomes disorganized, fragmenting into multitudes. Naming that you're fragmented is mindfulness, being able to be with the bare elements of the fragmented experience, stepping back from the disorganization, is also mindfulness. Concentration practices train the mind to focus on a fragment in particular, to orient in a direction and move toward something instead of getting lost in each and every little hurricane and tornado moving rapidly within the inner landscape. Both are essential. Name what's there, focus, and direct yourself toward steady ground.

The concentration aspects train the yogi to focus on each increment of time. Bringing attention to the breath as it contacts the nose, moves into and around the tip of the nose, flows inside the nose, down into the lungs, moving in and around the lungs, and then noticing each and every movement of the exhalation cultivates concentration. By returning over and over to the object of attention, witnessing without reacting to it, we develop two things: equanimity and the capacity to concentrate.

Being mindful, we observe the flow of sensations, naming the action tendencies to move toward or away from whatever we are experiencing. Both capacities are important: the ability to be mindful, naming without agenda what is happening, and the skill of focusing and concentrating throughout the day, which allows people to be more present in their everyday life. (We'll discuss this more in Chapter 4, on dissociation.)

What might be simple and easy for those who have not dealt with traumatic activation is one of the most difficult things for someone with a disorganized inner world. To concentrate on the rise of activation and only focus on that rise can be almost impossible when it feels as if piles of thoughts, feelings, and sensations are weighing you down. Learning about "Body Time" (Fay, 2007; Stapleton, 2004) offers clients a language of slowing down rather than maintaining their usual pace, sensing and being open and receptive to these differences. "Felt sense" is the word Gendlin (1978) used to describe internal bodily awareness, a meaning which the conscious mind is initially unable to articulate. The body processes at a different time and pace than our thoughts or emotions do. We need to school ourselves to wait as the body shares its experience with us (Ogden, Minton, & Paine, 2006; Miller, 2010; Stapleton, 2004; Weintraub, 2013, 2003).

INFORMATION PROCESSING

With spacious attention body experiences become messengers providing information about ourselves. Rumi's poem, *The Guest House* (Barks, 1995), invites us to see joy and depression ". . . as an unexpected visitor. Welcome and entertain them all! Even if they are a crowd of sorrows, who violently sweep your house empty Rumi suggests that the guest "may be clearing you out for some new delight. . . . each has been sent as a guide from beyond" (p. 109). The IFS model describes how each part holds a role that may be outdated. As we listen, be with, understand, and "unburden" that part, the client becomes less reactive, more accepting and inclusive of whatever that part was holding. The Becoming Safely Embodied™ skills (Fay, 2007) organize the mind by giving the mind tasks, focusing on bare noticing and creating distinctions in a morass of experience. Looking for and finding concrete building blocks in a disruptive moment, the mind starts to organize into a structure. What thoughts, feelings, and sensations are happening right now?

Information processing models describe the mind as a computer, which responds to stimuli, processing sensate raw data into working memory and logging certain information into long-term memory for future access. This top-down cognitive approach bypasses the overwhelming internal world of those whose body-mind are not organized and who are desperately trying to manage the raw, undigested packets of incoherent stimuli. Body-oriented psychotherapies like Sensorimotor Psychotherapy (Ogden, Minton, & Paine, 2006; Ogden & Fisher, 2015) and Somatic Experiencing (Levine, 1997) have shifted our focus in psychotherapy. Their models access "bottom-up" information coming from stimuli rather than using cognition as the starting point. Bottom-up processing integrates physical stimuli of heat, smell, sound, and light by processing stimuli into colors, shapes, and spatial orientation, and then into concepts. A top-down processing of cognition, concepts, understanding, and memory identifies those colors/shapes as an object.

For example, a client with dissociative identity disorder looked out her kitchen window one day and saw a snake. Terrified by snakes, she froze in place, concentrating on the snake outside the window, desperately afraid if she took her eyes off the snake it would move and possibly come into the house and hurt her. Seeing an object as shape or color (bottom-up), her brain took in the information sent directly to her amygdala, and sounded the alarm bell of danger. She was unable to account for how much time she lost watching the snake, yet at some point she remembered some of the Becoming Safely Embodied™ skills and brought in more top-down processing to organize this limbic activation.

One of the adages of the BSE skills is that if the experience is out of proportion (hyperactivated, frozen in place, unable to move, seeing the "snake") to the bare experience (in this case the experience was being in the house, looking out the window, and seeing something out there) then you can bet you're triggered. Living on the edge of high activation, the client drew on her top-down skills of thinking, sorting, organizing, and understanding, to recognize that a terrified part had activated in the amygdala and froze her in her tracks. By focusing on her frontal lobe (organizing data outside and sensation inside) she was able to look closely at the snake. Studying it, she realized it wasn't a snake but rather the branch of a tree that had fallen. With that top-down information, her body calmed. In this case, after all the work she had done on herself, she was able to simply laugh at herself, astounded at how these unconscious processes had taken over and hijacked her body.

KOSHAS: A YOGIC MAP OF THE BODY

Untangling the internal world, especially the more disorganized and chaotic it is, requires having an elaborate understanding of the body. The Sanskrit word for this multilayered organization, composed of body, mind, heart, energy, is the *koshas*, defined in the Yogic Upanishads as a map of energy and the physical layers of the body (Bryant, 2009; Feuerstein, 2013; Stapleton, 2004; Weintraub, 2012). It is through these interconnected sheaths of the subtle body that *prana* flows through everyone, everything, everywhere. Always present whether we're aware of them or not, these sheaths allow us to reconnect with the embodied soul, or essence, embedding in the bliss layer, the *anandamaya*. The sheaths or layers that envelope the body hold the imprints (*samskaras*) left by life experiences. These imprints (or knots or scars) are held in all layers of the physical and energy body. Rather than seeing the sheaths of the body as physical or static, the *koshas* orient us to the subtle body's felt experiences.

To give clients a sense of this energy experience I have them rub their hands together rapidly (like one does when warming them), then slowly pull the hands apart, palms facing each other. Playing with the space between, clients they generally describe a pulsing, a fullness, a something that they can't quite name existing there between the hands. Steve was surprised by the experience, saying "it's like taffy or something—I can feel it pull apart and come together as I move my hands toward each other. Pretty cool."

Let's explore this a bit further. Imagine holding an orange. Just a piece of fruit, right? Identifying the orange as an object in its gross form is what the yogis call *vitarka*. We're holding an object which we have a concept about: a piece of fruit we call an orange. Play with this a moment. Imagine holding this orange in your hands. Your mind is aware of it as an object. What happens if you drop any thoughts about it, letting yourself sense it through touch, smell, taste, sound, even as you also see it. Sense into it, instead of thinking about it. As your concepts and descriptions and explanations drop away, you may encounter something else, something harder to explain in words. Some might call this subtle energy. Yogis call the encountering subtle energy of the object *vichara*. There's more, though! Stay with the orange, letting the gross thoughts and concepts release. Open to experiencing whatever subtle energy (*vichara*) you may have found, and sense further into and around the object. Even as you do that, what are you aware of inside of you, around you, in the object, between the object and you?

The more we keep our concepts out of the moment the more likely we can encounter bliss (*ananda*) vibrating, engaging with the subtle form of any object. Sometimes at those moments we will experience a sense of identity (*asmita*) dropping away. We have an experience of no longer being separate. Training the mind

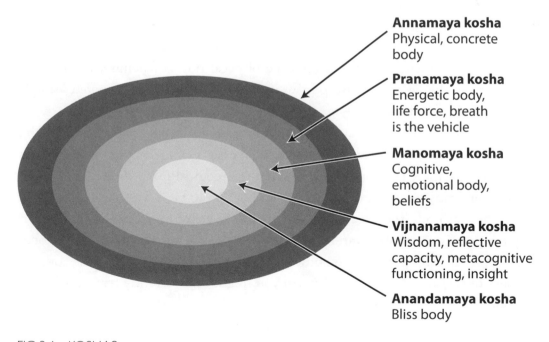

Annamaya kosha
Physical, concrete body

Pranamaya kosha
Energetic body, life force, breath is the vehicle

Manomaya kosha
Cognitive, emotional body, beliefs

Vijnanamaya kosha
Wisdom, reflective capacity, metacognitive functioning, insight

Anandamaya kosha
Bliss body

FIG 3.4   KOSHAS

to access different levels of attention can alter our experience of body, environment, and the moment-to-moment experience of living in the world. In her 2015 keynote to the Kripalu Yoga Teachers Association, Amy Weintraub said, "My belief is there is a pathway through trauma and the map can be the *koshas*. Everything we do affects us on all levels of our being. When someone is experiencing something in yoga class they're feeling it in their physical body—but also in every level of the body. The constriction prevents us from accessing the *anandamaya*. We can potentially release that constriction to reach the unending ocean of love."

In addition to our physical existence the *koshas* describe energy bodies that live fluidly within and around the physical body. The first *kosha* of the body is the *annamaya*, or the physical layer comprising the mechanics of our physicality—what we see, feel, and touch. The material elements of earth, water, fire, air are the "home base" for the other, subtle layers of the self (Stapleton, 2004). The Upanishads call the *annamaya* the "food body," describing our physical connection of being fed by the earth. For example, we know the effect a cup of coffee has on our body, some of us love that "oomph" that comes with caffeine, that boost of energy. Others find the caffeine too overstimulating. The *annamaya* is an entry point into exploring this first *kosha* or layer, the physical body. In hatha yoga, we become aware of the physical body, sensing the joints, bones, spine, muscles, skin, and into the organs and endocrine system. For people with a lot of trauma or attachment wounding entering the physical body, the *annamaya*, can be very difficult. They don't have the discrimination between the physical body as being separate from other layers of the *koshas*, resulting in an inability to be with the concrete, simple experience of being in the body.

For example, when I teach a simple breathing practice (Six Sides of the Breath), people can often be jettisoned into negative beliefs held in one of the other *koshas*—for instance, the *manomaya kosha* (beliefs, cognitions), when they feel the sides of their arms touch the edge of their body ("I'm so fat"). Instead of anchoring in the physical body they get swept into negative belief loops held around their body images. To cultivate awareness of this *kosha* it is helpful to have clients focus on the more neutral parts of the body (the tips of their fingers, the arches of feet, the lobes of ear, and the eyebrows) when you might inadvertently trigger a client's pain points held in this *kosha*.

Being triggered is always a possibility. It's impossible to cut out every possible trigger. Our goal is instead to titrate experience, to be able to hold and be with whatever is arising. "Accessing . . . *prana* happens by connecting our mental awareness to the tides of sensation as they ebb and flow through various regions of the body. In observing sensations as they pulse through the body the life force within the physical organism registers on the screen of our mental awareness." (Stapleton, 2004, p. 40)

Pranamaya is the *kosha* of energy and not just the breathing practices we call *pranayama*. Life force energy is the *prana* activated through breathing practices, creating a bridge to the senses and the physical operation of the body. Activating, harnessing, and training *prana* allows true nature to animate the inner world and ripple through experience in a smooth, organic way. Just as the skin is the bridge between the inner and outer world, *prana* is the bridge between the physical body and the still vastness of consciousness. If not "tamed," *prana* can churn the inner world, creating havoc. This can sometimes happen on intensive retreats when people reach for higher states of consciousness without being grounded in the physical.

Our clients know this layer well, at least unconsciously. Anyone with a chaotic inner world can feel overwhelmed by even the simplest breath. When the body's native defensive responses of fight/flight/freeze kick in to protect against possible danger, breathing patterns rapidly adjust. In response, their bodies have learned to reject consciously breathing. As a client learns to harness the life force through *pranayama* (breathing practices) they can modulate their inner experience. Years ago teachers often had clients "take long deep breaths." Seeing the complications for those with trauma, I suggest instead that clients take a tiny "sip" of breath, to titrate experience, slowly befriending their inner world, learning to actively have control over their experience. Simple skills like this teach clients how to use their breath, to have more or less activation as they need or want it. LifeForce Yoga teaches a "Stair Step Breath" which is a version of this same energy dial (Weintraub, 2012).

The third *kosha manomaya* is where we live most of the time, in our mental, cognitive, and emotional functions. (As an aside, for those used to other interpretations of the *koshas*, I add the basic building block of thoughts that float through the mind in this *kosha* as distinct from the discriminating mind of the *Vijnanamaya*.) We think about life, then explain and report what's happening in our bodies. We're overwhelmed by feelings—or we shut them down. In Sanskrit, however, *manas* (or mind) means something more than what the word means in English.

The Eastern traditions don't separate between body and mind, seeing the processing of thoughts and emotions through all sense doors. For those with trauma histories, untangling the physical and this *kosha* of the mental emotional level is the bulk of their training. This develops a map of their inner world, informing them of the raw data of sensations, feelings, and thoughts that complicate their daily moments.

Caught up in mental or emotional disturbances we become agitated. We need the mediating force of discernment and wisdom, bringing the capacity to witness and meta-process, to know, decide, judge, and discriminate between possible actions and ways of being. Knowing the wisdom that is larger than our thoughts and actions is the realm of *Vijnanamaya*. This sheath is veiled by the doubts and confusions that dilute access to our knowing of what would be the most "useful" way to encounter the next moment. As the word implies, it is generally a positive force, yet it too can be clouded by impressions and imprints of life experiences, making that wisdom difficult to access.

Anandamaya is the place every yogi wants to live from the bliss body. Not the hedonist pleasure principle kind of bliss, but the bliss that arises when there is no separation, when everything is welcomed, accepted, and embraced—even the most complicated, difficult, and painful aspects of life. It's in this sheath that compassion naturally arises, integrating mistakes, problems, and difficulties into the vast spaciousness of the whole.

At the center of these *koshas is* the eternal flame of *Atman* (Self), the consciousness that has never been born and never dies. This is the light that shines behind and through, despite whatever tries to interfere.

THE PRACTICAL PATH TO ENTERING THE BODY

Entering the body means encountering whatever is there, welcoming it, learning to befriend it without an agenda of what to do with it or to make anything right or wrong. Crossing the body's threshold is a curriculum in learning how to be, here, now. Thich Nhat Hanh (1999) urges us to enjoy walking without thinking of arriving anywhere. Every moment gives us a chance to pause. In this instance, even as you're reading these words, pay closer attention to what happens in your body. How do you respond when you read that there is no right answer? Or no need to get anywhere? You might have dismissive or distressed thoughts, or perhaps arguing, speaking back, or telling yourself I don't know this author or she does not know the particular dilemma with which I am dealing. You might also have had visceral responses or feelings of irritation or resonance. Yoga, meditation, and body therapies are about welcoming everything, even those thoughts, as information about this moment.

With that setting the stage, let's walk a bit deeper into the material. Your clients might say something like Dani did:

"I've barely begun to discover my body, because the feelings are so triggering. I use a lot of energy blocking out my body. It seems like the pain is coming from outside and inside at the same time. If I weren't so sensitive, I wouldn't have the pain. But the pain's not coming from the outside; it's already inside. It's a stored pain that's being touched. I know if I can heal the pain that's being triggered I can open up to who I am and embrace my sensitivity and learn to fine-tune it, so instead of seeming like a source of pain it becomes my safety and greatest strength. What I need help with is finding a safe pathway within my body to meet my hurt parts and to offer them healing. Often there's so much pain between here and there that I can't reach through it to help myself."

Many people want to feel alive, to enjoy a wider spectrum of feelings without being afraid or overwhelmed by their feelings. As a client shared with me, "I want to not only know what's happening in my mental processes, but below my neck, below my face." Or "I want to be able to name what my body feels. When I'm with my therapist and she asks me what my body's feeling, I can't identify it. So that is one of my intentions, to be authentic." Others have said, "I want to be able to speak, and when I speak, to be able to speak what is going on inside without falling apart." And, "I want to stay more present with myself. I want to learn how to be in my body when I'm feeling things, to know where they are in my body because I have trouble with that, too."

In Chapter 2, on shame, we explored the dual problem: wanting to heal, and also being afraid of healing. There's both the longing to have life be different, and at the same time a resistance to that very same healing. Normalizing this polarity identifies a key part of the inner territory. Practical, concrete skills make it easier to enter the body. Discriminating what happens inside at any given moment makes being in the body less threatening and overwhelming. When a person knows what's going on in their body, when they know what they're thinking, feeling, and what their body sensations are, they are more able to intervene when triggered, stressed, shut down, or overwhelmed.

A key element in this process is separating the story about whatever happens with a meta-perspective. For this, the details of the story are less important than discerning and being with the whole experience, as the story unfolds within. The more disorganized the person's internal experience is, the easier it is to be constantly distracted or hijacked, getting catapulted into old habits of thinking and feeling. The result is people feel stuck in patterns of doom and hopelessness. This hijacking process can happen instantaneously. In the beginning, most people don't know that they are hijacked or know how that happened. One minute they're fine, and then, BOOM—they're in it, overwhelmed by the experience. These moments don't happen out of the blue, but are part of a larger construct of internal experiences reacting to the internal and external world. This hijacked experience then feels like the "truth" of the situation. (We'll go over this in depth in Chapters 4 and 5, on dissociation and triggers.) As a person learns to parse apart that "story," they also open to the encoded memories held in the body. Having a guiding map (as developed in this chapter) makes it easier to navigate the process. Pieces begin to make sense. Triggered moments can be seen as reactive filters on a life event, not necessarily an accurate reflection of what is happening. This happens as the person learns to discriminate what the thoughts are, what the feelings are, and what the moment-to-moment body sensations of experience are. They grow in their capacity to intervene in the painful tsunami of a triggered moment, and shift it. We'll be exploring triggers in a later chapter, but for now we will investigate the building blocks of each moment.

The present moment, as we've discussed, is fresh, alive, ever unfolding. Painful moments and memories imprint onto the moment, creating filters, generally negative, on this pure moment, making it hard to experience the present unencumbered by past. Painful memories cloud the moment, reminding us to stay vigilant, protected against disappointment in the past or projected into the future. Mindfulness of the present moment gives a tool to walk respectfully into each moment, slowing down time, to witness and be with the body's experience with clarity and curiosity.

Each moment is made up of a number of basic building blocks. It's not just one thought or one feeling we are having, it's more like lots of thoughts and feelings on top of innumerable sensations. This seems to be happening at the same time, like a swarm of bees let free from their hive. In the swirl of it all it's hard to separate and identify the multitude of data points as discrete, small building blocks. Those moments, however, can be studied, noticed, and explored. In fact, the more familiar this internal territory becomes, the easier it is to shift and orient in the way that is most satisfying.

For most people the background noise and soundtracks of the inner world is so familiar that we take it for granted, no longer paying attention to the subtle fluctuations (Singer, 2007). Shutting out, numbing out, and compartmentalizing are second nature. Learning to manage stimuli is especially important for people with sensitive nervous systems. This chapter looks at the building blocks of each moment in practical and concrete terms, to help the client slow down and enter the body safely. Building this internal platform gives a person greater capacity to intervene when triggered (Chapter 5).

FACTS, FEELINGS, INTERPRETATIONS

Learning to be with bare experience is not a skill most of us learned. It's a skill meditators and yogis practice in intensive retreat experiences, watching the mind as it flits and changes and moves in fascinating directions, piling on stories, embellishing future possibilities and encrusted stories of the past. When our clients who have insecure or disorganized attachment styles tell us something from their life, their reflection tends to be full of reactions and activation, and sometimes doesn't make much sense. Facts, feelings, interpretations, and associations are all mushed together into an incoherent whole. We need to parse it out with them. As they learn to organize the overloaded internal world, they gain a sense of control over what's happening to them and in them.

A helpful tool is one I learned from Yvonne Agazarian (1997) creating distinctions between facts and feelings. First, a person needs to clarify what a fact is. Any journalism student will tell you facts are the who, what, where, when, and how the story moved from A to B to C. Facts are the observable data that we get through our senses: taste, see, hear, smell, and touch. They are the actual words that are spoken or the words that we said. When observed, facts are really simple. I am here, typing. As I say to my clients, facts are boring. There's nothing to cling to, nothing to embellish. By contrast, feelings give us the color commentary of the facts.

I'm a great fan of the Tour de France, which happens every July. Even the Tour can be seen in terms of facts and feelings. The facts of the Tour are that there are a certain number of teams, riding over a course that changes every year through various towns in France. Throughout this multi-week event, the facts are pretty simple. The fact is a certain number of men get on bicycles in the morning, and ride on a road or up and down a mountain. At the end of each day someone wins the Yellow Jersey. Day after day those are the facts. Some days there are mountains. Some days there are flat stages. Some days there are crashes. Some riders abandon the Tour. But generally, the basic facts stay the same. The Tour de France doesn't sound that exciting, described that way, right?

People new to watching the Tour think I'm crazy to be transfixed watching bicycle riding, day by day, week by week, up a hill, down a hill, up a hill. And perhaps if it weren't for the marvelous team of commentators, I wouldn't be as captivated. But Phil Liggett, Paul Sherwen, Bob Roll, Christian Vande Velde and Jens Voigt bring the whole event to life, telling stories, teaching the ins and outs of the rides and strategy, getting animated as crashes happen. This color commentary over the facts is what draws thousands of us around the world in year after year, expanding, diminishing, altering, shifting the pure (as with anything, rather boring) facts of cycling (riding up a hill, down a hill, spinning, braking, crashing) The feelings, interpretations, and associations not only enrich and enliven the bare facts, but can also skew them, expanding it out of proportion, by altering facts based on filters and schemas.

So, how does this apply clinically? In the beginning years of her therapy, Tabitha often got startled by noises outside my office window. I would ask her, "What are the facts happening right now?" Her blank stare gave me a clue on how much she was trapped between the present moment and the maze of dissociated compartments of her past. In the beginning I would prompt her on the facts, "The facts are, we were talking. Then there was a loud noise outside." Orienting her to the present moment, I would let that sit for a bit, and again repeat the facts gently and firmly, again and again, as many times as necessary until Tabitha's body eased, her head started to nod, and the glaze left her eyes. "That's right," she would say, "That's right." Over time we would add phrases like, "The fact is, you're in my office." "The fact is, it's 2016." "The fact is, right now, nothing bad is happening." or "The fact is, you and I are the only ones here in this room."

Naming the bare facts is a mindfulness practice. Concentration is developed by staying steady through the feelings and sensations. "The fact is there are sounds outside the room." Tabitha nods. "And as you heard those sounds outside you, something happened inside you." Tabitha nods. "Let's take our time. Is it a feeling? Or body sensations?" I might repeat the facts if Tabitha started to freeze, tense, or glaze over. If she wasn't able to focus on the body sensation in the beginning, I would wonder with her, giving her a menu, "I'm guessing you might have felt something inside? Maybe some tension? Or numbness? Or stiffening? Maybe a feeling of being scared? Or danger? Something else?"

In all likelihood your clients will do what any number of my clients would do—jump immediately to the heightened, escalated feelings, "I'm scared. I just knew something terrible was about to happen, but I didn't know what it was." "My heart is racing; I knew the noise was going to . . ." If the client continues to be activated, return to the facts, repeating them over and over, in a simple, clear voice until the client lands in the moment. At that point you can guide her once again, to name feelings and sensations. One person who was in one of the Becoming Safely Embodied™ Online Courses commented, "Now the pieces fit together! Facts are the facts of what happened, feelings happen around those facts or around the way we construe those facts. It's like seeing that from two different eyes. You know, getting that, I have some compassion for myself. I realized I can't change the past or the things I did. You know, I'll probably always have regret—but maybe I don't have to feel bad about having that regret, or even the guilt. What I'm seeing here, though, is that I don't have to wallow in that as I have been."

The importance of this simple skill was highlighted one year when I was attending a workshop with Allan Schore. Because of my participation in the workshop, I wasn't attending to emails as I would have on a normal day. Checking at the break, I found a flurry of emails from a woman in Africa who had taken a Becoming Safely Embodied™ Online Course. The first email was pages long, written without any punctuation at all, or any sentence construction. Much of it was apologizing to me, profusely, that she was writing and bothering me, interspersed with a painful encounter she had with her therapist and fears of being abandoned and discarded. The message was very difficult to read, not because of the content but because of the lack of organization. The second email was much the same. Somewhere around the fifth email there began to be some reflectivity as she linked the BSE course material in ("I guess the facts are . . ."), and then went rambling on. The seventh email started with her writing about the facts, naming the facts, and then going to a second paragraph (first time there had been a series of discrete paragraphs, in all of the emails), where she reflected on the feelings she had about those facts. It was astonishing to see how she organized herself bit by bit, by using the Facts / Feelings exercise.

Maribeth, another client, described the exercise this way, "Sometimes I have to do the exercise several times over. It seems that different parts of me have different feelings and interpretations of the facts. The intensity of feelings different parts have makes it hard to think or look clearly at the facts. I was surprised to find that as I stayed with the simple facts whatever I was feeling seemed almost irrelevant. The more I do this, it seems like different parts have such deeply held beliefs about situations. They hold so much fear, and can spray that fear through the system, immobilizing all of us [all of her parts] before any of us can look at what the facts are."

In a phone session, Mike couldn't find words to tell me why he was so upset. I asked him what he was feeling in his body right at that moment, asking whether he was on the high end of activation, or more shut down and numbed out. He described feeling a little activated.

I went through the facts with him, "So, right now the facts are, you're on the telephone talking to me, and there are other people in the area around you, right? Those are the facts."

He agreed those were the facts then said, "Well, I don't know if this is a fact, but I'm stuck in the past. Simultaneously, I get other thoughts in my head." In psychodynamic therapy we would explore that, yet for this skill building I returned to the facts.

"If we look just at the facts, right now in this moment you have thoughts about the past, including how you are stuck in the past." He was able to tell me he could hear birds outside the window, then looped a few times trying to engage me in other thoughts so I asked him about some very concrete facts. "Right now, in this moment, are you sitting on a chair or on a couch or on the floor? Are you standing up?"

He replied, "I'm sitting on a chair. Sitting at my computer." I repeated those facts back to him, adding, "If we hang out with those facts over and over, notice what happens: it's March 26, 2015, I'm sitting at my desk talking to you on the phone, you are there in (x) city talking on the phone while sitting at your computer. There are birds outside making sounds." We repeated those facts a few times, then I asked him, "What happens in your body?"

Taking a moment, Mike said, "The more I do that I get somewhat calmer. But the panic is still there, ready to rise any moment. If I don't focus on the facts the panic rises in my chest." Staying focused on the task of separating facts from feelings, I asked him what he felt as he was saying that. Mike noticed tension and how that contributed to the panic. "Let's just stay with those facts. Right now you're sitting on a chair in (city) talking on the phone, looking out the window at some birds, right? So let's just stay right with that. Right now you're sitting on a chair in (x) city, talking on the phone and looking at and hearing some birds. What happens in your body when you just stay with those facts?"

Taking a minute, Mike responded, "It's not charged."

"And what effect does that have on you?"

"It's calming. I don't feel the panic as much." In training the mind to stay focused on the task, free of the emotional valences, the body has a chance to calm. Staying with the simple facts can be hard but will eventually shift the state.

Clients will inevitably want to parse out the subtle distinctions, like Mike did with his panic. "Is the tingly sensation in my constricted throat, a fact? Is tingly neck, heat in my chest—those are facts, right?" This is where it's important not to get caught by the right/wrong debate. The exercise is designed to help people sort out what spins them into heightened or shut down states. What creates activation? What calms activation? Ultimately, they choose what experience they want to have. We help facilitate choosing what feels better, and invite them into a more nourishing state.

Providing ways for clients to find peaceful access to their body is important. However, there isn't one practice that works the same way for each person. Having a tool kit of exercises to offer allows the client to collaboratively explore what they need moment to moment. One practice that many find helpful in slowing down and entering the body is finding the Six Sides of the Breath, which is detailed in the practice section. When someone has disconnected from their body they won't have distinctions of the front/back, top/bottom, or right/left sides. This gentle *pranayama* (breathing practice) guides them to slowly access more of their internal body experience.

IMPORTANT CAVEAT TO KEEP IN MIND

If an experience feels overwhelming and too big, you can assume the person is triggered. If this moment feels too big to handle, it indicates that whatever is happening in this moment is charged with past undigested material. It doesn't mean that what's happening is wrong, rather that the body is taking the person to an old, triggered place. At those moments it's easy to feel lost, confused, panicked, and/or overwhelmed. Exploring how those moments are fueled by something undigested from the past helps to untangle what's going on.

THE BASIC BUILDING BLOCKS OF THE PRESENT MOMENT: THOUGHTS, FEELINGS, BODY SENSATIONS

Separating out the facts from feelings, we can then dive into the specifics of each moment in time. When life is in sync, our internal wave process is "coherent" (Elliott & Edmonson, 2005; Brown & Gerbarg, 2012; Servan-Schreiber, 2004), moving at a steady, even consistent, wave. In this steady, relaxed pace, thoughts, feelings, and body sensations have time to move and to integrate. When activated, the even, balanced, coherent wave pattern is disrupted, and may be an indicator for PTSD vulnerability (Shah & Vaccarino, 2015). Slowing down the body allows space for information to sort itself out, to organize, leading to more skillful restructuring of the inner world. This discrimination occurs with knowing how a thought, feeling, and body sensation are each different from each other. These building blocks form the foundation of the inner world. When someone has greater awareness of what's happening inside their body-mind-heart at any given moment, they have access to their inner compass. Once one makes sense of the building blocks of each moment it's easier to intervene more effectively with traumatic reactivity.

WALKING TOWARD EXERCISE

Having clients discriminate between a thought, feeling, or body sensation gives them internal control. It can also be a way to experientially notice attachment styles. As the body pulls away, or the person feels the impulse to move forward or grab onto, we discern a tendency toward preoccupied or dismissive styles. To do this, I have clients practice with me, or with others in a group, or on their own with an object in their house. Cindy did this at home, choosing to focus on a coffee cup that was across the room from her. Standing there looking at it, she reported, "At first there was no energy connected to it. I had the thought, 'There's a cup of coffee.' I took a step closer, didn't notice any feelings or sensations, but did have another thought, 'I need to clean the dishes.' I took another step closer, noticing a thought, 'I do not clean as often as I should,' whereupon I started to feel some guilt or shame, with another immediate thought, 'I am an irresponsible person.' I was rather surprised by this, and took another step, which brought forth pervasive thoughts, 'You always procrastinate,' feeling more guilt and shame, yet still no body sensations at this point. I took another step closer, and thought, 'Look at all the paperwork that needs to be done at work. You never get things done on time.' Now there definitely were feelings of being overwhelmed, and body sensations of tightness across my shoulders and lower neck that kept increasing. Another thought, 'At work you always say, I need to get this paperwork done so I can get it off my back' and then I realized that's the tightness in my shoulders. I had no awareness of this body sensation related to my procrastination, until this exercise."

Patty was in a Becoming Safely Embodied™ skills group doing this exercise with a partner. They both called me over to tell me that nothing was happening and they couldn't see the point of the exercise. I suggested they try it again, and I would watch. Patty's partner took a step toward her without any response from Patty. Another step, then another step. There was a slight flutter of one of Patty's fingers. I asked what was happening. Patty wasn't aware of anything, so I had her partner step back, pause, then step forward again. The little flutter happened again. Patty was still unaware of anything. So her partner stepped back, paused, stepped forward again. Attending to her hands this time, Patty looked up at me with surprise when she noticed the slight flutter. I wondered out loud what her finger was wanting to say with the movement. Playing with the finger movement Patty softly said, "I wanted her to stop. I didn't want her to come closer." We then did a series of experiments where Patty used her voice or a larger hand gesture to indicate to her partner to come closer, stop, or stay away. Years later I got an email from Patty, telling me how important that experiment was to her in being aware of what was going on inside her, helping her to make healthier choices.

The moments of life occur in our bodies as constantly flowing waves of experience, known in yoga as *vrttis*. Sometimes the wave is easy to ride, other times it grows bigger with tangled unprocessed material. A helpful way to be with these fluctuations of internal experience is when we can both be in the experience and still notice it. This mindfulness enables us to say, "Oh, I'm really triggered right now," rather than acting out the trigger. Dissociation is something done automatically, to decrease identification. Using parts language decreases identification, separating the felt experience from the one who is having the experience. Having psychological separation, the client learns to stay with what's going on, noticing it and having access to explore it. This experience of "dual consciousness" lets the person be in the experience, observing it and at the same time opening the door for integration.

Distinguishing between a thought, feeling, and body sensation gives greater skill in dealing with the inner world, and is the crux of the healing work most people have to do. Old habits of mind and emotion as well as old holding patterns in the body can easily hijack a client's attention into past interpretations and associations, without their being aware of it happening. Being aware accesses an inner compass to discriminate wisdom of what next step to take. Grounded in Self, it's easier to intervene in triggered reactivity and release shut-down tendencies, increasing the possibility for the process to move in a more organic and nourishing direction.

Interrupting this activated circuitry is something we'll work with in Chapter 5, on triggers, but for now let's explore how the body can be befriended. The primary perspective as a therapist (as well as for our clients) is to remember to trust one's True Nature or Self Energy. This helps our clients "unblend" (using the IFS parlance) from the multiple parts that fuel distress or separation, while holding the possibility of being with the underlying waves of physical experience that rise persistently and pervasively through even the most distressing moments of life. Developing wisdom consciousness, we begin to relinquish our identification with the thoughts and beliefs belonging to "me," thereby opening an access route to the higher synthesis of wisdom in which everything I need to know is already here, within me. Being able to mindfully observe the thoughts and beliefs and memories arising and passing away, we connect with the vast space of something more: the inner healer is revealed, directing the path home to the Self.

Thoughts

Let's break this down into smaller bits. Being able to name, identify, and conceptualize objects and life experience allows us to see what's there and what makes it different from something else. It also provides a type of shorthand in communication. When you see a table, you instantly have an idea of what a "table" is. You may not know what kind of table, or have any context of the table, but you know in its gross form what it is. In this respect, thoughts create identification. Another form of thinking reflects on the raw data (the "table"), making associations, judgments, and evaluations. This "thinking about thinking" is a metaprocess in the domain of theory of the mind, and is necessary for organizing the body/mind and providing a higher level of organization than just simple thoughts.

Basic thoughts are the vehicle we use to interpret the raw data of life; words that form sentence constructions, that describe and explain what is happening. Whether we're doing this explicitly or not, we are doing it implicitly as background, by processing all the time. These automatic and habitual interpretations of life start constructing experience. Developing the capacity to metaprocess gives the capacity to think about and reflect on those very words and sentences, and the implicit understandings and representations that are held within them. Both these kinds of thinking are essential tools for any person struggling with a history of trauma or attachment wounding. Strengthening the capacity to think and organize the inner world can put a brake on inner experience. This control valve of experience allows us to be able to have more of the experience, amplify it, slow it down, and even shut it off.

Engaging thoughts both as raw data and metacognition organizes and builds a sense of self. If a thought isn't concretized into body patterns or traumatic schemas it can be explored, developed, and shifted much easier than feelings or body experiences can. Cognitive Behavioral Therapy is predicated on this: change the thought to change experience. The problem for those with trauma, however, is that the body isn't always telling the same story as the mind. Bessel van der Kolk famously said "The Body Keeps the Score" (1994), describing the dark storage of traumatic memory. With trauma, people opt to live in their thoughts, explaining what's going on, constructing a world through words, as a way to separate and keep the big, bad, overwhelming pain in the background, or they split off through dissociation. In either case, to really enter the body, our clients need to cultivate a larger perspective, the "Self" to modulate inner experience. Thoughts are then in service to the Self, providing a brake to shut down or manage consciously instead of habitually. The person learns to slow down or stop the flood of experiences going on in their bodies. Our task as therapists is to help our clients mentalize their inner experience (Allen & Fonagy, 2008; Brown, Elliott, et al., 2016; Fonagy, 2001; Fonagy, Gergely, Jurist, & Target, 2002). This developmental task supports the ability to explore what effect thoughts, feelings, and body sensations have on experiences.

We do this by supporting our clients in developing a structure for their day, in predetermining ways to avoid anxiety-provoking situations, and by offering guidance in how to deal with any triggering they encounter. By doing this along with the client, the person develops a platform to organize their inner world, starting to trust that they can depend on themselves, or turn to appropriate safe people in whatever difficult situation they might find themselves.

Gaining reflective capacity creates clarity and a sense of control. Our clients find they are no longer victimized by their inner physiology. This is a form of mindfulness that helps them untangle the mess they feel they are in (or are avoiding), to focus (a form of concentration practice), directing their attention where they want to go. They learn they are in charge of their mind, body, and heart, instead of being at the whim of it.

We need to be aware as we sit with our clients of the tendency to shift from exploring inner experience to falling back to a safe position of thinking about, or overanalyzing what is happening. This happens when we use thoughts without sensate or affective information that the body is providing, accentuating the inner split between body and mind. All this can involve an obsessive quality preventing anything new to enter into the accepted formula, becoming repetitive and taking both the therapist and client further from the reality of the moment.

Feelings

Whereas thoughts can be abstracted, feelings are more closely connected to the body—happening *in* the body, and prompted by internal or external stimuli. Thoughts tend to be more ephemeral, allowing us to take flight from the physicality of the body. Feelings are more concrete than thoughts, locating us more firmly in the body, and operating at a slower pace than the quicksilver movement of thoughts. Interwoven in feelings are the even more basic building blocks: body sensations (which we'll get to in a minute).

There's much that can take our clients away from their felt experience, leading them to try to understand with their heads, drawing them into analytic explanations instead of deeper access to their felt experience (Aposhyan, 2007; Ogden, Minton, & Pain, 2006). The wave metaphor of the bell curve of sensation can make an easy visual to remember. Feelings rise, crest, and fall. Learning to ride that cycle of life allows entry into flow states.

So why, then, do feelings become such a dastardly, sticky muddle? Something happens outside or inside the body which triggers internal response: either a thought, feeling, or body sensation, which links in nanoseconds to an array of associations, memories, and interpretations which take the person out of the felt experience. Feelings tend to be like dust balls, accumulating lots of affective out-dated material the more affectively charged, the more the client pushes down the experience, or is thrown into associations and interpretations to those feelings. The felt experience of a feeling goes from a simple sliver of experience to one loaded and sticky with memories, associations, and beliefs—soon, looking like a snowball, gaining more and more dimension and weight as it rolls down the hill.

According to Patanjali, this stickiness holds the traces of memories encoded in the unconscious by past thoughts and actions carried out without thought or ques-tion. These unconscious patterns are the *samskaras*—the memory traces that remain as unconscious imprints. In the attachment perspective, these patterns are part of the Internal Working Model, embedded early, before there is any narrative mem-ory (Brown, Elliott, et al., 2016). Over time, as we repeat the same action/thought and have the same feelings, we produce a predisposition, an action tendency, habituating to these habit patterns, which yogis call *vasana*.

Our clients with traumatic or attachment histories know very well what "feelings" are. They definitely know what the stuck patterns feel like. For them this is something to be avoided, either actively, by numbing the feelings down (which is often the tendency for those with dismissive/avoidant attachment styles), or by being overly identified with the feelings, letting them run rampant (the tendency for those with anxiously preoccupied attachment styles). Our cli-ents may feel safer when numb, as they've effectively cordoned off the distress, the longing for something, putting it psychologically out of reach. For those cli-ents inclined to an anxious attachment style, learning to think about feelings instead of being immersed in them can downshift the plunge into overwhelm-ing anxiety. I've had many clients in individual or group settings who were stunned to learn they didn't have to have every feeling at full volume. Being able to titrate and tone down feelings to be more manageable allows the client to be able to be with the feelings instead of constantly flooded by them. On the other hand, those prone to a more dismissive/avoidant style can learn from oth-ers who are comfortable with feelings that feelings can be had without falling apart or being filled with toxic shame.

The *manomaya* is the *kosha* of feelings and emotions. *Mano* comes from the Sanskrit word *manas*, which describes the larger capacity of mind, not just cogni-tion, therefore the *manomaya* is the sheath in which we are interacting through our senses. Meet the mood," Amy Weintraub (2012), reminds us. Don't try to be where you aren't. Meet the mood as it is. When we do so, the door opens for the infinitely adaptable practices of yoga to embrace and heal the range of internal experiences. If angry, LifeForce Yoga therapists urge us to not flinch from that anger, but to welcome it and learn from it. Instead of talking about the issue, a LifeForce Yoga practitioner would suggest various breath, sound, or movement options to be with what is there, harnessing the energy and moving it in a new direction. In this way, yoga offers ways to receive the entire spectrum of emotions, beliefs, thoughts, not just one side of the positive/negative polarity. Instead of swinging between the various poles of experience or isolating on one end or the other, yoga repairs the opposites by first exploring one side of the polarity, then the opposite, then both sides together, simultaneously.

Sensations

Hafiz, the Sufi poet, empathized with us: "I know the voice of depression, Still calls to you, I know those habits that can ruin your life, Still send their invitations. . . ." (Ladinsky, 1996). His wisdom encourages us to "keep squeezing drops of sun" from our lives, even from the "most insignificant movements of your own holy body." Learning this is the practice of healing trauma through yoga. It is about squeezing drops of nourishment from the most insignificant moments of each day, and even in collaboration with the pain and anxiety happening over and over again. Taking time to sit with and be with those painful thoughts, feelings, and body sensations slowly turns the key to a new way of life. In time, they relax their dreary hold, and we begin to hear their important messages. When we can be with experience, even when there is a high level of discomfort, we open, and wisdom emerges.

This gives us a good entry point to explore body sensations. *Pranamaya* is the sheath in which energy moves, shifting and dancing through all layers of our energy body, inside and outside the physical body. This living energy, the life force of *prana,* is what animates our cells, fires our neurons, and saturates every level of our being. At the gross level it particularizes as myriad, infinitesimal micro-experiences, which we more easily grasp as sensation.

Being present in the body can be a particular challenge for people who have divorced themselves from their bodies. The dilemma is that sensations are intricately linked to feelings. Cut off access to feelings and it's difficult to contact sen-

	Wooden			
	Congested		Shaky	
	Dull		Trembly	
	Dense		Throbbing	
	Frozen		Pounding	
	Icy		Fluttery	
	Disconnected	Prickly	Shivery	
Tense	Thick	Electric	Queasy	
Tight	Blocked	Tingling	Wobbly	
Constricted	Contracted	Nervy	Bubbly	Tender
Clenched	Heavy	Twitchy	Dizzy	Sensitive
Knotted	Suffocated	Burning	Spacey	Bruised
Hot	Cold	Radiating	Breathless	Achy
Full	Numb	Referring		Sore
Sweaty	Closed	Buzzy		Tense
	Dark	Itchy		Tight
	Hollow			Nauseous
	Empty			

Sensations?

FIG 3.5   SENSATIONS

sations. The rhythm of Body Time helps slow down things enough to sort out felt experience from the myriad other things going on inside and outside the body. This entails learning a new language, a sensate vocabulary. Acupuncturists use this kind of language when they diagnose symptoms. When clients go to see Sheila Fay, an acupuncturist in Watertown, Massachusetts, and describe a symptom, Sheila asks them for sensate information about that symptom: Is it hard? Does it rattle? Is there pressure? How does that pressure happen? From inside? Or does it feel like it's coming from outside?

If a client is anxious, invite them to report how anxiety lives in their bodies. The pattern of anxious arousal is rapid fire, activating the nervous system whose alarm pathway is well carved. Learning to slow down is hard, but it becomes possible when the person is offered a sensate menu to help them describe felt experience (i.e., trembling, jiggling, wiggling, popping, glittering). Both of you are slowing the process down, and narrowing the field to explore smaller bits of information. Being slow, focusing on the moment-to-moment fluidity of body experience, puts a wedge into the sensate data pouring in at any particular moment.

SEATED MOUNTAIN POSTURE TO EXPLORE THOUGHTS, FEELINGS AND SENSATIONS

Using the Standing or Seated Mountain Posture in the practice section, clients experientially differentiate the basic building blocks of inner experience. To assist people in discriminating their internal world, I have them hold a posture, often a Standing or Seated Mountain Pose which has them raise their arms above their heads, or held in any way that feels comfortable. The body is always regulating movement by shifting even slightly to adjust to tensions; if we inhibit movement, experience will arise. As they're holding the posture, I ask the client to report out what comes out, without editing. I write down what they say, encouraging them to hold the posture as long as they comfortably can. The more "stress" there is the more they will have a variety of thoughts, feelings, and body sensations. When they need relief I invite them to slowly lower their arms, reporting what happens inside as they do that. What is the experience of relief? Even there we can find thoughts, feelings, and sensations which I write down. Afterwards we sort it out together. What makes a thought a thought? A feeling a feeling? And a sensation, a sensation? The more they can discriminate between the various levels of experience the more they will be able to intervene at those various levels.

CONFLATING CREATES DISORGANIZATION, DISCRIMINATING CREATES ORGANIZATION

Not having embodied distinctions causes problems as associations and stories conflate with direct experience. Being able to isolate and become aware of individual body sensations has tremendous benefits; primarily, there's less information to process in each moment. People who suffer from panic attacks can often find relief by bringing their attention to single sensations, such as their heart beating, instead of the larger clusters, or feelings of how scared they are or of how their thoughts catastrophized about a heart attack or potential danger. Helping someone to notice just the beat, beat, beat of the heart, concentrating on that and only that, helps anchor the mind on only one thing instead of all the attendant links to it.

The moment we become aware of a sensation, the mind links to something, importing associations, memories, or stories about the past, or predicting the future. This gets superimposed on the current moment. Rarely are we experiencing what is happening in this moment, free from interpretations and predictions of what's right/wrong. Trauma survivors tend to habituate to distressing associations, stories, and interpretations (van der Kolk, 2015). Once sensations are interpreted in light of the past, the current moment gets clouded; unbeknownst to us reality is skewed. For example, my client Tabitha was guarded against ever feeling what happened in her body, as she had lots of associations of being a child, trembling and afraid. Now that she's living in New England, her body gets cold in the winter and sometimes she trembles and has internal shaking. For years she conflated her cold response (normal in the New England winters) with being a terrified child, all of which would cause flashbacks, making it hard to leave her house. Over time we worked together to isolate the sensations from the stories so that she no longer has the instantaneous associations connecting trembling/shaking with fear/crying and actual danger. Tabitha was able then to practice staying with pure sensation, focused in the moment, while at the same time open to what was going on around her. With that she found that her options in those moments expanded. As her past loosened its grip on her, Tabitha was able to engage with the world in a more satisfying way.

BODY SHORTHAND: ANXIETY

Decoding these simple fluctuations in the body gives a person access to the basic building blocks of embodied experience. At any and every moment, something is happening inside our skin. Pulsing of blood, gurgling of digestion, throbbing of a headache, itching of dry skin. However, most of us rarely pay much attention to these sensations, instead clustering them in shorthand form to describe what's happening inside, when needed. This sensate clustering allows us to jump over the tiny building blocks of life experience to explain, describe, and illustrate what's happening in familiar psychodynamic interpretation of the experience we are in. We explain, instead of exploring (Agazarian, 1997). None of these sensations in and of themselves are good or bad, pleasant or unpleasant. Experienced yogis train themselves to notice and watch individual sensations rise, crest, and fall, in the now familiar bell curve. For them a tingle is a tingle, trembling is trembling, a twitch is a twitch. That twitch can be observed and sensed and moved with. Sensations are the felt experience which, we when we let go, opens the doorway to the stream of presence, *anandamaya*—entering bliss, oneness, the vast ocean of connection.

All of us have shorthand ways of describing our inner world. Instead of slowing down experience to study and explore sensation, which takes time, clusters of sensations get associated with feeling states or descriptions of what's happening inside. If, however, we take the time along the way to notice and create distinctions, we have a greater chance of being able to intervene when we're more stressed. To illustrate the points above let's explore the sensation of anxiety, a common enough state for most trauma survivors. I often ask people what sensations are there when they feel anxious and compile a list, which generally includes the following: fast heartbeat, butterflies, muscle constriction, difficulty breathing, shallow breath, muscle movements, and agitation. Would those be on your list? As you inquire into your own body experience of anxiety you may well come up with other sensations.

Let's compare that to excitement. What are the sensations you experience when you are excited? Generally, most people list the following: muscle impulses, butterflies, rapid heart rate, shallow breathing, and agitation. So, I wonder with them, what's different? And the answer is: the association, the shorthand label (the sensate shorthand) we place on the cluster of sensations. Once that association is made, whenever we feel a variation on shallow breathing and numb body, we're likely to think we're anxious. Perhaps the most nourishing benefit is that when we explore underneath all the thoughts, feelings, and sensations we open to the *vijnanamaya* layer. This subtle experience discriminates how life works better (or not) for the individual. It holds the energy of the heart, from where we sense what is true, what is essentially me underneath all the conditioned thoughts, feelings, and body sensations. Centered, we have intuitive flashes and understandings that occur in surprising ways. This is the area that IFS calls Self energy, and is the entry point in spiritual traditions for a vast knowing of who we are.

It would be simple to have a clear prescription for each attachment style. Clinically, clients (and their parts) will have a range of feelings. For example, our clients with preoccupied attachment styles, who appear to be emotionally aware, aren't actually "in" their feelings, or "having" their feelings. They are *run by* their feelings, without access to the intelligence the feelings are trying to communicate. Years ago I started calling this the "hamster on the wheel" experience. People would be feeling and feeling and feeling, without any resolution. On the other hand, it's easy to get caught up in a client's explanations of what's happening inside, especially if it makes a lot of sense. Psychologically astute, dismissively oriented clients who explain their feelings lose the chance to become more intimate with themselves and with others.

Over time our clients learn how being overwhelmed or avoiding feelings can interfere with becoming embodied. Certainly anyone whose internal world feels treacherous would gladly find a way to "get out." Clients who are more dismissively attached have been able to create distance from their feelings. Yet when our clients avoid integrating the wisdom of their feelings they lose the capacity to access vitality, sadness, creativity, wisdom, intuition, kindness, and compassion.

Safe Body Attunement Practices

PSYCHOEDUCATIONAL: SEPARATE FACTS FROM FEELINGS AND INTERPRETATIONS

Objective: *In this practice the client learns what a fact is, and how to separate facts from feelings and interpretations that carry an emotional charge. This helps our client be with experiences that make it hard to be in the body. Each component of turmoil is probably manageable by itself, but when they're all jammed together nothing feels manageable. This skill is a simple way to pull apart the myriad assorted components of experience and create some organization. Using thoughts to name and witness experience is one way to organize and create space.*

Instructions: There are three parts to this practice. It's important not to tell the client about the various steps of the process as they will try to do it "right," and miss out on the learning.

The second part has the client circle the facts and underline their feelings and interpretations. This engages the client in creating distinctions: What are facts? What are feelings? The third part of the practice asks the client to tell the story with just the facts, a few times over, and after each telling to notice their experience. Ninety-nine percent of the time the client is calmer.

1. *Tell the story as you experienced it.*

Take a situation that happened recently, something about a four or five on a scale of zero to ten. Nothing too triggering, but you also want some charge so your mind stays focused. Without censoring, either write down what happened, or tell the story to someone as it happened, from your point of view. Express yourself as fully as you can. Tell or write the story with all the embellishments, as if you were telling your best friend, including all the gory details of what happened.

Before we move on, notice your global body experience. How disturbing has it been to narrate the story? Rate it on a scale of zero to ten, with ten being the most upset or shut down you have ever been, zero not at all.

2. *Retell the story: Facts first, feelings and interpretations second.*

Now we're going to separate the facts from the feelings and interpretations. Circle the facts and underline the feelings and interpretations.

What are facts? Observable data is what you can see, smell, touch, taste; events that happened; words that were said; places in which the experience happened; body movements that took place; etc. Use this sentence as a starting point: "The facts are . . . [and fill in what the facts are]."

Take a moment to notice your global body experience now. What's your body like after doing this? How does it compare to before?

3. *How do you feel about those facts?*

Now that you have some space, how do you feel toward those facts? What's it like to know how you respond to them? Is there a connection between the facts themselves, and the feelings and interpretations you have about those facts? What do you think that's about?

One of two things is likely to happen. If the client is a more anxiously oriented individual, tending to become overwhelmed by feelings, doing this experience may create containment as it organizes what is happening. Conversely, if the client's main style is dismissive or rejecting, they will tend to go numb. Doing this practice offers them an invitation to have feelings from a safe distance while looking at the components of the experience.

"The facts are _____ and I feel _____ about those facts" and/or "The facts are _____ and that means _____"

What's your felt experience now?

If there is no change, try going back and repeating just the facts—over and over again (in a steady voice, if possible). For example, *"The facts are (I am here in x building, the phone just rang and it was (so and so)."* Take a breath. Repeat the facts again. *"The facts are _____"* List the facts. Breathe. Avoid going into the feelings (i.e., any embellishments related to interpretation). Anytime you catch yourself sliding into feelings or interpreting, go back to the facts. Repeat the facts over and over again until the nervous system calms down.

MEDITATION: SIX SIDES OF THE BREATH

Objective: *Focusing on the breath narrows the field of consciousness, to becoming aware of sensations/felt experience of the breath, moving up and down, side-to-side, front to back. This simple practice teaches concentration and equanimity*

Instructions: Learning to train the breath helps focus *prana*, and trains us in dealing with the turbulence that comes entering the body. Any and every time we bring attention to our bodies, we encounter something. Sometimes its pleasant feelings, sometimes its resistance. Calling this "turbulence," an ostensibly neutral term, decreases the negative valence.

In traditional meditation settings we focus on sitting a certain way, holding the spine straight, eyes closed or softly gazing, feet and pelvis positioned a certain way. In the 1990s, while teaching yoga and meditation to people on a dissociative unit at a major hospital, I found it essential for people to not worry about doing it "right." It is much more important to practice. Eliminating barriers to entry makes it easy to get the basics so clients will practice for one minute, or three minutes, stretching that where possible to five or ten minutes.

Harnessing and training the breath is what the yogis in ancient times called *pranayama*, the art and science of breathing practices, used to remove obstacles in the flow of the body's life force. The Sanskrit word for life force is *prana*, something we all have. It's the vital energy that animates every aspect of life, whether it's our heart rate, digesting food, or dealing with infections.

This intelligent life force actively participates in every moment of life, whether pumping the blood in your body, helping plants grow, or determining how the planets move through the solar system. *Pranayama* is the practice of tuning into this unlimited intelligence, aligning ourselves with the positive benefits of *prana* to physiologically activate the parasympathetic nervous system, shifting the fight-flight response, giving energy when we're depleted. Changing our body's nervous system alters our habitual psychological patterns, giving a sense of control. When we know we can regulate our breathing and our nervous systems, we have a sense of confidence that we can deal with life in a more satisfying way. Patanjali wrote that the goal of yoga is to remember and abide in our true nature—which is available to all of us. Activating and channeling *prana* helps support healing the body, mind, and heart.

Script: With that in mind, shift your attention from the busy contortions of the mind, becoming interested and curious about the workings of your inner physical world. We're going to start here with a simple, tiny extending of the exhale, training the body to rest. Then we'll do a simple breathing exercise, called the "Six Sides of the Breath," to gently allow oxygen to move more freely in the lungs and therefore the body:

Bringing attention to the breath (pause). Even now the breath is happening. Maybe you're taking little sips of breath, or you might be more comfortable taking deeper breaths. Whatever the case, let go of effort (pause), finding a rhythm. In the midst of this you may find your mind wandering, moving around—that's normal. Noticing that, steer your attention back to the rhythm of the breath.

I'll be leading you in a little guided practice. If it doesn't feel right, then tune me out, trust your own guidance of what feels right.

Sitting or lying comfortably in such a way that you start to settle in an enjoyable way. Allowing yourself to appreciate the possibility of easing and calmly relaxing.

Sometimes it is helpful to start with the concreteness of your body, wiggling around, feeling your spine and bones against whatever it is you are being supported by. If you like, letting your eyes softly close or perhaps just letting your eyes gaze downwards. Letting ease call to you, moving gently at the edges of your attention (pause). So that a wonderful sense of rest begins to sweep through your body and mind. Noticing your usual thoughts and feelings getting more distant, even as the air around you holds you gently.

Sensing inside your body, as you also feel the support of gravity (pause). Resting on the chair. Perhaps you can also feel inside your skin (pause). Becoming aware of the spine inside your body (pause) no effort (pause), no agenda (pause), no need to do this right.

Finding it infinitely reassuring to feel the strength of your spine right there with you (pause), relaxing a very deep part of you which comes to feel soothed and even more reassured (pause). All this happening in such a comforting way that you observe yourself quieting, and serenely resting, easily, like the calm clear waters of a beautiful pond.

If it feels right, imagine both the solid, steadiness of your spine (pause), and then imagine that there's a clear and open space right in front of the spine (pause). Then noticing your breath again, as you center yourself in your chest (pause). Making contact with your heart.

From there (pause), following your breath as it comes into your body (pause). Imagining it then moving up from your heart, moving up along the spine, feeling where the top of your breath is. (pause). Taking all the time you need.

Then coming into the center of your being, your heart, following the breath down (pause). Noticing the bottom of your breath, allowing it to move as it does, down from your heart then up again. Not trying to do it right, but discovering you in this moment, discovering how the breath moves in and out of you, up the top of you and down inside you.

Then breathing top to bottom, at the same time expanding. Grounded in your heart, as you breathe in both directions at the same time. Expanding to the top and the bottom at the same time.

Then feeling your spine on the back of the chair (pause). Breathing back into the chair making contact with the chair through your back (pause). Doing this a few times as you get comfortable with the breath moving into your back.

If you like putting a hand on your chest, on your heart, and breathing right into the warmth of your hand. Your breath on the inside making contact with your hand on the outside (pause), finding your own rhythm (pause). Then breathing front to back at the same time. Filling your center, including your front and your back (pause). Your hand anchoring your front, the chair anchoring your back.

Shifting slightly, breathing into your right side (pause), imagining your right arm being pushed away from your body. Letting the movement of your breath expand your lungs to the right, as if your breath is moving out to your right saying hello to whatever is there to your right (pause). Shifting once again (pause), your breath moving into your left side (pause). Effortlessly moving (pause), your breath, saying hi to whatever is on your left, your arm lifting away from your body with each breath. Then breathing left to right and right to left at the same time.

As you're reading, bring all six sides of the breath together, breathing like an umbrella opening.*

Top to bottom, front to back, side to side.

Then if it feels right, letting the breath expand even bigger (pause), if you feel comfortable letting your breath intermingling with others in the room if there are others (pause), sharing with them and offering to them a sense of kindness, well-being, connection, community.

* Thanks to Alice Rosen for this image.

Gently shifting back when you're ready (pause). Letting your eyes slowly open, moving. Shifting.

Riding the Bell Curve of Sensations

Using any one of the breathing exercises you've tried, start with watching your breath. Get as close as possible to each tiny moment of the inhalation, and as close as possible to each exquisite movement of the exhalation.

We tend to have shorthand for sensorial experiences in the body. Say you feel tight. That's one description. But is it accurate? Does it resonate completely? Is it tight? Or is it stiff? Strained? Tense? Thick? Bound? Constricted? Contracted? Dense?

Spend some time exploring your experience of sensations. How many of them are you aware of in your body at any one time? Spacey, fluttery, tense, constricted, tight, stiff, strained, slack, slow, soft, unstable, stretched, knotted?

Now focus on one particular sensation. See if you can "isolate" one and focus on it. Maybe it's a tingling, or a sensation of heat or coolness. Become fascinated with it. How does it shift and change? Watch as the sensation moves and alters with your attention.

Are you able to stay with one expression of this sensation? Try to follow it as the jittering in your spine (or whatever you are following) moves. Can you get as close to it as possible?

Notice how sensation has a life of its own. Can you see/feel/notice how a sensation rises, crests and falls? What happens in you as you keep track of these small movements inside you?

The more you notice the small movements the easier it will be to track the larger, more intrusive moments that inevitably happen to all of us.

PSYCHOEDUCATIONAL: GINGERBREAD PERSON

Objective: *Outlining the body allows the client to externalize internal experience, giving psychological space to intervene with symptoms. How energy gets held in the subtle body; map out tension and emotional turbulence inside and outside of body, training awareness of experience.*

Instructions: On a blank sheet of paper, draw an outline of a gingerbread person. (I deliberately use a gingerbread person instead of a person's body because of all the possible body dysmorphic beliefs that can easily arise.)

- Soften your gaze so you can turn your attention inward. What are you aware of? (You might want to give them a menu starting at nontriggering locations like hands, feet, shoulders, avoiding client's individually organized trigger points.)
- Are there thoughts? Feelings? Sensations?
- One by one find the location of the tension in the body arena (inside the body or outside the body) and color or write where it is on the gingerbread person.
- Allowing for as much time as the client needs or wants to.
- What happens inside you as you see the gingerbread person? How do you feel toward that drawing? (If a lot of negativity comes up ask the client to locate the negativity in or around them, and then externalize it through writing and drawing until they have more centered, grounded, or compassionate feelings.

YOGA: SEATED MOUNTAIN

Objective: *Creating a stretch that is just intense enough to activate thoughts, feelings, and sensations, the client enters into the posture while reporting everything that is going on to the therapist. The therapist writes down what's going on as it happens. Afterwards they sort it out together, inviting the client to become more aware of the subtleties that go on in the body.*

Instructions: This posture can be taught both standing and sitting. The idea is to hold the body in an appropriately activating form, so that the client can study the thoughts, feelings, and body sensations that arise while the therapist writes down in three columns whatever the client reports, to discuss the relationships between them afterwards.

Directions for the Standing Mountain Posture

Come into a standing position with your feet hip-width apart. Take a moment and notice what the ground feels like. You might even want to move around on your feet, feeling for what position feels most grounded to you. Roll onto your toes, back onto your heels; even play side-to-side.

Directions for the Seated Mountain Posture

Sit comfortably so that your legs are at a 90-degree angle and so the spine is tall without slouching. This might mean scooting forward on the chair.

Continued directions for both variations:

Come to a sturdy and balanced position. Bring your attention to your whole body, take a breath, and press up into the crown of your head. You might feel your head lift and your spine elongate. Keep pressing gently up into your crown and, at the same time, down into your feet. Notice the lengthening.

Gently begin to press down into your fingertips, as well. You'll notice as you do that there's a pull along your shoulders. If you can, also press up into your crown. Take a deep breath, and press down into your fingertips, slowly raise your hands up along your side. As your hands come up to your shoulders rotate your palms up.

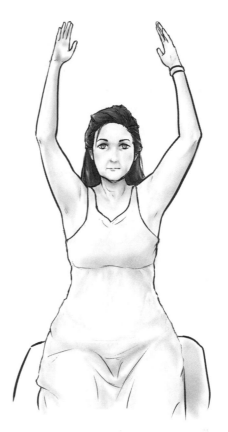

FIG 3.6   Seated Mountain

Press your shoulders down, and raise your arms straight up overhead. Pause when your palms face each other directly above your shoulders.

Take a long, deep breath. Relax your shoulders, press down into your feet and up through your crown. Let your bones—your structure—hold you in position, keeping your muscles relaxed and your breathing easy.

SUGGESTIONS FOR GUIDING THE POSTURE

With your client in the posture, remind them to breathe and to relax their muscles. You'll see some of them bring their hands down; some will lift them up again, and some won't. This isn't a contest. Whatever they do is "right." The point is to just notice. You'll write down whatever they report.

If you feel comfortable, you could demo the posture to your client for about three minutes, being transparent and comfortable about what is happening as you do it. I report out thoughts, feelings, and sensations. If you are uncomfortable about that, explain the process and let your client know to report out everything that they notice inside.

Often clients have censors in place to filter what they say. If there is a long slow period when the client says nothing you might want to prompt for thoughts, feelings, and sensations. If they feel numb or blank, ask them to describe what numb or blank feels like, where it is in the body or around them.

You can also ask them to scan the whole body to see if that experience is everywhere. Prompts include, "Is your right baby toe also blank?" "What about your eyebrows? Are they numb, or is something else going on there?"

When the client feels finished ask them to take a deep breath and, on the exhalation, relax their arms down, taking time to notice and report what's happening as they do this. Even when their arms are back down by their sides, have them report out the experience of relaxation. What's it like to savor that?

Then take time to talk about their internal experience, the notes you took, and what you experienced being with them.

MINDFUL PSYCHOEDUCATION: WALKING TOWARD

Objective: *The client walks step-by-step toward the therapist, with each step reporting out the thoughts, feelings, and sensations inside. This practice explores the intimacy and proximity issues inherent in attachment trauma. There have been many times when I have done this purely as an imaginative exercise, "Imagine taking one small step toward (or away from) me—what do you notice?"*

Instructions: In this exercise, the client has complete control, telling you where to stand, how far away, who takes the steps, etc. In groups I've had some members feel "trapped" by standing still, and they've experimented with being the one doing the walking. It's important for people to take on as much as they can, without setting themselves up for being overwhelmed. Encourage them to experiment with what's right for them.

This experience has one person (A) standing quietly on one side of the room while another person (B) moves at A's request, one step at a time toward B. Before the client takes a step or has you step forward, ask them to notice what's happening in their body. What thoughts are there? What feelings are they aware of? What body sensations? It's a version of the children's game, "Mother, May I?"

The goal is to have the client (and the therapist, for that matter) notice what happens inside, by slowing down the experience and gaining awareness of the tiny, subtle indications of information as they are flowing. B keeps moving forward as A notices what happens with each step.

Sometimes information arises as a flutter or a hesitation, without reason or context. Noticing these small things is important. Encourage closer study. Ask the client what impulses are there? To step forward? Or back? Maybe taking a half step or a step sideways. It can be interesting to see what happens when the client turns around and isn't facing you, or if the client asks you to turn around.

There's no right way to do this exercise. The only stipulation is to study the experience and have the client be in as much control as they need to be.

What we're looking to develop is a sensate vocabulary—tingling, pulsing, knotted, fluttery, cold, hard, and weak pressure—to describe their internal landscape. Often these sensations take time to study, so take the time needed to see what they learn. Invite and encourage them to play with the experience.

PURE EXPERIENCE: HEARING. SEEING. SMELLING. TOUCHING. TASTING

Objective: *Explore the bare facts of how you take in information. Yogic psychology tells us we have six sense doors through which we receive data. Through those doors there's almost an instant movement toward or away from that information.*

Practice: Freedom comes when we can interrupt that automaticity of grabbing onto something or instantly pushing it away

- Wherever you are now, hear the sounds around you. Can you hear without thinking? Without interpreting? Without embellishing? Be in the hearing.
- Let your awareness grow so that the sound is actually happening inside this larger space.
- What's that like?

- Try that with other senses. Taste. What is it like to taste before the "I want more" or "I hate this" happens?
- What about the other senses?

Instead of moving toward the emotion, in this meditation we relax our attention away from the feeling state.

It's not like the feeling is gone. You know it's there and at the same time you give yourself some distance. It's like you're standing on the shore, and a friend is out in a boat out in the ocean. You can see your friend in the boat, and you wave from the shore. This meditation gives you space from any intensity.

Start by noticing where the feeling is located in your body. Bring your attention to it, without being drawn into it. What will aid you in having some space is to consciously split your awareness—keeping part of your awareness attending the emotional state, while allowing the rest of your attention to expand into sounds around you.

You might hear birds chirping in the early morning, or a computer humming, or the sounds of the garbage men on the street. Let the sounds fill your awareness, even as you keep an attentional finger on the pulse of the emotion. You'll feel your energy expand to include this larger field of focus.

Allow the birds or other sounds to keep your mind focused and notice the effect this has on your body, and your anxiety or depression in particular.

CHAPTER 4

Disarm Dissociation with Presence

Denise was curled into a chair in my office. Arms tight around her, even as her eyes darted everywhere without seeing anything. As she struggled to speak, her head twisted continuously and into odd angles. Her therapist had come along with Denise for a consultation to help both of them work with dissociative states that hijacked Denise. They had been doing great work, that was obvious, yet the therapist, well trained in multiple treatment modalities yet not specifically in dissociation, was stumped. The therapist felt Denise was "getting worse" instead of better. When she broached the idea of a consultation Denise was hesitant but grudgingly open to it. Even as she was grateful for the chance for her parts to finally be seen, she felt more and more confused and disoriented. In the consultation Denise's eyes showed a trance beginning as the part took over. Then blending fully with the part, she was expressing the part's experience through movement and silent horror. Unable to find words, Denise was communicating in the only way she knew how. This part of her was holding something that she didn't know how to communicate in words so the communication came in movements, expression, feelings.

It's painful to dip this deeply into body memories. At the same time, it's important to know what's there, while not diving too deeply into the deep end of the psychological pool. Learning to titrate, taking slow steps into the material, allows the Self of the system to guide the course. Without it, integration doesn't happen; the parts stay compartmentalized.

These are tender moments for all of us. Sometimes, however, parts are so hungry for contact that they consume the entire session. Another option is to engage the present moment reality. The reality is (or we could say that the facts are) that Denise is 45, has a couple of children that she mothers quite well, has a solid career, and is recovering from horrible events in her history and in her adult life. As a society we need her to be in her life with us. We need her contribution, her vitality, her courage and determination. In therapy, we hold the polarity of her strengths and these nameless, voiceless parts of her, valuing the feeling states to come forward and be shared, while also creating space for Denise to be there with herself, to not be lost in the past.

As gently as I can, I remind her, "We're here with you, Denise, we know there is a lot going on inside." I watch her hand push out at me, pushing me away, rejecting this. This part of her wants to stay in this cocoon. Yet I know in the long run that cocoon will become a trap for her. She isn't only this despairing part. She is so much more than that. So I stay with her, "The fact is, we're here with you, in my office, on Massachusetts Avenue in Arlington. It took courage to ask for our help. We're here with you." After moments of squirming and pushing away, her body settles. That moment of intersubjective contact allowed Denise to begin to shift "time zones," time traveling back into this present moment, recognizing the larger reality instead of being caught in that one silo of subjective experience.

As therapists, we naturally want to help our clients. Our training supports this natural inclination, giving us the tools, treatments, and maps to follow when dealing with people's complicated inner and outer lives. We are regularly faced with our clients' unrelenting internal distress. They each acutely feel the staccato moments when they're unable to make sense of all that is fermenting inside them. They come to us, tormented with symptoms, which, as we learn to read them for what they are and interact with them, give us the felt subjective experience of their internal life. They're having symptoms, instead of memories. This is especially true when our clients have had any form of trauma or attachment wounding. As Rahima told me, "I wish I could come in with a broken leg, at least then I'd have a reason for the pain I would be in." Without external reasons for their suffering, our clients often retreat into themselves, isolating from others. They come to us vulnerable, disorganized in their inner worlds, asking us to enter into the broken states that consume them. Desperately alone, they ache for relief while at the same time pushing away the hope that it can ever be different.

We go there with them, willingly suspending the reality of the moment to enter into what Daniel Stern called the Intersubjective Matrix (2004), where the emphasis is on nonverbal, implicit contents of the present moment. The inevitable byproduct of this is to enter relational enactments (Bromberg, 2011) that are almost always "sloppy" (Stern, 2004) and are essential for healing attachment traumas. As well-meaning as any of us might be when we enter this matrix with our clients, we can be seduced into believing that the distress of the past they are expressing is the reality of what is happening now. Like Hansel and Gretel moving into the dark forest, we hope our breadcrumbs will guide both of us back to the reality of the present moment. Yet there are times we lose our way in this intersubjective matrix, as our client's felt experience becomes the dominant reality. Catapulted into a felt/psychic world, the person is disoriented, caught between this current moment and a wholly different time zone of psychological and body "memories." Both therapist and client become disoriented, grappling as the present reality collides with this subjective inner world of the client. Distressed parts located in the past time zone, affectively loaded and full of unprocessed "charge," become more real, more "true" than the current time zone, hijacking the client's awareness of their current age and circumstance. We can be drawn in, to join them in their helplessness and hopelessness, treating our client as the broken being their state is wrapping us in. Whiten (1991) reminds us that we, as therapists, are quite good at "mind-reading" despite our doubts and needs for reassurance and the fine-tuning of what we pick up. Being acutely aware of every micro-movement (Ekman, 2003), our clients scrutinize our face and listen to the tone in our voice, wanting us to join them in their inner "play." The unconscious fantasy is that if we can be inveigled into this world with them we can "retrieve them" from the past. They can then get what they couldn't get in the past. To do this requires some aspect of consciousness to be in the present moment.

INTEGRATING THE IMPULSE TO ESCAPE THE PRESENT

Untangling this, we meet our client's disconnected longing in the present moment instead of being pulled into their past subjective states. "We don't need all of the Self there. Five percent is enough," Richard Schwartz tells us (Schwartz, 1994). When grounded in reality, in this present moment, as we knock on the doors of exiled parts, our clients can go into the subjective past bringing Self and witness consciousness with them, opening the opportunity for healing. Without that, our clients are doomed to cycle through reenactment after reenactment, and we are often catapulted in with them.

Clients who live with dissociation rebel against this in treatment. They will demand, cajole, protest that "it" should come from outside. That someone should finally love them the way they want and need, that life should give them a break. That someone should do x, y, or z for them. That they should get what they always wanted, without which they won't release their hold on the past, or transition into the present moment.

As painful as this cauldron is, without wrestling in it, the person doesn't learn to encounter the patterns that shaped them and develop their own unique sense of self. The person has to face the painful reality that they didn't get what they wanted, certainly not back then, possibly not now, and in that confrontation with reality the possibility exists to shift from a life lived looking to the painful past toward one moving forward into the life they want to live.

Tilda's entire family has a history of dissociation and addiction, as well as physical, emotional, and sexual violence. She's the only one in her family who has sought mental health treatment. Tilda remains single, although she would love to be able to have a relationship. Currently, after 13 years of therapy, we are working with her being able to stay present with people she to whom she finds an attraction. I started working with Tilda after an overdose and hospitalization. It took a good year of working together before she told me what it was really like inside— that she was afraid she was crazy. "Really crazy, like schizophrenic crazy," she told me. External voices railed at her, coming from loudspeakers. She was terrified I would "lock her up" hearing this. Slowly, we began the process of organizing her disorganized inner world. Taking a number of the Becoming Safely Embodied™ courses she practiced consistently, especially the skills of deconstructing triggers, separating facts from feelings, practicing self-kindness and self-compassion. We drew pictures of her internal world, externalizing parts and voices so she could consciously be with them. Unblended from the parts we began to see how permeable her boundary was, how fluidly she oriented to "bad things" merging, taking them on. Tilda began to recognize when the past was intruding, when she was triggered, and how the voices were activated at those times. With time we cleared some inner ground, organizing the huge pile. Restructuring gave her a basis to stand on, to interact with others from.

Healing trauma holds the frame and dimension of this current time/space reality, while dipping into the past. Standing on the edge of the past we consciously turn the flashlight of consciousness into the dark past without falling in. If we don't keep some present moment awareness it's easy to slip into our client's subjective reality, losing the present moment connection that structures our meeting: we are here, in this physical space at this current time. We say to our clients, "In this moment I know you are experiencing pain and that that pain is connected to something in the past that is flooding into this moment. Can you feel me there with you, entering into this pain? I know you feel lost, and together we can find our way through." With that, we knock on the door of our client's time zone, the one in which they are lost and in distress, while staying in the present moment. Touching that state with them, we experience the felt experience they are subjectively in, entering the intersubjective matrix while staying connected to this present moment reality (Stern, 2004). Holding that dual consciousness (Corrigan, Wilson, & Fay, 2014b; Fisher, 2010; Ogden, Minton, & Pain, 2006; van der Kolk, 2015), we offer a lifeline for our clients to heal their histories and climb out of the past.

DISSOCIATION FROM AN ATTACHMENT PERSPECTIVE

Frank Corrigan, MD, a psychiatrist in Glasgow, Scotland, helped shape my view of dissociation, integrating an attachment perspective. Working in this way dissociation can be seen as a form of protest. The client's behaviors rail at the extreme disappointment of not having received what was needed as a child, of not being heard, valued, protected, and kept safe. Bowlby, and his colleague James Robertson, studied children temporarily separated from their families in the 1940s (Karen, 1994). The children were removed from familiar environments for a week or more, and placed in unfamiliar environments with previously unknown caregivers. Robertson and Bowlby observed their adjustment before separation, during separation, and upon returning home. Despite the variations in responses, they found three phases: protest, despair, and detachment (Bowlby, 1980). Protest behaviors began when the child felt a potential threat of separation, including tears, tantrums, anger, and searching for the caregiver. (Likewise, behaviors like desperately clinging to the therapist, frequently calling or texting, needing the therapist to help self-soothe, are the client's attachment system in action.)

When not responded to appropriately, the child fell into the despair phase, ushering in a hopelessness of anyone returning. Other indicators of the despair phase were diminished physical movements, obvious sadness, withdrawal from others, and, for some, hostile behaviors toward others as well as toward favorite toys/objects. At some point the child began to mourn the loss of the person (Bowlby, 1973). Bowlby cautioned not to misunderstand this phase as an adjustment to the caregiver's absence. If separation continued, the child entered the detachment phase, no longer pushing away substitutes. The most noticeable signal of detachment was when the primary caregiver returned, and the child showed little joy or enthusiasm, instead appearing disinterested or apathetic. Some of the children didn't recognize their mothers, and some walked away from them. In fact, some of the mothers later described their children as treating them like they were strangers. Some children vacillated between fear of imminent separation and a blank, expressionless faces. Others fell deeper into the despair and detachment phases, losing time, unable to regulate themselves or rejecting therapy or other people, burrowing deeper into isolation.

These relational patterns show up in the present moment as holograms from the past, projected into the present moment. Seen this way, they hold keys to repattern into an earned secure, stable self, if both the client and therapist are patient and willing to withstand the relational turbulence that ensues (Bromberg, 2011; Stern, 2004). Tronick's research with infants and caregivers described how "Stress Builds Character" (2007) when the caregiver-child pair successfully navigates though a process of match-mismatch-rematch. These "missteps in the dance" of therapy can often be "sloppy" (Stern, 2004) requiring creative attention and repair. "We [Tronick and Stern] both have commented that missteps are most valuable because the manner of negotiating repairs, and correcting slippages is one of the most important ways-of-being-with-the-other that become implicitly known." (Stern, 2004, p. 157). They emphasize how important it is that "sloppiness creates something that needs to be lived through and worked out rather than understood." (Stern, 2004, p. 159).

Even with the maps well laid out by trauma theorists such as Bessel van der Kolk, Judith Hermann, James Chu, Onno van der Hart, Kathy Steele, Elert Nijenhuis, and Giovanni Liotti, therapists find encountering the dissociative domain confusing and disruptive. We learn through trial by fire how sloppy and messy the process of healing is. This is confounded by our own unfinished countertransference material. In the midst of sitting with our clients and dealing with their inner worlds we can find our own attachment patterns activated forcing us into a parallel process exploring and remapping our patterns. Consultation and our own reflective process untangles and repatterns not only the client's nonnarrative patterns but our own.

DISSOCIATION AS PROTEST BEHAVIOR

Therapeutic change is fundamentally challenging even when the client actively wants the change. It inherently brings up resistance, especially when the lines between past and present are blurred. Embedded traumatic schemas give preference to perspectives from another time zone. Corrigan, Wilson, and Fay (2014b) write about the neurobiological residue of clinical despair, in which protest has more energy while despair has a spectrum of shutdown, depending on the amount of parasympathetic dominance.

"With detachment, a normal level of energy is available but the emotions driving attachment are suppressed or disconnected, or there is a state of low motivation and low enthusiasm for living. The primary driver to pathological dissociation is attachment disorganization in early life: when that is followed by severe and repeated trauma, then a major disorder of structural dissociation is created (Lyons-Ruth, Dutra, Schuder, & Bianchi, 2006). The nonavailability of the mother exposes the predissociative infant to a hostile/ helpless model of attachment. There are parallels with the fight/submit model of depression and anxiety, but in adults the fight/submit conflict derives from interactions with significant others and does not necessarily involve separation distress. In infants, it is assumed that any conflict engendered by the witnessing of behavior that fluctuates from frightening to frightened, hostile to submissive, would carry the risk of separation at least at the emotional level. As significant traumas often have feelings of lonesomeness at their core, it is likely that the circuits underlying separation distress contribute to the complex emotional residue of unresolved adversity; the submit state and the collapse despair state are overtly identifiable physiologically." (Corrigan, Wilson, & Fay, 2014b, pp. 194–195).

Clients respond well to exploring dissociation as protest behaviors. It makes sense to them that they are protesting being in the present. The part holding the pain fears that it will not be heard and tended to, protesting the separation from the past. For some clients, dissociation shows up in the protest phase as being angry and upset at not having their needs met, desperately seeking the therapist or others to fulfill their past needs. Clients holding tenaciously to their past traumatic stories express their protest by leaving treatment, while continuing to despair that change is impossible.

Judy was one of those clients who had been in many forms of therapy over the years, from analysis on the couch to cognitive behavioral therapy to Eye Movement Desensitization Response (EMDR) to Internal Family Systems (IFS) to Accelerated Experiential Dynamic Psychotherapy (AEDP). Coming into my office, she was determined to find a way to "beat her past" and make life better. Yet the hold of the past was uncompromising, and she eventually left therapy with me. Four and a half years later, Judy asked to resume treatment with me after having established a LifeForce yoga practice (Weintraub, 2013, 2012, 2003). Experiencing being in her body's discomfort taught her how to be with her body in a different way, tolerating distress, separating the past from the present moment. Judy described being in a yoga class wanting to leave her body as she was holding a difficult pose. Watching herself wanting to dissociate to get away from the physical pain and the associated memories, Judy remembered our past discussion of dissociation as protest. Realizing her pattern, Judy told me "I needed to see how stuck I was in my past, before I could use any form of therapy to change."

Dissociation defines not being in this moment; running the spectrum of simple daydreaming to complicated splits among the personality. Yet it's only in this moment that anything in life can be changed and integrated. We can influence the future or shift the past, but we can only do that when we're here in this moment. That's where integration happens. Helping our clients to be in their bodies, minds, and hearts provides critical assistance to being with the dissociative states that arise. As a client identifies the basic building blocks of their inner world, their thoughts, feelings, and sensations, they will more easily enter into and find their way out of dissociative moments. Exploring Body Time (as discussed in Chapter Three on Entering the Body) is different than the rapid fire world of thoughts, associations, memories, and interpretations they've grown used to. The body's wisdom is slower, taking a different felt language, disrupting the subjective realities and stories our clients have made up.

PARSING THIS MOMENT FROM OTHER MOMENTS

Separating this moment from all that clouds the inner space takes patience and perseverance. With our clients we peel apart the thoughts, feelings, and sensations that fuel each moment. We also parse out the psychological components, which is where Internal Family Systems therapy can be helpful. From a body-oriented perspective, "parts" are psychological representations combining thoughts, feelings, and sensations into discrete aspects of the larger whole. Normal in all people "parts" have various functions in the IFS model. The non-extreme intention of parts is positive, aiming to support the complexity of the whole known as "Self-Energy." These subpersonalities can become extreme, especially for people with dissociative features, where the part feels so "real" that identification is blended with that part (Schwartz, 1994). Being blended with a part is good when we want to fill up with a positive, nourishing, life-enhancing experience. If, however, as so often happens, a part is stuck in an unhelpful role with no way to change or be different, life becomes constricted.

IFS comes from a long tradition of therapies used to separate parts as a way of creating internal organization and integration. Fritz Perls, founder of Gestalt Therapy (1969/1992), had people sit in an empty chair, take on the role of a particular part, then moving to a new chair and new part, having a dialogue that embodies each part fully. In psychosynthesis, Assagioli, (1988/2007) developed the idea of subpersonalities in order to create internal psychological distinctions. Identifying and externalizing parts is a concrete way for clients to feel the difference between the physiological charge held in their bodies, and their Self. Simple ways of separating can be to write down the feeling, or role, or part, onto a sticky note or piece of paper, and move it somewhere else in the room (or out of the room, if more figurative distance is needed). Drawing the part, or writing down the internal dialogue by splitting a piece of paper in half, with different sides being different parts of a part, are other ways of externalizing parts. (More in the practice session for this at the end of the chapter.)

In sorting through this tangled internal web, we provide the necessary organization that our clients didn't previously build, laying down scaffolding to hold the slippery frames in place. Most clients find it helpful to know that they are living Parallel Lives (Fay, 2007), in which they are here in this moment with us while at the same time parts of them are living in a subjectively real, parallel life. Van der Hart, Nijenhuis, and Steele use the Structural Dissociation model, (2006) giving therapists a key to understanding chronic traumatization and treatment in which dissociation is not a random experience, occurring instead along existing "fault lines."

What separates this present moment from subjective and past states is a psychological filter, a dissociative barrier that keeps the past in the past, using tremendous psychic energy to keep it in place. The "blocked feelings" are kept out of conscious awareness through creative, yet often painful and self-destructive ways. The unnamed fear our clients have is that if that past material is allowed into the current moment, they will be overwhelmed by the crud of the past, becoming annihilated by it.

That pivot point out of dissociation can only happen in the present moment. This messy intersubjective space is hard to describe, even as it provides the key to the way out. We have to be with our clients in the dreadful reality of what happened while holding the truth that it's not happening now. (Of course, when a client is in a current traumatic environment, we must be attentive to that reality.) Clinically, dissociation is a creative solution to a painful experience that the person didn't have any other way of dealing with (Corrigan, Wilson, & Fay, 2014b; Fisher, 2017, 2010; Paulsen, Lanius, & Corrigan, 2014; van der Hart, Nijenhuis, & Steele, 2006). Simplified dissociation is a coping strategy that becomes a habitual pattern and way of being in the world. Neuroscience addresses this through the idea of neural pathways being laid down through habituation (van der Kolk, 2015). This path becomes familiar, as it is trod along over and over again. The terrain becomes known, landmarks recognized, the outcome predetermined. Protest, despair, and detachment patterns all become markers of habitual ways of interacting.

PARALLEL LIVES

This comingling of present and past is a simple way to define dissociation. For this reason I ask clients to learn the felt, experiential difference between being in the present moment and their experience of when the past intrudes. At first, these distinctions aren't obvious. Living in these blurred realities has been commonplace for them. For them, the past *is* happening now. Naming the body experience of the past invading the present, and how it shapes current reality, gives people a way to identify when the past encroaches in the present.

Living with "Parallel Lives" (Fay, 2007), our clients shape shift, traveling through psychological time zones. The therapeutic task is to have the client separate the past from the present moment. Together the objective is, "How do you know the here and now? How do you know you're in the past?" When in the present moment, we have access to our present moment wisdom accumulated throughout life, through all there is that has contributed to our getting to this point, with all its ups and downs. For trauma survivors, however, time becomes warped. The here and now time boundary gets blurred with memories, associations, and traumatic schemas from the past. For example, a client might be walking down a street. They are moving automatically, looking "normal," while their internal experience might be one of terror, panic, too much feeling, or no feeling whatsoever. Or a client like Denise, earlier in the chapter, gets flooded by the past while sitting with you in your office, eyes becoming unfocused, body shrinking into the chair, being pulled into the past. Despite the time zone warping reality, blurring distinction, the client has some sense that they are in your office, with you, in this time. They know at some level that their inner world is out of sync with what is *actually* going on outside. The facts don't correlate with internal experience. As I remind clients, when something feels out of proportion to the situation, you can be pretty sure that you are caught in a feeling/body memory.

When pulled into the past, clients consistently describe the past like this:

- Feel like I'm trying to survive.
- I have hopeless thoughts and feelings.
- My reactions tend to be really big or inappropriate or scary.
- Feel despair, depression, exhausted, paralyzed, hopeless.
- Have black and white thinking.
- Feel flooded, numb, hypervigilant.
- Always on the verge of binging or ritualized behaviors.
- Feel powerless.
- Really want something/someone to do something to help me.
- Feel obsessive and/or compulsive.

In contrast, clients use words like this to describe the present moment:

- Right-sized.
- Shades of gray.
- Centered, grounded.
- Able to concentrate, mind is clear.
- Can feel my body.
- Feel safe to express myself.
- Can deal with things changing instead of reacting or dissociating.
- It's okay to feel the feelings (any range of good, bad, or in between).
- Feel connected inside and out.
- Things roll off my back.
- Have a sense of spaciousness.

Think of there being layers of time, in any one moment. The more split off the charged material is, the more psychic energy it takes to keep the charged past out of the present moment. It's important to keep one psychological foot in the present while exploring the charged past. Step by step, this helps our clients learn that they are here, in this moment with us. At the same time (taking poetic license to help my clients easily conceptualize) I describe the "time capsules" of experience held in the past that are kept at bay by the dissociative barrier. Each time capsule is filled with thoughts, feelings, and sensations, wrapped into memories layered with associations, and stuffed into recesses of the mind to keep the present moment safe. When triggered, time capsules open or leak information, disorienting and rupturing the present moment. It's much worse when one (or combined) time capsules explode into the moment, catapulting our clients into a horrifying distortion of reality that feels absolutely real to them. With time and patience it is possible to learn how the felt experience of the past invades and intrudes into the present, bringing a greater sense of ease and organization in daily life. In yoga, as we've seen, we call these time capsules *samskaras*, imprints of conscious and unconscious impressions, perceptions and experiences.

Some psychoeducation is helpful for people. "You're in the here in and now. You actually can't physically or biologically be anywhere else. You are here. Your mind, or parts of you, might be someplace else, in the past, or in the future. The past is made up of a huge number of memories held in different time capsules.

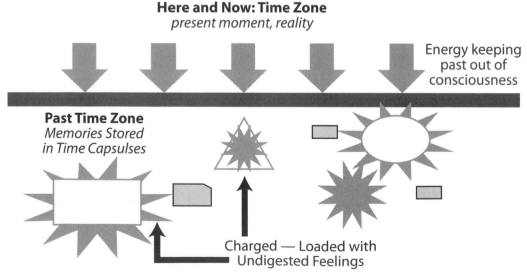

FIG 4.1   KEEPING MEMORIES AT BAY

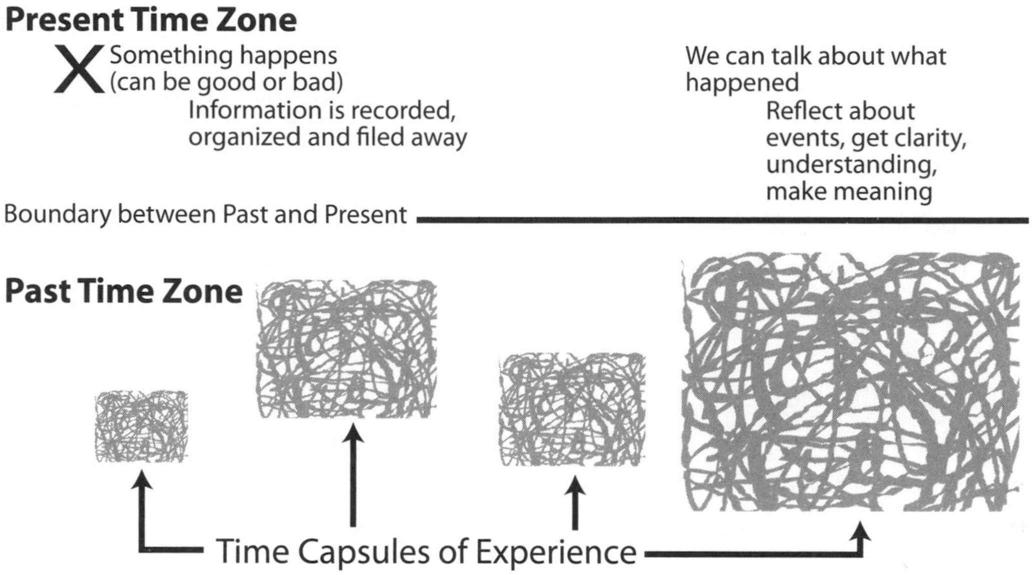

Present Time Zone

X Something happens
(can be good or bad)
    Information is recorded,
    organized and filed away

We can talk about what
happened
    Reflect about
    events, get clarity,
    understanding,
    make meaning

Boundary between Past and Present ——————————————

Past Time Zone

Time Capsules of Experience

FIG 4.2   PARALLEL LIVES WHEN LIFE IS GOOD

Remember the first time you rode a bike? That time capsule is made up of visual memories, feeling memories, different thoughts that you might have had, things that you said, things that were said to you, the way the bike felt to you, what it was like to be with or without training wheels. That's one cache of memories loaded into these time capsules. There are time capsules for everything that has ever happened throughout your life, the good things, the bad things, the indifferent things."

Having a drawing of the Parallel Lives model helps to make this more concrete. When life is good we move through life with more ease. We are able to be flexible and adapt, dealing with events as they occur, smoothly processing information, and storing it for retrieval in the future.

This overly simplified version of memory storage helps clients make sense of what happens. For example, if something happened at three years old, the experience is retained *as it was experienced*, not with an integrated adult perspective. There are reasons the three-year-old couldn't integrate that sensate data. Too much data flooded in for her, her brain wasn't developed enough, she needed help to contain the feelings and make sense of the arising sensate data. Without that the information is sequestered and cordoned off, held in escrow until some point in the future. When triggered later in life that three-year-old's experience comes blasting out of the past and into this moment. We call that a flashback. The past floods into the present, and these two parallel lives are merged into a chaotic whole. Not knowing what is happening, the person's internal experience vibrates with the old, undigested material from back then. As that time boundary dissolves in the face of this material coming up from the past; the client has the body/felt "memory" of what they weren't able to fully experience back then. The feelings that are too much *now* is because they were too much back then. In this present moment the client is reexperiencing what they were unable to experience as a three-year-old. It is helpful to remind the client of this over and over, and for the client to learn to say some version of this to themselves: "My goodness, this is so hard to be with now. It must have been unbearable back then."

Mary, one of the clients in a Becoming Safely Embodied™ group, described her own experience of dissociation this way: "It happens when this little part of me has taken over, and is extremely panicked because she can't manage an adult life at work or anywhere else. When she's in charge, you know, screaming, she doesn't talk to anyone. So that's what dissociation is to me. Dissociation is also very physical. It's like tunnel vision. That's when the panic has taken over. So I'm trying to work on that piece to integrate her, to let her feel good and know that I'm listening to her—or trying to anyway. She doesn't always have to take over when things are really bad. Like she can relax sometimes because I'm trying to speak up for her and take care of her. She doesn't need to live my life, because she's unable to at ten years old. She can't manage all that. I'm learning that I can."

Luke shared: "For me it's like a disconnect. It's like the heart . . . there's no connection between the head and the heart you know. Like I'm doing the motions but not really there. There's so many . . . something prohibits me from letting that vulnerable part of me out. You know, the . . . I don't—for many years as I've been in therapy, it's just like—I still check out. My body gets really tense and like frozen." Gretchen nodded as Luke spoke, finally able to speak as we neared the end of our weeks together, "I can disconnect in many different ways. Dissociation is sometimes different, depending on the situation. But I mean it generally involves a kind of numbness of some sort. You know, totally disconnected from my heart and my feelings, and you know, sometimes it can be a complete disconnection from my body to or, sometimes I can just feel like an observer. You know, a complete observer to the whole scene, but the one that goes through everything is just kind of that numbed, dazed, sort of. Sometimes when I have a cold it kind of reminds me of being disconnected, because it shuts off a few senses, like it shuts off, and you feel like you're one step removed from everybody. It actually feels comforting. I get relief from turning down the volume of all the stimulation that's going on. Such a relief."

Others like Colleen don't like the feeling of dissociating or disconnecting, "I don't like the feeling of leaving my body. But it feels like that part of me that I don't have control over, it makes me afraid. So it doesn't feel good, it doesn't feel protected, it feels scary like I don't know what will happen feels dangerous." Sarah agreed, "I don't feel safe. Period. I have different levels of being gone and absent, so it always feels out of control, and I don't want to come back because it doesn't feel safe. So there's a lot of frozen. If the fear is high enough then I get more and more frozen, can't move, don't want to move. Other times I will do these bizarre yelps and movements, all my muscles doing weird things. And—believe it or not—that, I only do this in private, this brings a lot of the stuff down."

SHIFTING OUT OF THE OLD FAMILIAR PATH

It helps to know the unique dissociative process of each person. Something triggers a cascading series of internal processes to cope with, which over time become habitual and with the same end point. This familiar path provides odd comfort, even while treading the bumpy and uncertain paths of life. Treachery might be behind a corner, but odd as it is, this treachery is better than the

Old Familiar Path

end up in old, familiar place
(usually doesn't feel that good)

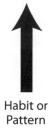

Habit or Pattern

- Comfortable even if it doesn't feel that good, like wearing an old pair of sweats.
- Behaviors we do on this old familiar path may help us feel better in the short term, providing relief.
- As we do the same thing, over and over again, though, we feel less soothed and more stuck.

FIG 4.3 OLD FAMILIAR PATH

unknown. In many ways this is what brings people to seek treatment. They come to us feeling stuck, in pain, and not knowing how to change. When there is dissociation involved, the client might have multiple parts engaged in a variety of habitual patterns, some of them conflicting. The internal cacophony that ensues makes it especially difficult to sort out the main ruckus. The person sitting in your office will tell you that they've tried other things, other models, other treatments, other therapies, none of which have worked, at least not long term. Often nothing has helped because the client has been fixated on changing the old familiar ways while being in it. There's something so seductive about being in the habit that it makes it difficult to change even while being stuck.

This is where it's helpful to name the protest. The dissociation, the lack of focus, the anger, the rejection, any pattern or behavior that a client manifests, I label as protest. They're saying, in the only way they know how, that "this isn't right!" "something's wrong!" "it shouldn't be like this!" Any expression along those lines is the unmet attachment needs being "spoken" or brought into relationship. We need to validate that protest, and engage with it, curious about what they are wanting us to understand.

Having a map helps navigate the territory. When a person knows there are steps to take that will (eventually) alleviate the pain, they are more willing to take those steps toward a more satisfying and nourishing life. The map is simple enough: know where you want to go, name it, clarify and anticipate the turbulence that arises on the way out of the comfort zone, slow down to find choice points to access with baby steps, walk one step at a time toward this new way of being, integrate the turbulence, while keeping the new end point in focus. This map builds on a foundation of what thoughts, feelings, and sensations pepper the psychological space, especially as the person stretches beyond what they know. Then break the process down, to find baby steps in the direction the person wants to go in.

INTERSUBJECTIVE CONTACT

Following this map in connection with a therapist whose purpose and intention is to affectively understand helps the client organize the multiple layers of experience into a more coherent whole. Daniel Stern (2004) writes about this intersubjective space: "Our nervous systems are constructed to be captured by the nervous systems of others, so that we can experience others as if from within their skin, as well as from within our own. A sort of direct feeling route into the other person is potentially open and we resonate with and participate in their experiences and they in ours" (p. 76). This intersubjective contact comes when we're not fused but differentiated, independent, and separate. Our clients, wounded and broken through relationship, need a safe, containing connection with us to return them back to themselves. The mutual rhythms that flow between therapist and client create solid internal ground on which the client can cultivate new habits and patterns that are more nourishing and satisfying than the old ways of being.

> *Mike would enter my office, and engage in an easy back-and-forth while he settled in. Then his body would twitch, or he'd turn his face away, or curl up into the chair—all signs that dissociative states were wrestling for attention. Although Mike was very well read in trauma and dissociation, knowing the theory didn't help, as he became swept up in the nanosecond communications of polarized parts imploring him to pay attention. I would say to him, "I'm right here. We're here in my office. And right now, nothing bad is happening." Mike's angry parts would scowl at me, communicating nonverbally how wrong I was and how little I knew. Gently, over and over, I would reassure him that we're here together and that these parts are wanting us to know something, things I wanted to hear and know about but if these parts took over then they wouldn't get what they wanted which is to be heard, known, understood. My stance was to be as reassuring and validating as I could, communicating my care in him, interest in him, my concern and attention while holding us both in the current moment. Session after session, we engaged in his subjective experience. Over time, Mike learned his own body time, created internal space, and found ways to hold onto himself even as the tsunami of the past threatened to take over.*

Intersubjective contact has the possibility of breaking the cycle of dissociative states in the present moment. You are there with your client, attentive, caring, reassuring, all qualities we can assume our clients didn't get in the past or don't have enough of now. Being interested in their internal world without being invasive (Fosha, 2011, 2000), or "looming" as Beebe, Jaffe, et al describe (2010) is a new experience for those who have been training themselves to push different parts of their experience out of consciousness to make life more tolerable. For those people who are uncomfortable with certain aspects of themselves or their inner world, it is important to develop ways to welcome and befriend them. Dan Hughes (1998), the attachment therapist who works with reactive children, suggests a "time-in" instead of "time-outs." Richard Schwartz (1994) says, "All parts are welcome." The iRest Yoga Nidra (Miller, 2015, 2014, 2010) therapist welcomes all that arises.

This welcoming stance creates an affective attunement. In matching the client's affect they are connected to their internal state. Being in the present moment, naming what's going on in their internal world, exploring their subjective states, we join our client in becoming more familiar with their internal landscape, validating the felt reality. The simple act of naming their inner landscape lands them more in reality of the past ("Yes, we know this horrible thing happened."), with the reality of this moment ("We're here in this moment, in my office, not back there."). While the client is caught in the intense whirlwind inside their psyche, by staying in the present moment we offer our client a subjective hand to grasp to help them climb out of the intruding past, inching their way into the present, co-creating a more nourishing present and future.

TWO ESSENTIAL SKILLS FOR HEALING TRAUMA

Mindfulness and concentration: two skills honed from yoga and meditation, are essential in working with dissociation—helping the body and mind to be clearer and more pliable. In doing so, the client learns to unlink themselves from the reactivity that comes with any kind of disconnection, eventually leading them toward a more satisfying way of living. To oversimplify this vast subject, mindfulness helps the client to name what's going on, while concentration practices develop the ability to focus, orienting to where the person wants to go, instead of being pulled into the cacophony of their inner worlds. Mindfulness practices help develop an ability to watch and observe without judgment (Germer, 2009; Neff, 2011), allowing the client to witness and observe the painful, or positive, experiences, and slowing down identification with these states. In the Becoming Safely Embodied™ Skills, mindfulness is developed through discriminating thoughts, feelings, and body sensations, as well as separating facts from feelings and interpretations.

Concentration practices, like self-compassion or loving kindness, help to direct attention into the body and mind in the present instead of being distracted into dissociative states. Focusing on one thing lets everything else fade in the background.

Changing our attentional focus deactivates whatever charge we have on the nonfocused object (Brown, 2013). For many people, developing concentration skills are their most powerful asset in navigating trauma recovery. Having that skill is especially beneficial when the nervous system is hijacked or overwhelmed with obsessive thinking, anxiety, depression, or flashbacks. "Narrowing our field of consciousness by selecting relevant cues is fundamental to organizing goal-directed behavior. If we cannot select what we give our attention to effectively, we may fail to notice relevant stimuli, or we may flit from one stimulus to another, with no ability to concentrate our attention." (Ogden, Minton, & Pain, 2006, p. 68).

DOWNSIDES TO MINDFULNESS AND CONCENTRATION PRACTICES

There are downsides to both practices to which we have to be sensitive. Mindfulness is an uncovering technique, allowing deeper access to nonconscious material. Willoughby Britton's Dark Knight of the Soul project addresses the complications of meditation (Rocha, 2014). When opened up too fast, people feel overwhelmed and disoriented as regressive states emerge. In extreme situations, on long retreats, people have had to be hospitalized (Rocha, 2014). Though, over time, mindfulness and concentration skills help slow down the instantaneous influx of sensory data that clogs the perceptual field. This sets the stage for people to learn how they got triggered, and how to deconstruct triggers.

When the dissociative impulse and behaviors are identified, it is necessary to slow down the process, becoming mindful of what's happening and concentrate on where to go. A useful map is through the process of "Carving Out a New Path to Look for Choice Points" (Fay, 2007) which includes these steps:

1. *Knowing the old familiar path.* Identify the habits and patterns that are so comfortable that, even when the person is tired of the pattern, they keep doing it anyway. "It's like wearing my old, favorite sweater. I know it's now grungy, but I love it. It feels so familiar and good that I want to keep wearing it anyway," Abby described. Training the person to inquire into the ingredients of the well-trodden path, we find thoughts, feelings, and behaviors that populate the path. When those thoughts, feelings, and sensations are outside their window of tolerance (Ogden, Minton, & Pain, 2006) the person has fail-safe deadening behaviors to manage them, such as overeating, restricting, overexercising

or not exercising, or a cadre of other self-destructive acts (Ferentz, 2014) or demeaning self-criticisms. The behaviors become shortcuts to move away from something that's percolating within. It's worked well in the past, laying down a neurological pathway to comfort and console. Unfortunately, over time the habitual pattern doesn't do the job in the same way, no longer soothing the activated nervous system. It becomes destructive, and the client ends up feeling stuck, trapped in the behaviors that no longer serve them.

2. *Mindfulness of Welcoming the Protest.* Being mindful, able to name the old familiar path that leads to the same place, externalizes the pattern, offering a choice point to explore something new. When the old familiar path is the only option, the person feels stuck, trapped, and like there are no other choices in life. "It shouldn't be like this!" is the simple, all-encompassing protest that shows up in multiple ways. However, the protest comes up, we welcome it; it is wisdom speaking. We now know what shouldn't be, so we can orient to what "should" be, what would be preferable, what the Nourishing Opposite would be.

3. *Choice Point – Nourishing Opposite.* Mindfulness provides the option to stop, look around, and choose. Sometimes the choice is to do the same old behaviors only to see the same result, feel the same protest. Over time, becoming more aware of the protest and all that it is wanting to express, the client learns to notice, to pause the action, to bring awareness into the process. Exploring questions like, "What is the Nourishing Opposite [of the protest]?" "What would that Nourishing Opposite look like out there? Feel like in here?" Practicing a new psychological muscle is difficult for anyone. With encouragement, clients begin to discover new options. Sarah, a client in one of my groups, said, "I am now able to allow myself to say no to others and to the parts who demand perfection or actions inspired through fear. I got this from practicing choice points and opening to the Nourishing Opposite over and over again."

4. *Turbulence in Leaving the Comfort Zone.* What keeps getting in the way? What creates that automatic return to the old, familiar, yet no longer wanted path? Whenever we step outside habitual patterns, our comfort zone, turbulence shows up, making mindfulness and choice points difficult to find. We need the balancing skill of developing concentration to focus and stay steady as turbulence is encountered. Anytime we cross an internal threshold, stepping toward something new, there will be turbulence. Yvonne Agazarian (1997) coined this phrase, teaching individuals in groups that whenever they face something

new or transition to something they are less comfortable with they will encounter turbulence of some kind. This is certainly true whenever we enter the body. We shift gears, we go from whatever is going on outside, to changing contexts and going inside. When the body has been the reservoir of discomfort, unease, turmoil, or despair, there will be turbulence in entering it. There will be some form of resistance, some unwillingness to do whatever it is. Everyone has their own unique signature of turbulence, combining thoughts, feelings, images, sensations, and memories.

You'll encounter this with your clients as you bring up the possibility of doing any of the practices in the book. The key to successfully navigating this threshold is to expect there to be protest of some kind. Expect resistance, expect there to be some form of "I'm not going to do this" or "What difference will this make? I'm still going to be with all this gunk inside." For some it might be overt, while others will present as if they are willing to do it but then gently dissociate themselves, letting their presenter parts take over while they stay safe in the background. Our task as therapists is to not be co-opted by the protest, by the resistance, or by the protector parts that are avidly keeping the pain out of harm's way. By gently leaning into the resistance we engage in "welcoming all parts," as Richard Schwartz so beautifully coined it in the IFS model.

To identify the resistance as it is coming up, it helps to first name the larger pattern, then drop the content so you can explore the sensations and bodily experience. Some clients find it helpful to name the turbulence as protector parts, designed to keep them safe in the only way they knew how. Noticing the resistance as the protest of what shouldn't be, separating from it even slightly, allows room for new expression, new explorations to arise. In IFS, we do this by asking the client to relax whatever protector part is showing up (Schwartz, 1994), not as a means of pushing the resistance away. The intention is to honor the resistance, acknowledging how valuable it has been, and letting it know that it can pop back in if at any time it feels too much is going on. We might say something like, "This resistant, protector part has all the power to reassert itself. For right now, though, would this part be willing to ease back and give you a little room? It doesn't have to do any of this. But what would it be like if it took a few steps back, for you to see what else might be possible?" (Schwartz, 1994).

Naming the psychological pattern generally gives some room for the person to explore the physical experience. Some people can more easily step aside, moving directly into the felt experience. What are the feelings? The sensations? Is it possible to ride the sensations, without getting tangled in the storyline? Having practiced having simple sensations in the body and feeling comfortable with these body processes makes it easier when more concretized patterns of sensation are then encountered. The body experience can provide a fresh and new experience counteracting the engrained mental and physiological pattern. Healing is about stretching into that new zone. As we progressively undo normal, everyday tension, we cultivate a quieter mind and body, opening receptivity to inner wisdom (Amelio, 1988–1994; Stapleton, 2015/2016). The more our clients practice easing these defenses, the more defenses soften, reducing barriers to whatever was exiled below (Schwartz, 1994). Part of yoga, meditation, or even psychotherapy is about opening a new embodied pathway to experience living the life most genuinely wanted.

With clients and in teaching workshops, I often describe turbulence as the electric fences people put up to keep their dogs in the yard. I describe a day I was walking with a friend, on a country road, enjoying the peacefulness, relaxing into the quiet conversation. We heard a dog barking, then saw it rushing toward us, activating in both of us a flight response, only to subsequently see the dog stop abruptly, barking madly but going nowhere. The dog had learned that stepping beyond that place would result in getting zapped. Our bodies calmed, realizing we weren't going to be attacked.

This is what happens when we encounter the edges of a comfort zone. We get twisted in place, barking madly, not wanting to risk getting zapped. Each person has their own form of getting zapped/turbulence. It might be depression, anxiety, fatigue, feeling disgusted, self-hatred, self-destruction, judging others, or anger. The choices are endless and unique to each person. The trick is not to get stuck in the turbulence but to see it as a way to reinforce the edges of secure space. Terry described the internal sense of pressure that came up when being compliant in his usual fashion, "I have to do it. The pressure to do it right is so strong. It's like I can't say something else—what if I don't say it right or what if I start feeling ashamed or what if no one understands?" Terry's old familiar path happened when he encounters anyone, especially his wife or boss, with a dismissive look in their face or eyes or making dismissive gestures with their shoulders or hands. The automatic cringe-and-despair vortex he falls into drives him into behaviors he later regrets. His longing for kindness and understanding seems so foreign to him that it's been unimaginable. Deconstructing each moment into its component parts helps to uncover what thoughts, feelings, and sensations are motivating action tendencies in one direction or another.

One caveat: turbulence does not feel comfortable! It's why we balk at engaging with it, preferring to return to the old, no longer satisfying path. It's in learning to navigate the turbulence that people come to feel stronger, more solid and more confident about themselves.

5. *Longing.* Everyone longs for more. It is a natural and native process, providing foundation for motivation to explore beyond what is already known. Stern (2004) describes the intersubjective motivational system to move in a new direction. In yoga, longing is prana pushing to return to the self. Wanting to be happy, to feel better, to be loved are each native, normal, and natural. Because they are so fundamental, but truncated or not encouraged, this motivational impulse gets distorted, building up beliefs that what we want is not possible. Under that defensive patterning, the longing for more is buried, creating internal chaos even as it's buried deep in the psyche. I'm sure you've heard this from clients: that their fear of failure, of disappointment in not getting what they want, is keeping them from finding choice points to endure the inevitable turbulence. It's like a garden that's become so overgrown you think it's impossible to grow anything there or to make it beautiful. Yet each time you do a little sorting and weeding, shifting and eliminating, the ground starts opening up. At first a mess, the garden is eventually cleared, becoming a blank slate, to be filled in however you want to, to beautify the area. With Terry, we had to consistently orient him toward his longing, which gave him a pathway to trust his own journey.

6. *Baby Steps.* We need to take small baby steps to move through turbulence, examining the thoughts, feelings, and sensations that occur. The impulse to take big steps and rush over the turbulence doesn't work. Big steps give the impression of getting somewhere, but if the internal ground isn't solid then we inevitably have to revisit those places, which leads to distress, and doubt that change is possible. When we fall flat or get scared, we hurl ourselves back to the safety of the comfort zone, not wanting to risk reaching out again. Learning to

go slowly, pausing, taking baby steps, supports building a strong foundation in which our clients learn trust and confidence in themselves, and in their capacity to move into the world knowing they can encounter whatever arises. Baby steps can happen in simple ways, like pausing, recognizing choice points, taking a breath, or counting to ten, to twenty, or thirty. Clients who take these new steps ultimately find themselves going in the direction that they want.

True to Bowlby's theory, when clients are given the freedom to explore without repercussions, they open up to something new. Often that new exploration is surprising or different than what was expected. The new path brings vitality and aliveness, even as it's turbulent. It's especially valuable when they have an experience with you in the safety of the therapy office. Or, if that safety is not yet established (and sometimes it takes a long while to do that—this is normal and natural in working with trauma survivors), we can invite our clients to imagine a new possibility (Brown, Elliot, et al., 2016; Falconer, Rovira, et al, 2016; Falconer, Slater, Rovira, King, Gilbert, et al., 2014; Gilbert, 2010), one in which they are seen with kindness and gentle goodness. Even with this possibility clients can find it hard to move away from the well-worn path that is so automatic to them. Dissociation often becomes a way to brake overstimulation, and turn down the volume.

Using drugs and alcohol was Gretchen's "go-to" way to turn down the volume, which worked for her sometimes despite the repercussions. It also felt horrible when it was so automatic that she didn't have a choice. She would find herself feeling unprotected when zoned out on too many substances, vulnerable in a different way. Recalling those moments, "I was realizing I need to be present and then I'm not, and it's like as soon as I think of it as sort of like fog, or like tissue that you're just trying to . . . trying to reach something or see something, and it just keeps on developing and I can't put it together. I can't choose, like I can't make a choice." This points to an important fine line, unconscious dissociation or using dissociation creatively as a time out, or a break from upset. The more people befriend their dissociation, the more choices they have. We don't want them to be dissociated at times when they need to be present. We want to help shift the client from automatic dissociation, where they feel there is no choice and they feel caught in helplessness and despair, to a place where they have choice, and can use "dissociation" creatively and in the service of their healing.

Yet moving into the present moment when being dissociated is not easy. The time zones are markedly different. Teaching someone their own unique telltale signals that slide them out of the present moment provides choice points so they can pivot as needed. As they realize that the time capsules of past material are what are making them panic or feel terrified. they'll be able to catch their breath, and gather some control over the physiological reaction to begin inching their way back to the present.

SOME PRACTICALITIES IN WORKING WITH DISSOCIATION: FIRST STEPS OUT OF DISSOCIATION

Everyone has patterns and ways of being that make life easier, more comfortable, and more enjoyable. Then there are those patterns that make us feel stuck. Caught. Trapped. Like life will never change or be different. These patterns are so comfortable that even when we don't really like what we're doing we continue doing it anyway. Some even describe it as compulsive, not being able to do it differently, like wearing an old, worn-out piece of clothing that we've had forever and which we don't want to shed. These strategies and ways of being can keep the demons away, keep the painful feelings out of consciousness. Mostly what these habits do, though, is keep us in relative psychological safety, in our comfort zone. Nothing is wrong with that, but if we want to change any part of our life, we will reach a point where that comfort becomes restricting, suffocating the new creative urge to develop. At their worst, these patterns lose their effectiveness, no longer soothing as originally devised. When they get stale, we feel trapped, stuck. We've forgotten we created the now constricting pattern to soothe us. Instead, we feel deadened. That's the point where we seek help, looking for a way to get out of the old stuck places. The first step, then, is to observe and explore the habits of mind and body that make the hated, stuck life so comfortable that the person is loath to change.

Prana, in its relentless quest to return us to True Nature, insistently flows and moves in and through the energy/physical body. Defenses, or *samskaras*, are psychically concrete, not easy for *prana* to move through or around. Caught against the *samskara*, *prana* pushes against it. Inside the *samskara*, the caught energy longs to be free of its knottedness. Over time, especially as *prana* pushes against the outside of the *samskara*, the ache gets louder; it's harder to push down or quiet the longing. The impulse becomes stronger, to break out of this old way, yet without something stronger calling to us it is hard to find a way through. The person reverts to the old ways of being. The longing is there, but caught in the stuck pattern. Unable to figure out how to get untangled or how to explore new options, the person reverts to the old familiar pattern. Sometimes someone tries taking a step or two outside the comfort zone but when their effort doesn't immediately yield a positive result they collapse back into the old. This reinforces the belief that reaching for something new is not only uncomfortable, but also subject to failure and disappointment. Thoughts and feelings of humiliation and distress percolate, gathering evidence from past experiences or inventing sorrowful pictures of a future remarkably similar to the past. In that conundrum it is hard to reach toward the new. The skills of unpacking the fast-moving states pauses the fluidly morphing packets of information that find the client set in patterns of experience. Slowing down the process, identifying small inroads into the rapid stream of felt experience, creates a way to identify choice points, allowing different pathways to open up.

Normalizing dissociation helps clients develop ease with its automaticity. Suggesting to the client that they can use dissociation in a positive way can pique their interest to explore ways to deal with traumatic schemas. Things like exercise, music, and watching favorite television shows are ways that clients already use to turn away from distress toward something else. Using another metaphor, I tell clients they can choose to can turn the radio dial from hard rock to classical or to talk radio—whatever they like. Encouraging this mental pliancy gives a foothold toward a more secure internal world. Hearing this in a session, Mady chimed in, "When I'm disconnected enough I feel like I'm wearing a couple of wet, heavy, wool blankets, that's what I call it, because my energy is not there. Choosing reading over drugs is obviously going to be the correct choice, but when I choose to read—well I guess what you're saying is, when I choose to read, I'm dissociating away from this feeling of numbness by reading. Interesting . . ."

As the client trains herself to stay in the here and now, they are better able to be with and withstand the blast of experience that pours into their nervous system in raw undigested forms. Reestablishing this time boundary happens when the client can be with any amount of stimuli without becoming overwhelmed. This happens as a matter of course, as the client practices staying in the here and now, observes what happened back then, and learns to offer themselves self-compassion for having experienced that in the past. They discover that when they are there with themselves they are no longer alone. Five years after finishing therapy with me, Dolores wrote about how she used what she learned. "I read a story in *The New York Times* about Afghan allies raping boys chained to the bed. I thought I would be sick reading it. I could feel a part of me shaking, another part wanting to sit in the corner, curl up, and disappear. I didn't know what to do. My body was both numb and shaking. Some small part of me remembered all we did. I realized I was dissociating. That gave me a thread to hold onto. I hated that this was happening to anyone. Slowly, I was able to realize I was here, in 2015, this apparently was happening in the world. It was happening, but not to me. I hated feeling helpless. Hated that it was happening. I was ashamed to know this was happening to anyone, horrified that I didn't know what to do to help. At the same time I was relieved that it wasn't happening to me. Separating facts from feelings helped me get some space. The fact is, I read this story in the paper. The fact is, this wasn't happening to me. The shame was a feeling, horrible, but the reality was I was safe, getting ready to go to work, nothing bad was happening to me right now. I held on tight, sat with my back against the bed, feeling my spine, trying to ground, to hold on tight. Practiced the Self-Compassion Break, felt the feelings of helplessness that this was happening to anyone. Sat with compassion for those children, boys, and for me. So horrible. I hate feeling helpless. At least now I know I'm feeling helpless, instead of being helpless. At lunch, I wrote emails, one to the *New York Times* thanking them for writing the article, then emails to all the politicians I could think of. Someone has to do something. Writing emails is what I can do. I'm not helpless."

GROUNDING IN THE SPINE

We often suggest that people ground through their feet. I have found focusing on the spine to be even better. The spine is the axis through which the nervous system flows. When clients are disconnected or dissociating, they often close their bodies down, often by pulling the shoulders forward, hunching, or collapsing around the middle. In this position, most people retract into younger, more vulnerable states. They'll describe trying to protect their hearts, belly, and tender places inside. Yet while doing that, they lose one of the greatest somatic supports they have. Orienting toward the spine draws people back away from the periphery, into the foundational column of the body. When under attack, or propelled by fears, people tend to leave their spine, draw into the fight/flight/freeze periphery parts of the body, clenching fists, twitching legs, and curling around something. Retraining the body to ground in the spine calls the person into the present moment.

In working with Wally for a year, much of every session was spent in helping him stay solid, in the flurry of dissociative impulses calling him to curl, twist, flutter his arms and legs. Currently in treatment, we've found it less important to deal with the content while he trains himself to stay grounded in his body and present moment. The spine does that, providing a focusing point away from the raging parts. At first Wally could only land for a few seconds, before parts disrupted his focus over and over again. Over time, he's been able to find his spine for longer and longer periods, returning more consistently to a calmer, centered place from which he could interact with his parts. "I'm starting to see why you keep coming back to the present moment thing. It kind of feels like I've got a new ground inside. When I feel myself starting to dissociate at work, I've been reaching back to scratch my back or lean up against a doorway. When people notice, I laugh it off, saying I have a really bad itch. Truth is, though, that it helps me stay centered. Who would have thought."

HARNESSING THE BREATH

Learning to harness the breath can provide ways for people to feel a sense of mastery over their body. The soothing sounds of *Ujjayi* breath can bring a sense of ease and centering into the spine. Adding in an instruction to gently welcome inner tension and conflicts suggesting to clients that the inhalation brings in new energy, cleaning and clearing the tension or conflict, while the exhalation flows the tension out piece by piece. Paul learned to harness his breath as a way to manage dissociation. Tracking his experience as he dissociated (which took some time), Paul began to notice that he started to dissociate in part by holding his breath on the inhalation. He played on his own with interrupting that pattern by holding the breath out at the end of an exhalation and concentrating on moving fluidly through the top of the inhalation. We never discovered any psychological content by slowing down the breath, but Paul found that pausing at the top of the inhalation and the bottom of the exhalation interrupted his dissociation.

Caroline's parts relentlessly hijacked her into panicked states. Her body would shake violently in my office, as tears of distress and panic flowed. We consistently practiced moving away from her extremity, grounding in her spine. This was made easier as she learned to harness the panicked breathing, holding on the inhalation and the exhalation until she could feel herself in the present moment. Maddie rebelled against having anything to do with parts that were sexualized, grandiose, and/or enraged. *Ujjayi* breath gave her a sense of calm. She then used the *So Hum* practice to make friends with her more extreme, scary parts.

ADAPTED SEATED TWIST

Others find a simple yoga posture, the Seated Twist, gives them a body-based way to explore parts of themselves that are activated. In a group, Ming felt a lot of fear in preparing for this particular pose. I asked her where she noticed the fear, and she pointed to her face, "Right down the side of my face. I'm going to cry." I asked her if she felt comfortable taking that part that was going to cry, and holding it in her hand. She struggled a little with it, so I asked her if it would be easier to put it on a piece of paper. "Yeah, that's probably better." Then Ming looked at me, "What do I put on the paper?" I offered a menu of word possibilities, crying, tears, or sadness, and also suggested that she could draw a picture of it. Having that freedom, Ming drew a little picture of tears. When she settled again I asked her to feel inside her body to see if there was another part that needed some attention. As she paid attention, she said she wanted to disconnect. Taking another piece of paper, I asked her how she wanted to represent that part. "Blank" she said as she wrote down the word. (There could, of course, be multiple parts activated in a client at any one time. For this experiment the goal was to give Ming a sense of success in separating parts, to give her room to explore.) I then asked her to feel into each of the parts and then place them on either side of her, slightly to the back of her. Having her feel the part as fully as possible, to access felt experience of the parts outside of her. After doing that I wondered with her what was happening in her heart, to explore if there was any movement impulse. Ming moved a little in her chair, while her spine lengthened and her shoulders lifted up slightly. She looked at me, smiling. I nodded and smiled back, suggesting that she take as much time as she wanted to enjoy this. When Ming was ready, I asked her to turn her head, letting her eyes lead her toward whatever side was pulling her. As she did I validated her, "Yes, that's right. Turning to see what's there. Seeing that part, while you feel yourself grounded in the length of your spine (pause). Letting yourself enjoy the sensations of stretching and moving. When and if it feels right, see if you can connect with this part in a way that feels just right, not to fix it or change it or even process what's there—just to be there (pause). Right now you're seeing this part and offering it a blessing of curiosity, or kindness, or compassion if that feels right (pause). Then relax, stretching, allowing your spine to uncurl, grounding again in your heart." As she settled in, she twisted to one side and then went back and forth a few times, noticing the differences, feeling the twist. When she was done, she laughed. "Well, at first I couldn't even think of what parts there were, but then they came to me. As I twisted back and forth, they had a little bit of a dialogue . . . yeah, between me and between each of them. Yeah, I don't know. I just went with it. It was better than I expected!"

Helen chimed in, "As I did it, I felt a real clearing. I just felt so much better. I felt like just the heaviness that was on me kind of moved, so I was so much better. At first I had this part that didn't want to do it, so I called it a "wanna go home" part [laughs]; I just wanted to get this over with. But then as I did it, it was kind of nice having both there, and that there was some separation. I was there with them. I could feel the separation. I definitely feel better. I feel more cleared."

Madeline, who was in the same group with Ming and Helen, said, "First, I thought, oh those parts. I know them already. I felt getting close to them would be overwhelming. So I did it somewhat reluctantly. It wasn't overwhelming though. First, I like just kind of sitting out there in the void. It's like, I don't know what to do with them. But then I came up with some things that worked. But really it doesn't feel like it's me being with them. I know I'm not the ages they are but emotionally, yeah, it's me. Because that's where I live. I fought against every instruction you gave but you know when I put those parts to each side I started feeling a bit more grown up. I almost felt like they're not alone—but that's kind of weird. Like I'm there with them? So the little part that feels like she's always got to be an adult when she isn't—well I put her to the side. I told her to go ahead and be a child. It's okay to be a child. You don't have to say you're a little adult any more or that you're going to handle things because you couldn't and you can't. I will. And then I did the "God bless you" even though I didn't want to and then kind of spontaneously I said to her, "You're going to be fine. You don't need to show up. You need to help me still be a kid inside so I have you there but I'm here with you. Then I told her, you're not abandoned anymore."

In an individual session, Serena described her experience. "I have a lot of trouble tuning into these child parts. It's like a magnet, if I feel them there I become them. I turn into them. And I lose a sense of me being grown up—and I drive a car! [laughs] I feel like I don't know where I am going to go. So I thought this was very calming. I was really surprised at how it's like, 'Wow' two at the same time. I'm feeling myself here and I've got those two parts over there and I'm staying here. I'm just saying hello and just sort of recognizing they're here. I didn't go there. So that felt really different to be able to do that."

Harry acknowledged parts of him holding fear and regret by using the Seated Twist. "I was able to say to the regret, 'I acknowledge and accept you.' And to the fear I was able to say 'I acknowledge you' and I wanted to be able to say, 'I accept you' but I wasn't able to." I asked him what happened in his body when he could accept one and not the other? I wondered if that increased any tension or holding. "Actually the reaction to both sides was somewhat similar. There was more tension when I was trying to say to fear, 'I accept you.' And I realized that was a falsehood, and then the tension went away. And then what did I say, I said 'I acknowledge you and know that you're there and hope to be able to accept you or work with you.' Then the tension left my body for a little bit. It feels very empowering to be able to acknowledge these parts and to know that they are separate and that they are not everything."

This form of acknowledging or honoring or blessing has been significant, as people learn to turn toward a more hopeful way of being. To complete the Seated Twist I offer the option for people to twist toward each part, offering a quality that feels just right to them. Sometimes people use the *metta* (loving kindness) practice (below) as a template from which to jump off.

After honoring the different parts on either side, the person comes back to the center noticing the experience in the spine, shoulders, arms, while looking for any moments of goodness that can be replenishing and nourishing. Encountering positive emotions can bring up unexpected feelings (Germer, 2009; Gilbert & Choden, 2014; Schwartz, 1994. For Serena it was, "I'm okay . . . whenever I say that it just brings up a lot of sad. I live in so much denial that I'm moving along just fine, and then I say that, and I feel it, like yeah, I'm suffering. I'm not living with ease. But it feels good. in an odd way. Kind of like a purification or cleaning me out." Others have said, "Integrating. I feel I've taken my parts and integrated them back into me." "I felt honest saying it to myself, but I was kind of struggling with saying it to parts because they're not at peace, they're not happy. So it seemed like they didn't know how to. Well, I guess it was a wish. Maybe it was too hard, and didn't seem like a fit."

PRACTICING SUBJECTIVE SOMATIC INQUIRY

Learning to listen to the body, discriminating what "feels right" and when something "doesn't seem like a fit," is an important, attuned attachment response, whether with others outside or our own internal experience. Knowing something didn't work instigates an inquiry of what might work, what would work better? (Emerson, 2015). Holding an open inquiry draws forth a willingness to explore, again activating positive attachment. Abby reported, "It took me some time to find the right phrases. I started to get close. Once I did get close enough, I could feel it when it resonated as 'right.' I found myself trying different things until it really felt right. Kind of like, 'May I accept myself as tired' and 'May I relax into this tiredness.' Because at that point I realized the tired part doesn't want to be tired. I don't know, there was a lot of angst in there. So it was kind of like finding the right phrases, 'May I really relax into being tired.' Sometimes the other part, the one that wanted to lead, which is a familiar part to me, it's kind of a bother. It just wants to get through whatever I'm doing because for some reason I'm uncomfortable in some way. When I did it, it felt right too. I said the basic, 'May I be happy, May I be at peace' just for me. [laughs] They seemed to fit for me, myself, but those phrases didn't seem to fit really with the parts!"

One of the women who had acquired the Becoming Safely Embodied™ Skills Manual from her therapist wrote to tell me of her process. Living in a remote part of the world, she turned to the BSE manual often when there was no other way to structure her internal world. "This part of the course about dissociation is the most exciting and most challenging. It is where I am in the manual, and never moved beyond. The concept of choice points was huge when I was working with the manual. It opened the thought that I can potentially choose what area of feelings I will let flow through me and which feelings I can acknowledge and let go of. I haven't achieved this much yet, maybe three or four times in the past year. I know continuing to use the BSE practices will help me be able to do this. Carving a new path is an exciting hope though incredibly difficult. I've learned that as we carve a new pathway the turbulence may be experienced in several different ways by several different parts. I know it is possible as I have changed some old patterns and begun new paths in several areas. Mostly I hear from other people about how much I've changed, how much more real I seem."

Belinda reported, "Now I'm seeing a new kind of turbulence—when people notice me changing and really don't want that. They want me to stay the same. They keep trying to pull me back into the old pattern. I've felt a lot of pain when people reject this me that isn't a victim. It feels more me in a good way, but then they say I'm selfish for basically not doing what they want me to do. I'm starting to see that guilt is my turbulence, guilt that I want to be me and don't want to be who they want me to be anymore. It's really hard."

BASIC SKILLS THAT MAKE IT EASIER TO BE IN THE BODY

The following basic skills make it easier to be with overwhelming or shut down moments in the body. Practiced over and over again, when not in the midst of being captivated, the skills become second nature.

Slowing Down: The body changes when dissociation begins, contracting or tightening in an attempt to contain or keep away an experience that isn't wanted. Slowing down time makes room for tiny choice points wrestling control from the dissociative entrainment. With these subtle moments the body's muscles can ease a bit, the tension softens instead of galloping away. As the body relaxes the muscles around the tension, the frontal lobe has more space to come online. Unconsciously, the client hopes that tightening up creates control, keeping the bad things at bay. The fear is that relaxing or easing will give up control, making things worse. The skill is learning to let the body fill up with sensation rather than shutting it down. For many clients, it is a revelation to know they don't have to be caught up in the intensity. This means trusting that intensity is reduced when not jammed into an ever-shrinking space.

When the client enters states of overarousal, overstimulation, hypersensitivity, or any traumatic states they feel they are taking their hands off the wheel of their life, losing control instead of gaining it. Slowing down trains us that our body doesn't go from 0 to 60 without going from zero to one, one to two, two to three, etc. Slowing down, the client begins to experience life unfolding instead of being immediately catapulted into disaster. They learn the relief and enjoyment of having their hands on the wheel; they get to steer themselves where they want to go.

Concentration and Focus: Slowing down is the precondition which allows focus on where you want to go, concentrating on a goal instead of being repeatedly distracted by the myriad distress signals coming from thoughts, feelings, and body sensations. Without the ability to focus on the pinpoint they want to follow, it is impossible to gain internal ground. Even when we ask parts that are distracting to step back, the fluidity and complexity of the inner world can subsume the client's tenuous hold on Self. Meditation and yoga practices (or basic arithmetic or counting, for that matter) help the client defocus on the traumatic uprising, turning instead toward less affectively loaded material. Some clients use strong hatha yoga to root their attention in the physicality of taking on a posture, harnessing themselves. Others find intense physical postures difficult, but can count while they are walking, one step, two steps, three steps, and so on.

Staying Open, Welcoming, and Becoming Fascinated: Being able to retrain the body to not instinctively shut down offers one of the great physical pleasures—having more space inside. Often, when any of us are in the grip of something new, we can become blinded by the fear of the unknown. Learning to stay open, holding a welcoming stance, allows us to look around and be fascinated by the process. With a secure ground we can explore with enjoyment.

Yoga can help our clients do something similar. Taking on a new physical movement means initiating physical sensation. Focusing on sensation over time develops concentration. As the sensation increases and becomes uncomfortable, the automatic tendency is to release the movement. Encouraging the client to stay open, welcoming sensation, learning to surf sensation, lets the muscles encounter what is there without interpretations and associations. Less caught by the intensity of sensation, there is a wedge into felt experience, allowing the client to become fascinated with the trembling, shaking, and vibrating going on. All the practices below, such as the practice of Reaching Out, Opening Up, and Drawing In, are designed for this purpose.

Practices for Disarming Dissociation

FINDING AND GROUNDING IN THE SPINE

Objective: *Clients tend to curl into themselves, closing off their front as they move into disso-ciative spaces inside themselves. It's as if they are trying to get smaller, no longer filling up their adult 'here and now' bodies. The function of the spinal cord is to protect the nervous system. Upward extension and motion are secondary. This practice offers them a felt experience of 'here and now' reality, grounded in one of the powerful structures of the body. Psychologically, finding and grounding in the spine connects to our core column, developing confidence.*

Instructions: There are two ways to do this practice, on your back, lying down, or sitting in a chair that has a back. [My instructions will be for sitting.]

Sitting in a comfortable position, bring your attention to your back. Often when we turn our attention to our back, we naturally start shifting and stretching and moving a bit. Go ahead and do that, noticing how each movement affects you.

Sometimes the back and spine is tired, and needs movement to bring blood, bring in new energy, invigorating the spine. Take the time you need to feel your way into this, rolling your spine on the back of the chair, curling up a little, arch-ing the back (pause). Can you get a felt experience of the long tube of your spine? Perhaps you can sense how your spine is connected at the top to your head, rock-ing gently on the top of this long column (pause). You might find it helpful to feel the base of your spine, as you sit. Take all the time you need to do this, letting the breath enter the lungs and expand along the spine.

Where does the breath go? Can it flow easily through the length of the spine or does it get caught at some point? If it does get caught, hang out there, not push-ing or trying to change it at all—practicing being with whatever is there, welcom-ing it (pause) opening to it.

Does it feel grounding to notice these parts of the spine? Or are you noticing activation? If you are, make space for that, taking time (pause). You might also want to explore if there is a part of the spine that is more comfortable than another to be in touch with, and bring your attention there instead of to the places that are uncomfortable (pause).

Now sit and notice—feeling into your body as a whole. What effect did this have on you? (pause) Do you feel more connected to your back? (pause).

If it feels comfortable, open to the natural bubble of quiet that's at the center of any movement.

As you become more familiar with your spine let a part of your attention rest on your spine, while you also attend to the space in front of your spine. This may take time and practice. Most of us are used to connecting to our body with broad strokes, dipping in and moving quickly on.

Gently and slowly feel your way along the front of your spine, letting this be an adventure, without a definitive way to get "there." Let go of any fears of doing this wrong. The beauty of the practice—any practice—is to move slowly, attuning your focus, your attention, to gently noticing what's there.

Softly noticing. Waiting with kindness. Expecting your inner world to welcome you back. Continuously tuning your focus back to this space in front of the spine.

What kind of space is there? You may encounter a wide space (pause). If so, relax into it. If you don't have a sense of that, welcome whatever comes, staying open, relaxed, inviting whatever is there to come forward.

If it feels right, imagine a column of energy gently, calmly moving in front of your spine. It might have a color, it might not have a specific shape, allow it to let you know about itself. These subtler experiences might only come with a deeper relaxation.

Being with the breath, flowing up and down the column along the spine (pause). Not manipulating any part of this. Breathing in and out, swimming on the breath. Allowing the breath to breathe you.

Notice when you feel resistant, upset, or angry, turning your attention back to this simple flow. Reorienting yourself, finding the spine, letting go of the concept of the spine and feeling into this column of energy. Resting in it. Bathing in the light, vibrancy, vitality.

When you feel you have had a good long drink of this good friend, open your eyes and look at the world from this place. Notice what happens? Do you lose contact quickly? What happens to the quality of the world around you? How do you experience your body? Notice any sense of vibrancy, and relax into it, reminding yourself over and over again that you are safe—that being alive and in your skin allows you the greatest chance of happiness, healing, and ease of being, relieving you of stress, anguish, discomfort.

Can you maintain this connection? What would you need to have this connection more solidly there for you, during your day?

MODIFIED UJJAYI PRANAYAMA

Objective: *Turning toward experience and taking little sips of it, the client practices taking in difficult emotions, to puff out, recycling tension or restriction then filling up with more positive qualities. The client experientially learns they are not stuck, that difficult internal energy can be shifted.*

Instructions:

- *Making contact.*

Take a moment to notice where the distress or discomfort lives in your body or around your body. If it helps, put your hand on that area making contact in a way that feels really right. (pause). If you can sink into your body making contact with the cells, bones, muscles, where this discomfort is. What happens when you do? Is it possible for the breath to reach this place? Flowing in and around whatever tension or holding is there. (pause). Taking all the time you need.

- *Ujjayi (see instructions page)*

Starting *ujjayi* breath and connecting into this place. Riding the waves of *ujjayi* (pause) , connecting the breath with this place inside. Seeing what color the tension or discomfort is, what shape, size, vibration. (pause).

- *Cleaning and recycling*

Starting with either the next inhalation or exhalation, imagine inhaling/exhaling out some of the tension. (pause) As you inhale/exhale, seeing the color, shape being released. (pause) Then imagining what quality you would like to have touch or move or fill this space (pause), bringing that in on the inhalation/exhalation. Perhaps gently holding the breath, pausing, internally cradling it. (pause). Then letting it cascade and flow in and around the tension, (pause).Exhaling a bit more of tension (pause), inhaling what feels good and right.

- *Cleaning. Clearing. Recycling.*

PRACTICE: WELCOMING AND INCLUDING— SO HUM/HAMSA VER 2

Variation – also in Chapter 2

Objective: *Dissociation happens from splitting off experiences that were too difficult to include. This adaptation of the So Hum (I am) practice offers a way for clients to embody what has been extruded.*

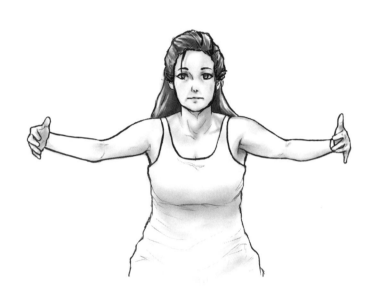

FIG 4.4A—SO HUM 1

Instructions: Externalize whatever part or experience is feeling complicated either through your imagination or writing or drawing it on paper. Imaginatively or concretely place what you are externalizing wherever it feels safe in the room or outside the room.

Using the mantra *So Hum* (I am) quietly sense into your spine, landing in your body, ground in your feet, centering yourself. I am. *So hum*. Right now you are here. Right here.

As you feel yourself in your body open your attention to this externalized part or experience you have been exploring. Open your arms in a gesture of welcoming yet only including as much experience as you're comfortable with. *So Hum*. I am this too.

Taking all the time you need

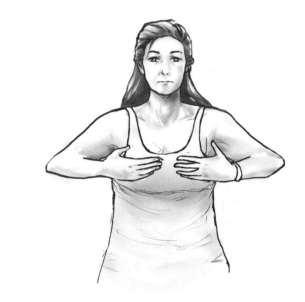

FIG 4.4B—SO HUM 2

make contact with this externalized experience, hold a posture of welcoming what is there, *So Hum*. I am this too.

Being true to your own timing, staying in contact inside your body, as well as keeping in contact with this other, slowly draw the energy toward you, *So Hum*. This too is me. Continuing to draw the energy to you as long as it feels comfortable. No need to push or force it to happen. Keeping with an attitude of exploration and welcoming.

PRACTICE: UNBLENDING AND EXTERNALIZING PARTS

Objective: *This practice offers a gentle opening to receive here-and-now data points keeping the client more regulated in the present moment. Simple, concrete ways are below: Gestalt Empty Chair technique and writing body experiences on paper and putting it around the room (or outside the room).*

Gestalt Empty Chair technique: Notice inside whatever part is most active. Then imagine putting that part away from you in another chair.

- Staying in the chair that you are in, look across at the other part that you have designated in that chair. What does it look like? If I were to see if what would I see? How old is it? It might just be a blob of color or a shape. Letting however it shows up to be perfect.
- What happens in you when you are separate from it? Have some space from it? How do you feel in your body in this chair as you look at it? How do you feel toward it?
- When you feel grounded in yourself in this current time and space literally go over and sit in the other chair. Feel what it's like to be this part. What thoughts is this part thinking? What feelings does it have? What body experience? What does it want to say to you?
- Come back and sit in the here-and-now chair. Let the part's experience ease away from you. In this chair what is it like to hear what the part wanted you to know? What effect does that have on you?
- As you feel comfortable, have a dialogue with this part, shifting chairs as you take on the experience of each side.

Writing/Drawing technique: Notice inside whatever part is most active. Then take some pen and paper to write or draw that experience on paper. It might be a shape, or scribble, or color, or a word. Let yourself be creative and not think about what you are putting down. This is a perfect way to take whatever is roiling around inside and externalize it on paper.

- Take a look at what you have drawn/written. What response do you have to it? Is there something more to add to it?
- How do you feel in your body having externalized this to some degree?
- Take that paper and put it somewhere else in the room. It can be as far away as you like. Some people also find it helpful to put the paper outside the room. Whatever you do, notice what happens in your body, mind, and heart.
- Keep doing this until you feel more settled and comfortable in your body.
- If you want, you can then interact with specific parts.

Journaling technique: There are two ways to do this. You can either split a page from top to bottom or write sequentially.

- Write from either you, or from this part, that you want to (or feel a need to) communicate with. Let each side have a say. Then respond. Let the conversation flow as it does without editing, censoring, or judging what comes up.

PRACTICE: ADAPTED SEATED TWIST POSTURE

Objective: *Moving and twisting the body to look over each shoulder, the client moves from the frozen state that comes with being triggered. Client is asked to orient to what he/she sees over each shoulder, facilitating moving out of a triggered state.*

Instructions: Bring to mind any part that has been active lately, maybe a frozen part, or an angry part, or a lost part; you know your parts so see which ones are most active. Taking time to feel and notice where these parts live, in your body, or around your body.

After you make contact, find a way to externalize two of the parts you want to engage with today whether through your imagination or writing or drawing the part or imbuing an object with the part.

Then bring your attention to your body, sitting in your seat, begin to gently move first your spine and then your body one way or the other, to your left, then to your right. Allow your neck and spine to move freely and easily.

As you have a sense of your spine, grounded below through your seat and moving with ease, begin twisting the body to look over each shoulder. Feeling the movement, where the movement begins in your spine (pause) How does the twist want to happen? What is it like if the twist starts in your neck (pause)? versus when the twist starts in the middle of your lower spine? Play around with it and find what feels right to you.

Then, coming back to center, making contact with two of the parts either through your imagination or in the concrete form you created earlier. Twisting slightly feel which part needs to be on which side (pause). It might not matter or you might get a sense of which part feels more fitting on the left or right.

Twist to place these parts on one side and then the other (pause), feeling the twist to one side (pause), coming back to your core (pause). Then twisting again to the other side (pause) noticing what is there doing this.

Explore what feels right (pause). Does it feel easier to do with your eyes open, twisting to look at the part? Or does it feel easier or more right to close your eyes and visualize? Let the movement be gentle and kind, playing with tiny nanomovements each step of the way. Taking time (pause). Letting enjoyment be the guiding principle.

As you move through the twist orienting to what happens through bare noticing (pause). Twisting over one shoulder (pause). Then grounding in the center before moving to the other side. Letting this centering in the core facilitate connection to this present moment (pause). Then moving to the other side.

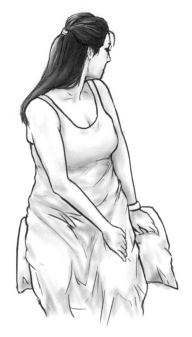

FIG 4.5A   SEATED TWIST #1

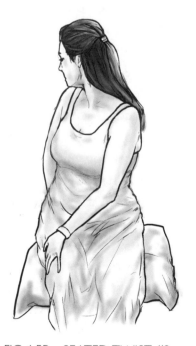

FIG 4.5B   SEATED TWIST #2

Welcoming each side to interact with you, inviting it into the here and now (pause), perhaps having it look through your eyes as you turn forward or twist to the other side. If a dialogue wants to happen, invite that to happen (pause), taking all the time you want and need.

PRACTICE: DEVELOPING CONCENTRATION THROUGH METTA (LOVING KINDNESS)

Objective of skill: *The past looms large for trauma survivors, overshadowing the present moment, which requires concentration, the ability to focus and move in the direction you want to go in, instead of being hijacked by the disruptive past patterns. It also means being able to steer the mind, heart, and body toward cultivating positive experiences instead of ricocheting and reinforcing what doesn't work and doesn't enhance life. Cultivating concentration practices helps clients live in the present, able to let the storyline of the past recede, so that new experiences and choices can be developed.*

Teaching Points:

- Learn to concentrate on one thing while letting everything else fade into the background.
- Focus and concentration deactivates whatever charge we have on the nonfocused object.
- Concentration is one of most powerful skills trauma survivors can learn. With practice, it helps calm hijacked limbic systems, antidote obsessive thinking, anxiety, depression, or flashbacks.
- Receiving anything (gifts, cards, and verbal messages) has frequently been humiliating, disappointing, upsetting, or negatively charged for trauma survivors. As a result, most have doubts and feel hopeless about anything positive, predetermining unsatisfying outcomes.
- Survivors of trauma are generally afraid of being overwhelmed by feelings, as they're laden with past schemas. Fraught with danger, they don't feel safe opening to feelings or body sensations. Contracting, however, reinforces the old, outdated experience of life in which they are not able to deal with life safely. Even as it protects it also keeps nourishment out.
- To offset this habitual pattern of keeping something out we need to:
  - develop capacity to focus and direct energy.

- cultivate space for internal kindness and begin to see the possibility of a kinder external world.

Buddhist practices of *metta*/loving kindness are easily adapted, as are practices such as saying the rosary or chanting, singing, saying a mantra, or centering prayer. Simple arithmetic also serves the purpose of developing concentration and focus.

Benefits:

- Concentration opens the door to blissful states.
- Heart/mind/body gets focused, reducing disorganization and scattered attention.

Drawbacks:

- Since internal boundaries are relaxed there may be a tendency to feel out of control, uncertain of where each person begins or ends.
- Regression can happen as psychic boundaries are relaxed.
- Self-hate can intensify to protect against self-kindness, or self-compassion.

Instructions:

To do *metta practice* you'll need three or four benevolent phrases that invite a positive internal experience. The traditional *metta* phrases are:

May I be happy.
May I be at peace.
May I live with ease.
May I be free from suffering.

Some people find that these phrases don't quite fit for them. If that happens to you, choose a different set of phrases—a mantra, a simple centering prayer, a few nurturing affirmations, or a structured prayer with prayer beads. Clients have reported it's best to choose a phrase or word that allows them to focus without getting entangled in the associations to the word. If the phrase, "May I be happy" brings up too much internal commentary (ex: why you should never, ever be happy), then it's going to be too disturbing to walk or sit with. That won't help to build a sense of quiet inside! Making it your own, adopt phrases from your own spiritual traditions or phrases that have meaning for you. Over the years, people have chosen phrases like,

> May I be happy someday.
> May I be calm.
> May I be gentler with myself.
> May I be free from self-harm.

People often use the phrases while walking or moving in their daily life. They can easily be adapted to waiting in line, driving, or anytime when you find yourself crowded by negative internal noise. Directing the mind to where you want to go instead of where it's prone to go is always a good thing.

Instructions for sitting:

Once you have your phrases in mind, find a quiet space and sit in a comfortable position. Take a few long breaths. Letting your eyes softly focus on a spot in front of you, or close your eyes if that is more comfortable.

Begin saying one of the phrases you've selected—slowly, with intention. Say the first. Let that settle in.

Then say the next, or even repeat the first. Breathe deeply and let each settle in before moving on to the next.

Over and over, for as long a time as you like, repeat the phrases, allowing yourself to resonate with the qualities as well as your intention to become aligned with those qualities.

If your mind jumps to the opposite of what your phrase/intention invites becoming too distracting let go of the practice and come back to it at another time.

The next time, limit yourself to one to five minutes of practice. As it becomes more comfortable to stay with your intention, gradually increase the time.

Remember, there is no right way to do this. It's a practice to find the softest, easiest, most comfortable way to develop concentration. Don't push yourself if it doesn't feel right. Just try it again another time.

If, for whatever reason, you find you are beating yourself up, remember compassion! And focus on your desire to feel good (another kind of concentration practice) instead of feeling bad.

OFFERING *METTA* TO PARTS

Objective: *Meditation Loving Kindness to Parts. This classical version is adapted to working with parts of the self, practicing how to be gentle and offer kindness to ourselves. Life can deal some pretty hard blows. We are often even harder with ourselves. The habit of being critical or blaming ourselves is carved deeply into our psyches. When we wonder, "Why isn't life changing?" it's important to remember how long we have been hard on ourselves. When we stop to consider it, we realize we've been harder on ourselves for a lot longer than we have been kind to ourselves. Reversing this pattern is the practice of metta. These practices are about reversing that trend.*

Instructions: In this, as in all the practices, turn toward inviting in softness, gentleness, and kindness. You may find you have parts that resist this or get angry at the suggestion. These are often protector parts that are hell-bent on making that sure you don't get hurt or disappointed by something not working yet again.

If possible, welcome any reaction with interest and curiosity. It's important not to lose sight of what these practices are doing. We are practicing training the mind to go where you want it to go.

Meditation is the art of becoming familiar with what is. When you practice, you're exploring feelings or internal experiences. It begins the gentle, often unfamiliar practice of "being with" yourself. This is a soft and vulnerable practice that might take time to get used to.

Using the same approach as described in previous practices, these practices add the psychological component to an internal experience. They begin as the anxiety practices begin: noticing where the anxiety is and becoming interested and curious about it. Then you'll take it in a different direction.

Offering *Metta* to Parts - Steps:

1. *Ask the anxiety to separate.* Gently asking the anxiety to separate from you allows you to learn more about it and help it to heal. Sometimes it can be help-

ful to imagine the anxious energy moving out of your body, possibly moving into the chair opposite you (see previous Gestalt empty chair practice). This can make a difference over time. All you're doing is creating a little psychological space so you're less caught up with your immediate experience. You can also try making a physical representation of the internal experience. Try drawing or writing it down on a sticky note or sheet of paper. Then put the paper in your lap or across the room.

2. *Now that it's externalized and a little more separate:* Offer it metta/loving kindness. Even if you don't know how to do that, let this part know that. "I don't really know what I'm doing but I want you to know I'm trying. I want to offer you kindness . . ." Or let it know that you wish it some peace. "May you be at peace. May you be free from suffering. May you be happy." Be as honest and authentic as you can be.

3. *Take a moment and notice how the part is responding.* What happens as you wish for this anxious part to be free from suffering and to be at peace? How does it respond?

   Take some time to integrate the anxious part's response. Then continue sending it metta. Let it take all the time it needs to absorb the healing energy of metta.

4. *Reflect on what happened.* Write about what worked and what didn't work. Were you able to separate the part? Did you have a sense of distinction between you and the feelings? What worked best for you? Were you able to draw out the part/feeling? What happened when you did that? What was it like for you to feel for this part that is holding all the feelings of pain/suffering?

Carving Out a New Path: Teaching Points Inquiry into the Old, Familiar Path, Finding Choice Points, and Opening Up to Where You Want to Go

Objective: *To help the client identify how the past is intruding in the present moment. Gaining a sense of control the client can sort out and ground in the sensory experience of present experience. Learning the specific ways the past clouds the present moment gives the client affective, perceptual, and behavioral cues to shift the slide into dissociation.*

Teaching Points:

- *Dissociation barrier:* The mind has a wonderful means of survival in order to deal with horrific experiences: it compartmentalizes. It takes the horrible experience and puts it behind a barrier, keeping the painful material out of your awareness. This dissociation barrier operates like an affect dial, muting or completely shutting out pieces, or the full experience.

  For some, the barrier becomes more permeable over time and traumatic material leaks through as body/mind symptoms. For others, the barrier is breached in rather dramatic ways. Sometimes the person is not aware at all of what created the breach. This helps explain why someone could be doing well, enjoying life, showing no overt signs of trauma, then be catapulted into flashbacks, intrusive memories, nightmares, and disturbing body sensations. Working with the Parallel Lives approach helps sort out what is happening in this moment and what undigested material is presenting itself.
- *Time Capsules of Experience:* A key point to make is that if the experience is too big, feels unmanageable, is overwhelming, and/or we have the impulse to shut it out we are almost certainly dealing with past, undigested materials.
- *Past Flooding the Present:* It feels like it happens without any precursors or warning, yet the client can learn the alarm bells that spin them rapidly into overwhelming experiences. By using the Parallel Lives model (and Carving Out a New Path) clients can re-land in the present, and use curiosity to explore what part of the past is exploding into the moment. When the relationship to the past is established there is often a relaxation in the nervous system.

Inquiry with Clients:

- *Past:* How does your body respond when you're in the past? What do you see? Feel? Think?
- *Present:* How do you know when you are in the present moment? What are the cues? What do you see outside of you? What happens in your perceptual field? How does your body let you know you're in the present moment?
- *Blurring the time/dissociation barrier:* Can you track how the past invades the present? What happens first? How does this quicksilver process happen?

• *Charged Time Capsules:* What time capsules of experience tend to be the most loaded with charge? How can you identify them ahead of time so you'll be more aware of the charge they carry? Naming them helps to see them more clearly when they are activated.

Carving Out a New Path: Practice Steps

Objective: *At any moment there are multiple options and choices yet we're habituated to choose what we're most familiar with. This practice helps you explore what other options are there, exploring what the benefits and drawbacks would be to take the various choices.*

Instructions: There are different kinds of patterns everyone has, some helpful, others not. These different habits can feel like reality. Take a moment and list some of them without worrying about doing this right. This exercise is to raise your awareness so you can have more attention on what you decide is reality, offering a wedge into experience to see where there's any room to change.

There are many ways to do this exercise: a) as an imaginary exercise, b) writing or drawing (so have some paper, pencils, drawing materials nearby; often it's easier to do this without a computer), or c) physically by standing, moving, orienting, and taking small steps pausing to write as the movement exploration brings up insights. Some will find it immensely helpful to physically move. Others find movement and physicality too challenging, and are more comfortable writing or drawing.

Carving Out a New Path - Practice Steps:

1. *Focusing on a pattern:* What kind of patterns are you working with right now? It doesn't have to be the best, or perfect, or right pattern. It's just a pattern you are choosing to explore now. These patterns are the kinds of things we take as truth, as reality. It could be fear of speaking in public, fear of conflict, or ways of socializing that you don't understand, what happens as you reach out. Perhaps it is feeling trapped in being nice or not feeling able to say what you mean. Maybe it's doing the same thing when you get home, tired at the end of the day. Or perhaps behaviors you do when you feel overwhelmed, shut down, or want comfort.

Bring to mind that experience and way of being. Let it live in full living experience in your body, entering it as if you're entering that felt experience in your daily life. What do those moments feel like in your body? What's the experience around you? What kinds of thoughts do you have? What happens in your body? What feelings come up? What gets stirred up? What behaviors want to be acted out? Imagine or actually walk down this path, taking one step, then another, experiencing what's there.

When you are in this pattern, going down this old, familiar path what is the end result? Where do you end up? How do you feel when you've gone down this path?

Take all the time you need to do this. Letting it come to mind, filling up with it.

2. *Orienting to the new:* What would you like to have more of? What would you like to move toward? Is there something that is calling to you? Something you would rather have than what you do have? Knowing this path is no longer satisfying, what would you rather have? Do this slowly so you can feel what happens in your body as you go through the exercise.

What's calling to you? What have you always wanted but had to shut down or push aside? What have you doubted is possible? What thoughts are there? Feelings? Body sensations as you do this? Slowly notice the small little things. Watch for how quickly you deny yourself what you want.

What is your heart's desire? What makes your heart excited, opening your heart? What makes you want to be happy and alive in the world? What would you like instead of this old habit?

Watch how quickly you might want to push this away. Can you slow it down to catch a glimpse of what you want?

You might want to externalize the old way, turning instead in a new direction, your body moving away from the old way of being.

3. *Turbulence:* What gets in the way? What kind of turbulence do you encounter as you find yourself wanting more?

Always, whenever we reach for something new, we experience turbulence. Alarms get set off, distress signals flood our bodies. The old way is cautioning us, "You can't—you better not go down this new path."

What comes up for you as you do this? What turbulence is there as you reach for this new pattern? What forces you back into the old path?

Some people find it helpful to literally stand in the old pattern, looking toward this new path, this longing, this hope. What thoughts are there telling you not to move forward, not to go in this direction? What feelings come up as you attempt to step in a new direction? How does your body feel? What sensations arise? You might even feel body impulses to move toward, or to cringe away (pause).

You might even want to look back at the old path and notice what happens.

4. *Choice Points:* What kinds of choice points might there be? Where are small moments in time or in your thoughts, feelings, body sensations when you might be able to shift in tiny ways rather than being caught in the web of the old path? These small baby steps help us encounter and move through turbulence to find more satisfying ways of being.

Slow down as much as you can or as you need to. Where is there a choice point? What gives you the wedge into the experience where you can feel the old path telling you not to go away—as well as the new path calling to you. This choice point is present in all moments yet we often overlook this opportunity to pivot.

Play with this a bit. Notice the old path, the old habit, and way of being. You might want to nod in acknowledgement to it and then turn to the new path. Right here in this moment you are in a choice point.

Now, take one actual or imaginary step toward this new path. What happens? Anything? Maybe nothing. Take another small baby step onto this new path. Does anything come up? Maybe a thought? Feelings? Body sensations? Perhaps some cautionary memory or worry? Turbulence can come up in lots of different ways, memories of bad things having happened or fears about the future? Voices in your head? Critical comments (pause). You might start feeling depressed or anxious or worried (pause). All these things can be seen as turbulence, ways that your body is cautioning you to take care.

5. *Baby Steps:* In your imagination, or through drawing, or actually standing and taking steps, lean toward or move toward this new experience. We need to be able to know what turbulence will arise, what your particular flavor will be, how it comes up. Knowing it well helps navigate it with greater equanimity.

The best way to do this is to take small, little baby steps (pause). slowing down the movement so that you become so familiar with the ground you are covering that you don't get thrown off (pause). Breathing into any distress signals that any turbulence sends with rapid fire warning (pause). Slowing down your breath (pause), staying present to the process without getting hijacked by the turbulence.

As you do this noticing what might help you move toward and through the turbulence? Noticing each and every little tiny step in the process (pause), developing your focus and concentration as you slow down and pay attention to how this is unfolding.

What happens as you take the small step? Only taking that small step physically, emotionally, mentally (pause). What thoughts are there? What thoughts would you rather have? What feelings are there? What kinds of feelings would make the process easier? What kind of body sensation would feel just right and soothing as you take some of these steps?

What might help you move toward and through the turbulence? What do you imagine would make the process easier for you? It might be a thought that you would rather have, or a feeling that would make it so much easier? What kind of body feeling would feel just right—soothe you in just the right way as you took the next step?

As you're doing this paying such close attention that you can easily remember later on what helps take each small step (pause). Reinforcing how it's just one step (pause) and the step seems simple and easy (pause), effortless when you're only taking this next step.

Sometimes taking one step teaches us so much (pause). Hanging out there (pause). Witnessing this courageous act of having moved away from the pattern (pause) moving toward what you want one small step at a time (pause), without getting lost or caught in the distress. If it feels comfortable, congratulate yourself (pause), then notice what it's like to feel proud of yourself (pause) noticing what it's like to have me proud of you (pause). Taking in only the amount that you can digest at this moment (pause), another way to take a baby step.

Before we end let's explore what you could take from this that you could practice in simple, easy ways a couple times a day. How can you reinforce what you learned today in your daily life?

CHAPTER 5

Manage Triggered Responses

Sitting there, doubled over, terrified, hands pressed against her face, writhing, Carol's cries were agonized. She's been telling me how she is in her forties, successful in her work and home life, having worked on healing her trauma for years—yet here she is, once again in this dreadful place. She describes how real the agony is. When she's triggered, the trigger is so enveloping it's hard for her to realize she's triggered, telling me, "It's so horribly confusing," Carol groans, "It feels so real. It feels true! My stomach is tied in knots; I can't think, I'm terrified—and it wasn't even a big thing that happened! I just want to sink into the earth and disappear."

Our job as therapists is that of a midwife, helping our client shift triggered moments brought on by stimuli in the here and now, while disidentifying from the excruciating physiological symptoms so the memory can be explored separate from the present moment enactment. As long as Carol's body is physiologically consumed by the past in the here and now, she will be racked with somatic upheaval, feeling like life is not worth living and wanting to do anything to shut off the pain.

I remind her, as I have many times when memories have overwhelmed her, that when the feeling is so intense and out of proportion to the experience we can almost guarantee that she is re-experiencing a time capsule of past experience, something put away at an earlier time because it was too much to experience back then. The memory comes to life, exploding open a sequestered time capsule, filling her body with sensations and thoughts that it would be better to die—anything to get away from this feeling.

Carol writhes in the chair, telling me how the nerves in her body are burning and hot. Slowly, using the skills she's learned to disidentify from the intensity, we acknowledge that this might be a body memory held in this time capsule. I ask her if she can be with the body sensation, and I remind her we can take our time. We've practiced over time being mindful of thoughts, feelings, and sensations allowing her to concentrate and attune to her body. She's learned to get close to sensation. Now we're practicing the yogic skill of intensification, learning to harness the pattern's energy. We take the time she needs. The burning intensifies. Her body trembles some. I can see the contraction begin in her torso as her body quivers. We breath together. I feel my body connected to her as she groans, struggling to stay soft, creating room inside, learning to shift gears inside.

I watch her body relax, her eyes open and look at me. It's easier, she reports, but still there. I nod. Sometimes it takes some time. She takes a big breath, looks at me with tears as she connects the body experience with something nascent, a felt experience, inchoate, not fully formed. We can guess, I suggest to her, that your body felt this way at some other time, Carol. You didn't have the means to experience it then, your mind couldn't make sense of it all; it was too big a shock to your nervous system. Perhaps as we sit here together your body is letting you remember what you experienced at some time when it was much too hard to hold this. Carol's belly shakes again and she starts to cry. I ask her what's happening. Just tears she says, no story to it.

Many clients with trauma and attachment issues will come into therapy having little narrative memory of traumatic events. Their bodies, instead, tell the story (Fisher, in press; Ogden, Minton, & Pain, 2006; van der Kolk, 1994, 2015; van der Kolk, McFarlane, & Weisaeth, 1996), shaking, clenching, moving with no attendant content. Pat Ogden et al (2006) and Peter Levine (1997) have helped many of us to find ways of being with these bottom-up body processes. Others, like the Maine-based therapist, Deb Dana, use Porges' Polyvagal Theory to help people tone and strengthen their vagal nerve. Having a map, an explanation, a reason for why traumatic responses affect us in the way they do helps people deal with being in the body. Explanations and maps make meaning out of confusing and disorienting "stuff," making the experiences digestible. Explanations, even as they report and describe an experience, don't always give access to the felt, unnamed experience. There are times when our clients don't know the story or content; other times protective parts and implicit patterns have deliberately kept the information away. Those are the harder times for our clients. They feel like they're floating in a vacuum.

In order to manage the triggering trauma, a person lives alone inside their psyche, separate from others—but also separate from themselves, disconnected, isolated, working hard to keep the distress from arising. Their energy is spent keeping old undigested experiences out of awareness. It was too big to bear back then, and the fear is it still is. Perhaps my client Estrella can illustrate this for us. Not only is Estrella a high-functioning executive in the world with a horrendous personal and familial trauma history that she manages by constantly working, she also is a spiritual teacher in her tradition, leading retreats around the world, often getting caught in dangerous traumatic reenactments. Estrella made a drawing which beautifully illustrates one of the inner legacies of trauma: compartmentalization. In the drawing her brain is divided into silos, color coded. The drawing speaks of the order Estrella created to manage the internal chaos caused by her history. She was often in affairs with married men, living multiple lives supported by the imported skill of compartmentalizing—one part not always knowing what the other part was doing, saying, or experiencing. Over our years of working together, and in her own work on herself, she has been able to learn about having boundaries outside herself so that her internal compartments were able to soften and get the support she needed without acting out the internal story through messy reenactments.

Triggers Require a Whole Toolbox

A trigger is the lever one presses to discharge a firearm. With PTSD, triggers come when stimuli in the here and now cause neurons and synapses in the brain to fire instantaneously, connecting to stored associations. The trigger is in the moment, evoking thoughts, feelings, or memories that surge up. The person then "remembers" (in flashbacks) unpleasant, horrible, disturbing, frightening, or repulsive experiences.

Learning how to identify and intervene in triggered responses builds an internal platform for recovery. Janina Fisher reminds us that our clients have symptoms instead of memories. From this perspective, triggers, albeit dreadful, also hold the key to unwinding the embedded traumatic schema. Triggered responses provide a hologram of the past presented in this moment. "Visiting the past in therapy should be done while people are biologically speaking, firmly rooted in the present and feeling as calm, safe, and grounded as possible. Being anchored in the present while revisiting the trauma opens the possibility of deeply knowing that the terrible events belong to the past. Therapy won't work as long as people keep being pulled back into the past" (van der Kolk, 2015, p. 70). As the client learns to be present in this moment, they have options to be with the triggered experience instead of being hijacked by it. This gives the client a measure of control and ability to intervene in the physiological onslaught. Balance is restored. Life in the present moment then feels in proportion to what is happening.

Making this shift is difficult for our clients. It is hard for them to psychically untangle from their past, which lives so fresh in their present moment experience. As therapists we need to stay grounded in the present even as our client morphs into a young child (or other self-states) in front of us. With our clients frozen, shaking, or furious it can be hard not to get pulled into their subjective reality. Holding the dual consciousness of this moment with our client, while attending to the affect swallowing the client from the past, is an essential skill for a trauma and attachment therapist. It's not about being swallowed by the past but rather staying in the present while exploring the past with compassion. It's about knowing that "it" was the felt reality back then while feeling "it" now. This connects the past with a full heart and body while staying located in the present.

Triggers crack open implicit time capsules of memories that explode (or leak) in the present with the feeling experience *as it was encoded* in the past. That's the key thing here. Whatever is held in that time capsule is loaded as the felt experience *back then*. As real as the sensorial impression feels right now it doesn't have to be the historical reality—what's essential to stay grounded in is that triggers open up implicitly encoded experience. When the sensorial impression holds good things, it feels nice to remember it, we like it, and the time boundary is maintained. If, however, and this is where the mind is absolutely amazing, if it was something that we didn't like, the mind has all kinds of ways to shut out the material so that we don't have to deal with it. It gets put aside in one of these time capsules.

In the last chapter on dissociation, we explored how helpful it is for clients to know that their inner torment might be a form of memories of a previous time in their lives, imprinted before their brain had developed enough to make sense of what was happening. Making sense of all this requires safe ground, usually in the form of a safe therapist skilled in trauma to help deal with the nascent feelings, and to process experiences. Without the underlying support that organizes implicit experience, people feel that life comes at them "out of the blue" often without context. Life is then disruptive, disorganizing, and chaotic. They find themselves lost in feelings and body experience that they attribute to this present moment reality. When triggered, it's dreadfully difficult to parse out "reality" from intruding body memories and traumatic schemas. It feels impossible at those times to do what body-oriented therapists teach: get close to felt experiences without shutting off or being overwhelmed by the body's reaction.

This is what Carol has been practicing, learning to welcome sensations instead of reflexively shutting off. "Unbelievable," she says as she shakes her head, "this is so intense." It is. And if it is this intense now, I say to her, imagine what it must have been like when you were little. If it's this bad now, it must have been impossible to experience then. No wonder you set it aside for another day. It's actually a really smart strategy.

She nods silently as she lives more fully in her 46-year-old body. "Holy shit," Carol says, shaking her head. "This is hard." Yes, I acknowledge. It is hard to enter those spaces if those memories, feelings, sensations, and parts take over. Entering the body is hard when it's chock full of undigested information. Carol knows this well, having spent the last two days tortured by the triggered symptoms before she had a chance to come in for a session.

With the trigger less excruciating, I ask Carol: What happened? What happened before the trigger? It was really quite simple, Carol said. She went to visit a friend who was really busy. This was a very good friend for many years who had taken a new job a year ago and was working really hard. Unfortunately, this meant the friend didn't have the same time for Carol. On the surface everything looked fine between them; however, they hadn't had time for deeper contact, relying on texting to maintain the friendship. That was really hard for Carol. They were finally able to have a long talk, which left Carol feeling much better. That made it an even bigger surprise when she her found herself raging on the way home.

With the here and now facts in place and her body less crippled by symptoms, I asked Carol what she thought accounted for what happened. "It feels so intense I could throw up," she tells me with her eyes closed. Is it okay to stay with this, I ask her?

Carol nods. "It's here," and uses a hand to indicate where it is in her chest. I watch her shoulders relax and soften and know, without hearing from her, that something has shifted. She reports that she has an image of herself holding this little swaddled child, wrapped in blankets. Carol says it feels like it's burning up.

How do you know that, I ask her? She says, "I feel it in my body, but it feels like it's hers. It's weird." Okay to stay with it I ask?

Nodding, Carol murmurs to me, "I'm just telling her it'll be okay. I'm here." Carol's attunement with this image lets her know that the child didn't feel wanted growing up. No one wanted to be with her, hold her, care for her. Carol's face becomes beatific as she stays inside, then tells me that she's letting this child know that even if no one else wants her, Carol wants her.

I watch this internal scene unfold, seeing Carol's body soften even more, tension leaving her shoulders. I know, and I will remind Carol, that this internal part of her needs to be tended to frequently. The triggered symptoms are this part trying to communicate in the only way it knows how. The huge explosion of feeling is a time capsule of experience of this young part of Carol who never felt loved and cared about in the way she needed. She's letting Carol know how alone and terrified she was. Carol's attunement to herself held in the safe container of our connection reinforces the secure base we've created to enter the intersubjective matrix together.

Often, as therapists, we have no idea what is historically accurate. Even the client may not. That's not what is most compelling in these situations. What is important is for Carol not to be crippled by these triggers. This has been happening for years. As we traced it later in other sessions she was able to stitch together triggers with times when she needed to feel loved but was too ashamed of that need to do anything about it. Learning how to interpret her body's alarms gives Carol clues, putting the puzzle pieces of her life together. In the past she needed attention and love. In the present she needs attuned connection with herself while she also finds ways to share her need for connection with others.

As this process unfolds clients generally find that the part holding these feelings will either not need as much attention, or won't be there at all. In IFS language that part will have "unburdened" itself, freed to no longer hold that role. Using self-compassion or the Becoming Safely Embodied™ skills, clients will spontaneously say when the past integrates that "I don't know how it happened but the part seems to have grown up. It's not there anymore in the same way."

The Inner Pinball Machine of Triggers

Being in the body of unresolved trauma is akin to being in a pinball machine where the ball ricochets from one lever to a barrier, then to another lever and barrier. Any number of stimuli (a simple gesture, word, color, shape) can trigger the client into re-experiencing the traumatic past. Intruded upon, at times persistently, with a strong somatic expression our clients reel with out-of-proportion reactive moments. When these triggered reactions happen, clients are catapulted into saying and doing things that are ego dystonic, perhaps haunting them later with shame or humiliation, or leaving the client reeling with terror, panic, paranoia, or numbing out. Inadvertently, their behaviors express their inner distress and give us a felt experience of their traumatic inner working models. This notion of persistent re-experiencing of the past intruding in the present moment is one of the generally accepted consequences of trauma (Brewin, Lanius, Novac, Schnyder, & Galea, 2009; Lanuis, Paulson, & Corrigan, 2014; Michael, Ehlers, Halligan, & Clark, 2004; van der Hart, Nijenhuis, & Steele, 2006; van der Kolk, 1994, 2015; van der Kolk, MacFarlane, & Weisaeth, 1996).

Simply said, triggers happen when some unintegrated piece of history gets activated in the current moment. The past intrudes into this moment in the form of kinesthetic, auditory, and visual flashes, hence the term "flashbacks." It doesn't feel like it's the past intruding—it feels like it's now. Flashbacks are horrendous to experience. Reality is distorted and confused. Mitigating and unwinding the residue is essential. Time traveling into the past happens automatically especially in the beginning of the healing journey. As difficult as it is, flashbacks are often the biggest clue to the traumatic aftermath that percolates inside our clients. Separating these undigested shards from the present moment allows the client to become here in the moment, witnessing, and being with instead of caught in the quagmire.

The great problem is that the body continuously re-experiences stress which cements the past trauma into the present. This blurred boundary between past and present insures the client's suffering will continue as the brain doesn't make the distinction between now and then. Bessel van der Kolk describes in his book, *The Body Keeps the Score* (2015, p. 66) ". . . as long as the trauma is not resolved, the stress hormones that the body secretes to protect itself keep circulating, and the defensive movements and emotional responses keep getting replayed. . . . Most people may not be aware of the connection between their 'crazy' feelings and reactions and the traumatic events that are being replayed. They have no idea why they respond to some minor irritation as if they were about to be annihilated." Clients report feeling overwhelmed with emotions or body sensations, going numb, spacing out, caught in terror, panicking, feeling crazy, like a bomb went off in their bodies . . . and any other range of experiences.

Daniel Brown, PhD, told those of us training with him in attachment focused therapy, to consistently and persistently invite the client throughout the session to notice how much the person was in the present moment; that in turn helped the person organize their present moment experience. Using the idea from the Subjective Unit of Distress Scale used in Eye Movement Desensitization Response (EMDR) I began asking clients for a Subjective Unit of Presence (SUP). "How much are you here on a scale of zero to ten (or one to 100 percent)?" helps a client reflect on their current state. Yvonne Agazarian, in her Systems Centered Groups (1997) asks, "Are you more here, less here, or about the same?" These easy to pose questions ask the client to break the trace of the captivating past to be here, in this moment.

As mentioned, triggers can be seen as a hologram highlighting the past in the present moment. Our clients, naturally, are terrified of the intrusiveness of triggers as the trigger opens the door to flashbacks that swirl the client into excruciating holes of terror. The stress hormones experienced over and over again carve these memories deeper into the nervous system (van der Kolk, 1994, 2015). An activated nervous system makes everything feel real, as if the danger is happening now. The result is life gets organized to avoid as much of this traumatic intrusion as possible. Because the trigger isn't always obvious, people's response may seem (to themselves and others) to be crazy. Whether the reactions are external or internal the person feels out of control, irrational, "nutty." Often, to manage these disorganizing feelings and behavioral responses, people will hide their reactions, blame others for what happened and why they are responding this way, over eat, over sleep, over exercise, under exercise, restrict....do anything to manage their symptoms and/or pretend that things are okay.

The consequences of being triggered leave people lost, confused, wanting to shut life out. Some of the greatest suffering our clients have is being alone with this pain, unheard and disconnected. Safe Space Radio, the radio show by the psychiatrist Anne Hallward, is dedicated to finding ways for people to reduce stigma and offer hope about places where they have felt silenced. In talking about traumatic silence and its effect, Hallward (2011) cites research on the subject of "telling." Even if just one person hears and understands a person's distress there is a huge reduction in subsequent symptomatology (Pennebaker, 1990).

Even before telling the story, though, the first step to recovery is knowing the traumatic loop that occurs, sensing how it happens inside, anticipating and naming how it tends to happen (van der Kolk, 2015). The Parallel Lives model discussed in Chapter Four describes how the brain instantly responds to the here and now, associating to experiences in the past. To summarize the intricate process for clients, here is a proposed description: thoughts, feelings, and sensations surge up from the past, breach the dissociative barrier with somatically and affectively charged material, distorting the present moment. Many in Western cultures have difficulty being with positive emotions. For those who have dissociative defenses even pleasant material can be extremely disruptive. As one person wrote, "Having heard about your site from my therapist and looking through it I was wary of the kindness shown on the site both by your writings and also the concept of kindness to oneself. I've been scared to death of people being kind to me. It's never worked out well in the past. Kindness would trigger a cascade of terror keeping me in bed for days. I had to relearn this all over again, which I was able to do using the skills you have taught me."

After taking a course Sally reflected, "This made so much sense, informing me about my triggers, which I am not always aware of, let alone being able to sort them out. That intrigues me and helped me look at what happens in my life. I can get really reactive or other times I can't leave the house. People don't know what to do with me. I often times feel like I'm living in a crazy land, boomeranging all over the place. Being in my body has been impossible. Your course is showing me that it's possible to make sense of all this. My therapist suggested I take a course with you to help me deal. As I result I've learned better ways to be with myself when I'm triggered. Thank you for putting this together."

This input emphasizes the need to have a foundational understanding of what thoughts, feelings, and sensations are, how to separate the facts from feelings and interpretations, as well as learning attachment language to meet internal experience with matching words and tone. Paul Gilbert (2009a, 2010) repeatedly says the mind can be a tricky thing. If we don't know the workings of the mind we easily warp "reality" to fit our fears. Clients respond to simple maps that help concretize the traumatized inner world they live in. The Parallel Lives model from Chapter 4 assists in making sense of their inner world, describing a dissociative barrier, how memories are encoded as Time Capsules of Experience, and illustrating how the past is separate from the present moment. Expanding the Parallel Lives model to identify triggers and how they manifest, then how to deconstruct them, and developing skills to be with them so they have less effect, are the practicalities of this chapter. Employing self-compassion calms and soothes threats (Corrigan, Wilson, & Fay, 2014a; 2014b; Germer, 2009).

THE TRIGGERED MOMENT

Carrie began to put some of these pieces together. She realized she had body memories of being a small girl, trained to be a good girl, taking care of the men in the house, making sure their needs were met without their having to ask. Her now grown-up consciousness knows that she shouldn't treat all men this way, but she kept finding herself acquiescing, especially with dominant, nonrelational men. It drove her crazy. Over time, she realized she had a three-year-old part that had retained those memories, undigested, living in a separate silo in her mind. When dominant men were around, the three-year-old part of her took over, making Carrie crazy. She didn't know how to stop it. As she sorted out the automatic behaviors into feelings, thoughts, and sensations, she came to see how these feeling and body memories were held in escrow until she was triggered. Then the three-year-old's experience came blasting out of the past and into this moment. Labeling these body experiences as flashbacks instead of crazy behavior made a world of difference for her. She was then able to identify the experience as it was happening, naming it as old, undigested material from the past, and not something she needed to act on in the moment. In therapy we were able to integrate the three-year-old feeling memories in slower, manageable ways so they didn't hijack Carrie, causing her to behave in ways that she later found despicable. Self-compassion was a natural outcome as Carrie realized how her time boundary rapidly dissolved in the face of this material coming up from the past; having her experience what she wasn't able to experience back then. Her practice evolved, to where she could stop in the face of a trigger, telling herself, "This is so hard now—no wonder it was impossible to feel back then."

Carrie's example shows that when our clients can train themselves to stay in the here and now, in the present moment reality, they can withstand the blast of experience that is being poured into them in it's raw, undigested form. Reestablishing the time boundary happens as the client stays present without becoming overwhelmed or needing to shut down. What sounds like a huge proposition happens as the client learns the distinction of being in the present moment, allowing them to stay in the here and now observing what happened back then. Cultivating self-compassion facilitates this process of having had the experience.

ATTACHMENT TRIGGERS

Being triggered by traumatic intrusions is a common problem (van der Kolk, McFarlane, & Weisaeth, 1996), propelling the client to get away from the traumatic past or the fear of future trauma. A subtler form of triggering exists for those with developmental trauma which activates the attachment system of longing/wanting/needing. When those native needs are unattended to, ridiculed, or dismissed, protection and defenses were, and are, built to cordon off the evolutionary need to attach, to be protected, to be seen, valued, and cared about.

These native attachment needs are encoded early in life, before narrative memory is in place (Brown, Elliott, et al., 2016), occurring in the body as dislocated feelings and sensations. Trevarthen (1979) described the emotional communications that happen between caregiver and child, also characterized by Buck (1994) as ". . . spontaneous emotional communication [that] constitutes a conversation between limbic systems . . . a biologically-based communication system that involves individual organisms directly . . . constitute . . . a biological unit. . . . The direct involvement with the other intrinsic to spontaneous communication represents an attachment that may satisfy deeply emotional social motives." (p. 266) "The limbically connected dyad translates this spontaneous communication . . . activating emotional preattunements . . . [whose] meaning . . . is known directly by the receiver." (Buck, 1994; p 266).

Making these nonnarrative communications available to present moment reality is the task of psychotherapy. In the activation of attachment, AEDP uses the therapeutic dyad to reorganize internal representations (Fosha, 2000). No matter what model of therapy we use, projective identification (Klein, 1946) as the unconscious co-creation of therapist and client comes into play, through various parts of the self projected onto the therapist. Philip Bromberg (2011) describes enactments as core components of the healing process that happen in the therapy hour, especially with trauma and attachment wounding.Triggers can give a laser pointed somatic flashlight on body memories being pushed into consciousness. An attachment focused perspective looks for the unmet relational distress as a means to help decipher the trigger.

Different parts hold undigested needs, sequestered out of conscious awareness. Getting triggered breaches the dissociative barrier in painful and disruptive ways, both small and large. The therapist's task is to help take that huge, undigested, previously unintegrated experience, and metabolize it, collaborating with the client, so the client can organize their intersubjective matrix and make sense of it all; and through this spontaneous emotional communication, we, as therapists, signal safety, understanding, connection, and compassion. As our client's attachment system gets activated, the attachment therapist consistently and persistently trains the person to notice their protest, feel safe having needs and wants, then turn toward that for which they've always longed. This collaborative task remaps the internal working model.

Recently, I was in a session with a client who is also a psychoanalyst well-versed in his own psychology. Triggered by the loss of the person who had sexually abused him, my client became so disorganized he wanted to take an extensive leave from his practice. Some models of psychotherapy would suggest moving deeper into this loss. Having given the client an Adult Attachment Interview, I knew his attachment history. Instead of going into the loss, we discussed using the attachment protocol developed by Brown and Elliott, et al. (2016) to remap his obsessive ruminating. At first skeptical, having gone into his history one too many times without feeling any shift, this client ended up responding positively to this new approach. Session after session, we collaborated on imagining new scenarios: one in which he was, and is, loved, cared about, safe, heard, and understood. This model of treatment initiated a quieting of his nervous system. Within a few weeks this client turned to me and said, "I'm calmer—that's surprising."

Turning toward positive attachment nourishment reshapes the larger psychological space in which people live. Even as our clients long for kindness and compassion, they often fear receiving these, resulting at times in backdraft (Germer, 2009). Paul Gilbert (2009a) has done extensive work in exploring the fears people have of compassion. Having a force field of positive attachment in place gives the client a greater capacity to discern when the past material is leaking/exploding into the present. Separated from the panic, terror, or numbness, the client is better able to catch their breath, slow down their physiology, and begin walking themselves back into the present. The basic skills described in earlier chapters are intended to help in those overwhelming moments. When practiced repeatedly they become second nature, when in the heat of the triggered moment. To counteract these fears of compassion, concentration practices of *metta* and compassion can be powerful skills. The practice part of Chapter Four describes a simple version of a loving kindness *metta* meditation (Salzberg, 1995).

APPLYING YOGIC PSYCHOLOGY TO A TRIGGERED MOMENT

Given all this, it's easy to see how being in the present is a convoluted experience for our clients. The layers of psychological and somatic conditioning are their reality. Patanjali gives us a way out of this in his Second Sutra, *"Yogas citta vrtti nirodha"*: Yoga is the stilling of the fluctuations of the mind. Yoga is integration (Feuerstein, 2013; Stapleton, 2015/2016, 2004) which happens as the changing states of the mind are stilled (Bryant, 2009). We are conditioned by previous experience, and out of that conditioning arise the *vrttis*—thoughts, feelings, and sensations—that form the perceptions of what we see and know. We unconsciously embellish with imagination (the color commentary we make about life), sleep (which for trauma survivors tends to be disrupted, often the land of nightmares), and memory (especially the time capsules we've talked about) that cloud remembering of our true nature. Caught in these constantly shifting states, our attention is drawn away from pure nature. The inner sea (*citta)* of our being is churned by tumultuous waves (*vrttis*), which Patanjali tells us can be helpful or detrimental. The detrimental *vrttis* are ignorance, ego, grasping, aversion, and resistance (Patanjali I:1–5). As our clients learn to harness their thoughts, feelings, and sensations they gain focus and internal concentration allowing the fluctuations of *citta-vrttis* to begin to still. Whenever we encounter something with our senses an impression is formed. Throughout our lives, we are imprinted with a spectrum of often undigested sensorial data points, ranging from the mundane to the dramatic.

Trauma is imprinted as detrimental *vrttis*, obscuring the person's perception of themselves and of life. Becoming absorbed in these impressions, the client identifies with the fluctuations, forgetting that the *vrtti* is imprinted on the original nature, or what we would call in IFS "self-energy." Patanjali (Bryant, 2009; Feuerstein, 2013; Stapleton, 2015/2016) stressed that we can't control the fluctuations of the mind without practice and dispassion (Yoga Sutras 1:12). His next sutra reinforces the need for practice in order to gain stability (Yoga Sutras 1:13), which happens only when cultivated properly, and for a long, uninterrupted span of time (Yoga Sutras1:14).

In adapting Patanjali's Yoga Sutras to being triggered, a three-pronged approach is necessary: understand the map, deconstruct the trigger, and develop skills and cultivate practices that ease the body, mind, and heart. Those who experience trauma don't have the embedded felt sense of a relaxed and easy body/nervous system. Luckily these skills can be learned over time, changing the person's relationship to their body. Especially important are learning the benefits of play and body easing practices that help develop a solid sense of self inside. It is an Olympian task to countermand the onslaught, when triggered. Just like an athlete, however, the more a client practices between sessions, the more they support their own healing.

Someone emailed me:

"It was about three months of peeking in and out of the site, when I began to realize that my whole being ached with longing to be allowed to explore the things I was reading. One of the most important things at this stage was the explanation, by Deirdre, that the BSES [Becoming Safely Embodied skills] were something that could be used in between therapy sessions. All the hours between were a disorganized struggle just to survive, the thought that there might be a constructive practice I could work with on my own was a hope that I learned to put into practice over time."

In the therapy hour, we validate the natural need they had in the past, and still have in the present, to be cared about, protected, and reassured which activates the client's attachment system. We teach them as a child would have been taught in a secure environment, that even when they are feeling the hurt, we're there with them, that they're not alone. We help them digest whatever experience they are having, and make meaning of it in a way that promotes integration. As Don Stapleton (2015/2016) reinforces, "Learning something new produces chaos and confusion. That's normal." It can be helpful for someone learning how to deal with new experiences to say to themselves, "I don't really know how to do this, but I'm trying. Even when I make mistakes it's because I'm learning and trying. That's why I'm coming to therapy, to learn how to do this differently."

Learning that it's okay to take tiny micro steps—and even more, that it's okay to make mistakes—normalizes being in a traumatized body full of stress and contraction. Important in this, is educating clients about the tightening and contraction that happens in the body. There was a point where this tightening once served a good purpose. It was an attempt to contain the experience, and keep out feelings, thoughts, memories, and other intrusions. Tightening the muscles helps us prepare for taking protective actions. Relaxing muscles is frightening, as it countermands this protective function, resulting in fear. How can we do this in a more manageable fashion? Instead of requiring clients to "take a breath," or shift their state, have clients learn to titrate what is happening, opening up the channels of experience, instead of tightening and rejecting internal experience. The adage I frequently invoke is that "There's no right way, and there's no way to do it wrong." This gives the client space. Such effortless acceptance, with concrete pointers on how to manage internal turbulence in body, mind, and heart, gently urges the muscles to soften, inviting an opening, when and if it feels right. During this process, the client becomes aware of the intense amount of energy they've used in order to push experiences out.

NO LONGER ALONE: INTRODUCING COLLABORATION

Collaboration with the client is essential in repairing attachment wounds. As much as a client may wish to do everything by themselves, the repair needs to come with a safe other (Tomasello, 2010; Brown, Elliott, et al., 2016; Germer, 2009; Gilbert & Choden, 2014). Different attachment styles need different kinds of collaboration. For those with more of an anxiously attached style, collaboration includes tempting the client to become fascinated with their inner world. This opens the door for attachment repair for those who either were ignored or were projected into. Those who formed more overly dismissive attachment styles need to have a collaborative respect in entering the body, curious about how their body and mind are organized, then following the client's lead, gently inviting an exploration while attuned to the toxic shame that comes from being humiliated from wanting connection. There is no single prescription or treatment protocol to plug a client into. Sensitive attunement means using our entire wealth of clinical experience to collaborate on what this person needs right now, which might be different from the last session. The suggested practices in this book are meant as possible guidelines with which to experiment. The interaction between you and the client provides the matrix to discover possible ways to mitigate the intensity of these attachment and trauma triggers.

Because attachment wounding is embedded in the body, soothing, caring practices invite the person to land inside their skin. One possible way is through finding imagery, sounds, tone, and words to offset the triggered response, and mitigate the fear that comes from feeling out of control. The intention is to explore with the client ways in which they can hold experience in their bodies, opening them to what is moving in them, instead of contracting away from it. When triggered, people pull into their bodies, withdrawing even as parts of them explode in rage, or respond with a desperate panic. Learning to make internal room for the difficult felt experience, instead of contracting into smaller space, allows the person to feel more spacious, reducing arousal. Their experience is no longer being jammed into an ever shrinking space.

As you recall from previous chapters, this requires entering into Body Time (Fay, 2007; Stapleton, 2004), training the mind and body to slow down. This is another form of collaboration—albeit, intrapsychic collaboration. The person develops the capacity to be with themselves, rather than disconnecting. Relaxing a pattern of holding tension in the body is a learned process, and one of the tenets of Self-Awakening Yoga (Stapleton, 2015/2016). Slowing down the breath, or focusing attention on smaller and smaller increments of time or sensation, gives the body the space to stay with the felt experience, as it is unfolding. Over time, this creates a sense of mastery, of being with the body instead of feeling victimized by it. Cultivating the capacity to be curious, deepening concentration and focus, becoming fascinated with *how* "this" is happening, helps our clients to further create space. How exactly does their body go from zero to one? And then one to two? Concentrating on this little moment of time and what happens in it can become absorbing. Focusing the mind exactly in this tiny moment slows down time, changing the felt experience of time, and giving room for the body to unwind more. In yoga postures, the practitioner grapples with how to shift small muscles, so that the next movement can more fluidly occur (Stapleton, 2004).

Cindy shared about her process of using the Becoming Safely Embodied™ Skills manual by herself, and then later doing the Embodied Practices online course. "I spent years learning about containment, trying to feel my body. I was always frozen inside, despite what I was doing on the outside. I go easily on auto-pilot, while the fear runs crazy fast in my body. It's especially hard for me when there are sounds and noises around me so I tend to isolate at home. I'd listen to your audios or the videos and have to listen 20 or 30 times to make sense. I started writing down what you were saying, I guess as a kind of concentration practice. I think that helped me make sense but more than that to hold onto what you were saying. When I watched the videos of you making a movement, it would take me, oh, I don't know how many times of watching you, to learn the different movements a person *could* make. It was like I didn't know how to move my own body. I had lost the signal. I got better, because I would play the video so many times and then I started moving with you in the video. I kept focusing on the mechanics so that I wouldn't listen to my mind telling me about how stupid this was, and how I was going to get in trouble, just by moving."

IF IT'S OUT OF PROPORTION TO WHAT'S HAPPENING, IT'S A TRIGGER

Triggers are kept alive when the person believes in the triggered reality, becoming locked in the memory state. When Cindy practiced encountering and exploring triggered states, instead of reacting, she developed insight into her own experience. Tracking her inner experience moment to moment, over time, helped her see the implicit pattern. That kind of mindfulness is very difficult when the body is reactive. Deconstructing triggers (the practice is described later in this chapter) builds a buffer zone of ease, to establish a larger view, giving space for the triggered sensation to relax, even if only a tiny bit. Slowly a structure is built within the self. Translating the trigger out of felt experience gives room for perspective taking, allowing the experience to be digested, assimilated, and integrated.

In my early days of working with trauma, I tried to minimize my clients getting triggered in any way I could. That proved to be impossible. The more I studied the phenomenon of getting triggered, the more I realized there was no way around it. We all get triggered. People with trauma and attachment histories will get triggered more often, and in bigger ways. The question, then, can't be to completely eradicate triggers. Instead, we look for how to exist with the triggers, how to de-construct them, so they are learning tools, becoming keys to healing trauma. Now I remind clients, "You will be triggered. We need to expect that. Here's the secret code that will help: If what you're experiencing is out of proportion to what is happening in reality, then you can guarantee something is triggering the past."

Keeping this "out of proportion" idea front and center has helped clients in individual therapy, as well as in groups, workshops, and courses. "I watched the decreasing reactivity video on your website. It was a novel idea to me that one does not have to respond to reactivity. The problem is that I hardly ever know what is triggering me. I can kind of get what my thoughts are, but the triggers? I have a long way to go with that. It's interesting though—that triggers spin me off into behaviors—I guess I always thought that might be a possibility. The challenge is learning those triggers, but more than that how to behave differently around them. The concrete examples in the video helped."

HOW TRIGGERS CAN POINT TOWARD HEALING

All this leads us to a possible conundrum—that triggers could be a way to heal. Clients with trauma and attachment histories have cut off access to their innate needs, wishes, and desires. For them, triggers are like explosives, blowing open the attachment scars that might not have been visible. The natural impulse people have is to shut down the churning turbulence with as quick a fix as possible. When triggered, it doesn't matter to the conscious mind that it's a temporary fix. Soothing the suffering is primary. Developing a capacity to slow down, to discover what's held inside the trigger, provides a road map to a more satisfying life. That requires, though, that clients are open to the exiled attachment needs that lie underneath the trigger. The triggered reactivity doesn't go away immediately, but begins to be met, experienced in some way, and integrated. Attending to a need and learning to provide positive nourishment grounds a person deeply. Confidence and self-worth arise from this ground.

HOW THEN TO STAY PRESENT WHEN TRIGGERED? CONCENTRATION AND MINDFULNESS

Clients will tell you that having the map helps. The more they recognize that they are being triggered, the more they are able to stand back from the triggered experience, without being swept under the tsunami when it comes. A cognitive map, like the Parallel Lives Model, describing what happens in a triggered body, helps. Yet the map alone will not make a difference, unless it's applied to felt experience. Two important skills are needed, culled from the yogic and meditation traditions: mindfulness, and concentration practices. Being able to witness and observe what's going on is what we call mindfulness. Focusing the mind on an object, being able to stay with it despite distractions, develops with concentration practices.

Noticing, naming, and identifying bare facts have been part of all the early skills presented in this book. They help develop the fluidity to observe, without getting caught in the emotional muck. Imagine how helpful it would be to be able to notice what's happening, without getting swallowed up by it? That's the benefit of mindfulness. All trauma survivors need this ability, to watch what's coming up, observing the huge experience as it's happening, without getting lost in it. Chris Germer (2009) writes in *Mindful Path to Self-Compassion* that he uses Guy Armstrong's definition of mindfulness, "Knowing what you're experiencing while you're experiencing it." Chris continues, "There's freedom because paying attention to the stream of our perceptions rather than interpretations makes every moment fresh and alive. Life becomes a festival to the senses when we're mindful" (p. 38). To live in the fresh present moment provides a balm for the painful patterns of cringing and withdrawing from life.

Practicing mindfulness offers clients a training ground to increase their ability to distinguish between thoughts, feelings, and body sensations, strengthens their capacity to watch, observe, and notice without getting hijacked, encourages disidentifying with whatever is coming up, while supporting ways to befriend symptoms, feelings, and parts of themselves that feel overwhelming. As their internal world becomes less disorganized, they gain awareness for their own internal structure, further allowing their inner world to continue to make sense. Mindfully attending to internal noise assists the client in discerning smaller and smaller building blocks of each thought, feeling, and sensation, frame by frame, moment by moment. Slowing down time like this opens gaps between impulse and action, creating choice points, both psychologically and behaviorally. As internal understanding builds, clients develop new perspectives and internal freedom from what dominated them previously. "Examining our life experiences with such discrimination develops a mental muscle that begins to slow the reflex to act on every desire that surfaces in the moment. In slowing down to discern the possible outcomes of a given choice we can suspend the reflex to fulfill that desire immediately" (Stapleton, 2004, p. 41). Mindfulness develops speed bumps between stimulus and response, giving time to explore what's happening, instead of being caught in the automatic, habitual away of reacting.

As with everything, though, especially with those with trauma, dissociation and attachment complications, there are cautions. Mindfulness, as it is traditionally taught, is an uncovering technique which can open the door for unprocessed material to quickly surge to the surface. If too much comes up too quickly, it can bring on regressive and even psychotic states. Cultivating choice points helps in this regard. If the client is feeling uncomfortable, scared, overwhelmed, or out of control, they need to be able to stop. Often they need to simply change their focus, and do something different. At the same time, it is also important to remember that getting triggered is not necessarily a reason not to practice. What is important is learning to titrate experience, slowing down, and moving gently. For many, this might mean mindfulness for 15 seconds, or taking a longer sip of breath rather than a full, deep, three-part breath. We're much better off helping our clients take a thimbleful of experience at a time, like a tiny a sip of breath, and learning to digest that small fragment rather than going headstrong into healing the deeper wounds.

The mindfulness practice, of observing and being with what happens, creates a wedge in the huge tumult that the body and mind sometimes experiences, giving the client access to stay here, in this moment, and holding the boundary between past and present. Concentration practices, on the other hand, allow the client to stay focused in the midst of the emotional and physiological tsunami that occurs, especially when they're triggered or caught in dissociative states. Our clients need to focus on getting back to safe ground, rather than being hijacked by flashbacks of any kind. Concentration skills hone the capacity to stay in the moment, this tiny moment; focusing on one thing to the exclusion of all else is concentration practice in action. Developing concentration skills to focus the mind, then staying with a point of focus, makes it easier to navigate triggers, without getting caught in the scary, ever-present flashbacks that are pressing in. Simple concentration practices are counting from one to ten, doing math equations, focusing on an object, or using singing, worry beads, or a mantra. How many of your clients look at your bookshelves while talking to you? They're often orienting, focusing, using an object to ground in the present, helping them to stay with you. There are other concentration practices that I'll describe in the practice section at the end of the chapter. To summarize a longer discussion (you can find more on my website), the benefits of concentration practices are huge, and can, with steadiness of mind, move someone from disorganization to incredible states of awareness. For our clients, to be able to not get plowed under by raging triggers is a huge accomplishment, and worth everything. Concentration practices narrow the field of consciousness, reducing the amount of stimuli racing from the amygdala to the cortex, initiating a brake so that the body can gently begin to ease (Damasio, 1995; Porges, 2011).

Concentration practices can have drawbacks, however. Focusing on one thing reduces hypervigilant defenses, making the dissociative barrier operating in the background more permeable, allowing more noise in the system. Concentrating, which gives rise to positive experiences of relaxation, spaciousness, ease, joy, and bliss, opens up a spaciousness that can be frightening. Concentrating on one thing, if not titrated, can overload the system with too much energetic stimuli, making it hard to keep the mind/body steady. If our clients are in a fragile place or have a permeable self/other distinction, they can get confused, not knowing where they end and others begin. Without structure, people can be besieged by stimuli, ending up feeling out of control. Becoming overwrought, it's easy to be overtaken by a self-destructive urge, or to intensify self-criticism and/or self-hatred.

What to do? When concentration opens windows and doors to negative stimuli the client can shift to a more supportive internal state. One way to work with detrimental states is to practice balancing the negative with the positive opposite. I discovered this in the 1980s on a long silent retreat. On the way to the retreat, I had stopped in New York City to visit a friend for dinner. Coming out of the restaurant, I found the window to my car had been smashed open and all my suitcases were gone. All my clothes. Even worse, all my favorite shawls and pillows that I had bought in India and Asia over the years were gone. I arrived at IMS, the retreat center in Barre, Massachusetts in shock. Sitting on my pillow, my nervous system in chaos, I found myself saying *metta*. Yet the phrases, "May I be happy" sounded ludicrous! I was in agony. I didn't want to deny that dreadful state I was in. Obviously I wanted to be happy and at peace, but I was a long way from that. Getting there seemed like an impossibility. Not wanting to contradict my inner state, I started balancing out the painful state with a simple "and" statement. "I feel terrible, *and* may I find peace." "I hurt everywhere. I'm in physical pain, *and* may I be free from suffering." The simple addition of "and" allowed me to bridge incongruent polarities to come to balance and move into the flow. As a therapist, I've taught this balancing to my clients, urging them to acknowledge their reality while providing an antidote. Balancing "I'll never be at peace," with attuned phrases like, "*and* may I find a way to be free of that." This isn't to deny the negative experience, but to balance it by bringing an antidote, the opposite experience by including "and." Rather than staying stuck, we open up the possibility of turning toward more nourishing states. Hearing this story, Jeremy started using as his mantra, "I'm here in this moment *and* I'm getting triggered."

Celeste gives us an example. Despite struggling with dissociation, Celeste recently had a fleeting sense of pride brought on by a colleague's acceptance of her work which triggered attachment wounds, rattling her for days. Everyone longs to love and be loved, that's normal. If, however, that longing was rejected or shamed, the psyche cordons off the longing, in toxic mental mines. This is what Celeste had to deal with. Being proud of herself as a child brought on physical and emotional violence. Reclaiming her natural need to be proud of herself, to feel like she belonged, required Celeste to be mindful of all the thoughts, feelings, and sensations that crowded into her awareness. She then had to focus on what she felt and believed. That it was okay, even good, to feel good, to feel proud, to feel connected. Welcoming in the positive, as she was focusing on the good, instead of what triggered her. The triggering past then started to recede, as over time, with practice, Celeste felt more solid. She was able to stay in the present, and we were able to process the traumatic memories with more ease.

This gift of being able to focus—to be concentrated on where you want to go—when things are pushing into your attention is a critical component, especially in working with triggers. It takes time, but the body will come to a greater sense of ease. Many years ago, as I was healing from my own trauma history, I remember being triggered for some reason that I can't recall. I walked for an hour before the triggered response eased. I kept repeating to myself that this was all that was happening right now. "I'm triggered." When the attachment system is being activated, clients won't necessarily have a narrative to describe *why* they are triggered. At this point, the content doesn't matter. The goal is to deescalate the amount of sensations the body is processing. After the hour of walking and focusing my mind, I could still feel the effects on my body, but was better able to engage with my life, like I was back in myself. Telling this to clients helps them to know that change is possible, and that they are not alone.

GROUNDING IN THE SPINE

As touched on earlier, most grounding techniques focus on the feet counting on gravity to ground. Being with and watching clients who struggle with being in their bodies I've watched people curling up, closing the front of their body. Clients, especially those with dissociative states, tend to pull in, around, and into the front of their bodies, exposing their back. What is protected? The heart. And for women, their breasts as well. Our backs are generally stronger, have more muscles and bones. Central to the back is the spinal column which houses the core of the nervous system connecting the brain with the rest of our body.

As you're reading this, notice what happens when you make contact with your spine. Can you feel the long tubular, fluctuating presence that contains the nervous system? There's so many different aspects to the spine. Focus for a moment on the base of your spine, where you're sitting. Perhaps rolling slightly on the sitz bones. When you have a feel for that gently press up through the crown of your head, lengthening your spine even as you're seated. Holding those two points, the crown and your sitz bones, what happens as you breathe down the length of your spine, moving gently? Engaging your head, perhaps twisting a bit.

When I did this with Lolly she was able to feel the crown of her head but couldn't figure out where it was connected to her sitz bones. I wondered with her what might happen if she wiggled in her seat. Did that affect her spine? It did, although she didn't have words to describe what happened. Then we tried pressing up and down at the same time, experimenting with what happened. As she played with her own spine while sitting in the chair her breathing eased. As I commented on it Lolly became aware of her internal focus. At some point she naturally rolled her head forward, then to the side, enjoying sensations. For some clients this is all they need, to feel their spine. Sometimes I have them place small pillows at different spots on their spine to feel what happens in them. When clients are activated and triggered I have them place hot water bottles or heating pads on their back, resting into the sensations of heat soothing the nervous system.

When Lolly was ready I asked if she wanted to try something else. When she nodded I suggested she try the Assisted Tree Posture that I do with people to connect them even more to their spine while at the same time giving them a felt experience of "having their back" or support. Moving over to the back of the office door I encouraged Lolly to feel the door at her back, rolling her spine against the door. When she felt connected to the door through her spine I wondered what would happen if she felt into her feet, the crown of her head, and her spine. When she felt sturdy in that we played with shifting weight to one foot, letting the other foot carry less. That tiny balance was possible as she kept contact with her spine against the door. Her focus intensified as her body found the tiny movements to keep her balanced. When she was ready I wondered with her what would happen if she brought the relaxed foot up to the standing calf or inside of her knee. To do this she needed to keep focusing, pressing down through her left foot. I also suggested she be aware of her crown while doing this to hold her spine sturdy. She held that for a moment focusing on keeping herself steady by leaning into the door. When she was ready to let the posture go I invited her to notice what relaxation felt like. Was there some release? If so, where and how did that feel? "What I found was in doing it, supported, against the wall, allowing myself to do that, I could take away the fear and anxiety of whether I am going to do this right or fall over! I realized all the obsessive thinking I have when I'm in a yoga class. Doing it this way I could just relax into it. I compare myself to other people who don't need to hold on, which is of course, why I hate taking yoga classes! So doing it this way was great. I could feel the door against my shoulder blade which gave me confidence or something."

SOOTHING TRIGGERS WITH SOUNDS

One practice that clients find soothing is to use sound whether internal or out loud. In groups or in individual therapy I suggest to clients to try any of the primary sounds that are native to primordial languages everywhere (Weintraub, 2012). Making sounds, though, can be complicated for many clients with trauma and attachment wounding. They may well be aware of internal sounds but to bring the sound into consciousness? And it can be even harder to make the sound audible. How then to stimulate the natural balancing sounds that soothe a baby or the sound of lullabies to quiet a child? The brain stem is one of the first developed parts of the brain, responding to vibration and sound. Philippa laughed thinking about lullabies, saying she can't sing but she can certainly hum, which is what she did with her children. Sounds create vibration. The more we harmonize with the vibration we attune our nervous system. Kyle, who is a musician, knows the value of music and sound. Despite that he squirmed at the idea of making a sound toward his depressed nervous system or parts inside. Although he scoffed he gave it a try and was quite pleased at the result. "It seemed easier to offer a sound…. well, it's not tangible or psychological. It felt like I could focus rather than trying to think about it. It made it easier to stay with it." Celeste who had been quiet for most of the group piped up. On her daughter's recommendation she went to a workshop where the leader used crystal bowls to attune the chakras. During the early phases of the workshop, Celeste's skepticism won out and she felt it was all "malarkey." Yet by the end of the workshop she described a "release of tension that was other worldly" as if a relaxation entered her body that she had never had before.

Humming is grounding and balancing, something people can do anywhere, anytime. In a group where I taught humming as part of the Embodied Practices for Healing Trauma, Pat told the group how he used humming when he woke up in the morning feeling dissociated. He initially started humming to ground himself and bring the fear down. I suggested he hum to the part that was dissociating or afraid. He later reported that humming to the part would bring reassurance and dialed down the fear even more. Together the group played with humming out loud or humming internally using the practice at home. Many of the members later spoke of how they found it frightening at first to hum out loud, "just hearing myself real in the world was scary but then strangely quieting." Another told us how the sound was deep inside her and bringing it to mind was one thing but to make the sound out loud didn't feel safe. Her practice was to soundlessly hum feeling the vibration in her throat without making a sound. Another woman reported that it felt good to make sounds out loud because it distracted her from the internal upset that was going on, soothing her, giving her something to hold onto while she felt rattled inside.

Laura described feeling frozen and unable to separate from that frozen part of herself. In an Embodied Practices group, I had her hum at whatever sound level she wanted. I asked her then to explore if the internalized vibration could meet the frozen space inside. The larger group held the space for her as Laura soundlessly sounded. We literally saw her body relax its tension. Not saying anything we waited for her to open her eyes. Looking around, Laura told us she started to feel warmed from the inside.

Dan was triggered and let me know in no uncertain terms as he walked into my office. He couldn't sit he was so distraught. I asked him if he was willing to try something. Knowing me, he rolled his eyes but was willing. I suggested he put his triggered response (some people don't like to use the word "part") in the middle of the room while he and I would hum and make soothing sounds directed at that "part." An adventurous sort, and being so triggered he didn't know what else to do, Dan agreed. Filling the office with soft, gentle sounds made a palpable difference. Dan's shoulders eased, his voice lengthened, and the tone become more solid. Then we were able to sit and deconstruct what the trigger was all about.

For those clients who find it difficult to "separate" from the felt experience, sounding/humming can bring ease. First bring attention to the body as a whole then find a sound in whatever pitch and tone feels right. Even if only an internal sound, vibration can shift the felt experience. By tuning into the felt experience the client has a nonnarrative body sense of what is needed. Clients report "hearing" internalized sounds of their bodies or parts (if they use that language) to which they then "respond" with a soothing, reassuring internalized or external sound. Tuning into the sounds that various distressed or traumatized parts are making can be too activating. Generally, the best approach is first to respond to the activation with soothing sounds reminiscent of lullabies. David Knoerr, a body-oriented psychotherapist in Watertown, Massachusetts, often makes simple "hum" sounds as the client shares difficult material. His clients describe it as comforting and joining, feeling attuned to by him.

Katie shared that her constant cynicism often came to the fore when I suggested practices like this. She decided to meet her cynic with a sound that would have her cynic feel understood or appreciated. I waited patiently, wondering what was happening, as I watched her, the energy in the room softening. Opening her eyes, Katie exclaimed, "I couldn't believe it. The sound moved *with* the cynicism, rolling with it. It felt like a dance! Like we were dialoging together but without words." Elisa Elkin Cleary, a trainer of the Comprehensive Resource Model, talked with me about how making sounds (called toning) can assist people in attuning to their internal awareness, bridging the distress and "resourced states." Toning to the distress allows the person to see and hear their inner experience without words and overt meaning influencing interpretation of the tones/sounds. This allows the inner state to be acknowledged and understood. "The implicit memory of the dissociated, or otherwise overwhelming, experience encountered through a sensation, feeling, thought, or explicit memory, can then become conscious (co-conscious) allowing the opportunity for change. Toning the internal resources promotes a deeper connection to that which supports trauma release and healthy expansion. In The Comprehensive Resource Model, the different uses of toning are developed from the needs resulting from the client's distress and the creativity of the CRM Therapist. However, the aim is always to ensure that the toning comes from an increasingly regulated, rather than abreactive, state so that the individual remains fully present while processing the selected material." (Schwartz, Corrigan, Hull, & Raju, in press).

REACTIVE VERSUS RESPONSE CYCLES

The problem for clients is learning to do this on their own outside of the therapy hour. Giving clients the skill to deconstruct triggers, learning about their reactive cycles and how to shift into response cycles, allows the client to feel a greater sense of mastery. Breaking apart these triggered moments, step-by-step, moment-by-moment, so that we can learn about what happened; what the experience was that was so big it had to get pushed out of awareness. As clients learn about the biphasic trauma response, the window of tolerance (Ogden, Minton, & Pain, 2006) and how they move in and out of it they start monitoring when they are in their window of tolerance, when they are present. When they are present they are able to digest what was so disruptive. As a child, through no fault of their own, they weren't developmentally able to organize or make sense or understand what was happening in them and around them.

DECONSTRUCTING TRIGGERS

Deconstructing triggers (Fay, 2007) happens by slowing down time just as we would in making an animated storyboard. Describing this process as graphic novels, cartoons, or an animated movie gives clients a mental picture of the slowed down process of seeing one image, then the next, and the next. These many separate vignettes are bound together to create a larger story. Animated storyboards isolate images that happen so rapidly in a movie that our mind and senses take in the whole rather than seeing the individual pieces. This slows the process down, enabling a way to peel the story apart frame by frame. The fluid whole is deconstructed to see each piece of the storyboard. Discriminating what each thought, feeling, and sensation is becomes grounding, giving the person a chance to notice how each moment is different while also conjoined. This is a way to put a brake on the intense action, giving time to explore loaded moments that have undigested fragments of life experience communicated through thoughts, feelings, body sensations, and impulses. From a yogic perspective the intent of such powerful energy moving in the body is to move toward integration, to clean whatever is blocking the free flow of pure energy. Psychologically, we're learning to digest life experience which results in feeling less blocked.

Deconstructing triggers has two entry points: starting before the trigger and moving frame by frame toward the triggered moment; the other way in is to start at the triggered moment and slowly, frame by frame moving forward or backwards in time. Either way entails noticing the tiny little moments that happened within the exploding frame. I've often mentioned to clients to slice the moment very thin, so that it's transparent. In that frame, what was the thought, the feeling, the body sensation, and were there any impulses? Then, move to the next frame either forward or back. In that moment, what was the thought, feeling, sensation, or impulse? You're looking for the tiny miniscule moments to slow down the triggered response. Yes, the bomb blew up *and* we can track how that bomb blew up second by second as if we were slowing down the animated movie. The actual stimuli that triggered the inner tsunami may have been instigated by someone else, either what they said, or body language, or even what they didn't say. It could come from a color, shape, sound from outside and it could also come from some internal experience.

STEPS TO DECONSTRUCTING TRIGGERS

Jennifer came to a group triggered. Rather than have her sit there falling into a black hole and affecting others in the group I asked her if she was willing to explore what was going on. To help her deconstruct what was happening I suggested we start at the beginning, before she got triggered and work our way toward the moment she got triggered.

1. *What was the context?*

    I explored with Jennifer who was there? And what state she was in. At first Jennifer couldn't tell. She only knew she was stirred up. So I began exploring with her trying to locate the beginning of the trigger, asking her "When you came to the group, were you, what were you thinking? What were you feeling? What was going on?"

    > *Jennifer:* I was coming to group and everyone was in the waiting room talking. I wasn't in a good mood. When we started talking about triggers I thought to myself, this is a stupid topic.
    > *Deirdre:* What were the thoughts?
    > *Jennifer:* How dare I try to help myself? *%^&&@ and Deirdre's a @ ($★#&^ as well.

Deirdre: What was the feeling?

Jennifer: I'm shut down. Well, I guess there's a lot of agitation.

Deirdre: And what's happening in your body?

Jennifer: It's hot, pulsing, flashing.

[We continued with this moment by moment.]

2. *What happened next?*

Deirdre: If we pay attention moment to moment, what was happening next?

Jennifer: You're talking about triggers.

Deirdre: Yes, and when I talked about triggers, what was the thought you had?

Jennifer: [more swear words] and I also had the thought that don't you know how lucky you are?

Deirdre: What were the feelings?

Jennifer: I felt bitter, angry and afraid.

Deirdre: Did you notice any sensations? What was going on in your body?

Jennifer thought for a moment then said she felt shaky with a sense of falling, no ground. She felt cold and tired.

Deirdre: Okay, what happened in the next moment?

Jennifer: I had a thought, "just stop all this darn {swear, swear, swear, swear, swear.}" And another thought of telling myself to pay attention.

3. [We acknowledged the conflict going on but rather than going into it I asked, "What were you feeling?"]

Jennifer: I wasn't aware of any feeling.

Deirdre: What was the behavior?

Looking down as I asked that Jennifer notice her hands were pushing against her legs.

Jennifer: I'm trying to push . . . push some feelings down.

4. [We could see something changing in her as she was doing this and speaking. I asked her what was happening.]

Jennifer: I'm feeling smaller and smaller—as if the sounds are getting further away. Feels like I'm going down a tunnel.

Deirdre: Are you aware of any thoughts?

Jennifer said, Help is good. Maybe I can do it. I can't do it on my own.

Then Jennifer spoke another thought: This is going to hurt. PROTECT!!! I have got to protect myself.

Sitting a moment longer, Jennifer described: I want to feel closer to everyone, to Deirdre, but I'm afraid to be seen.

Saying this, she realized her body felt shaky. But she felt bigger. She was no longer going down that tunnel. And as a result then she could reenter the group and be present, less withdrawn and irritated.

Sorting out triggered moments can occur by investigating small little moments or larger more complicated events. For this experience in the group, Jennifer was surprised that she felt less withdrawn, irritated, more relaxed, and willing to engage with the group as a whole

The objective is to take something apart, slicing an overwhelming experience into smaller and smaller pieces. Look for: What's the thought? What's the feeling? What's the body sensation? Breaking the large moment into smaller bits slows down time, gives room to interact with the confusing moment. Our reactions happen so quickly that we're generally not aware of it. It's like the body goes from zero to 100 in a second. The metaphor I use with clients is going to the deli counter to get some sliced meat. The deli person will ask how thick you want it. For our purposes in deconstructing triggers we want to slice the moment paper thin. We want the information transparent, so thin we can see right through it. Natalie asked me, "What do you mean by interacting with the trigger? That sounds potentially horrible." As we deconstructed her trigger she had an "aha." "I think what we're talking about is that if you get sucked into the past, like you're in the middle of that feeling of the past, it's really hard to look at it because you're in it. So if you can get a little bit separate and remind yourself of being in the present, then you can actually have some way to interact with that, in some way. It feels different, like I'm here. Yeah, what was good was looking around because when it happens I don't even realize that I'm gone. It's just where I go."

To illustrate how to slow down time and enter into smaller and smaller segments to deconstruct triggers I've included some examples that are composites of what generally happen in a group (or individual) session. This next composite illustrates what happened with a client when someone touched her:

Deirdre: In that moment, when somebody put their hand on you, what happened?

Sandy: Danger.

Deirdre: Was that a thought, feeling, or body sensation?

Sandy: I thought I've got to protect myself. Tough shit. I'm scared. I guess the feelings sometime came first. Sometimes when I'm moving around and bang my foot I instantly feel assaulted, like I've been punched or something. I then have all these feelings, without any thoughts at all. Just feel assaulted by somebody.

Deirdre: If you slow it down what's the feeling in your body?

Sandy: I'm just like kind of stunned and like you would feel if someone turned around and decked you. You just are like "Whoa."

Deirdre: Perfect. Slowing it down you realize there's more going on in each moment. Let's explore this as one of those little storybooks that you flip through. Each page has one scene and then the next scene. Let's look at each page individually. What happens in the first one?

Sandy: I whacked my head.

Deirdre: When the whack happened, what was the thought, what was the feeling, what was body sensation?

Sandy: Hmm. I guess there wasn't a thought, but there was first the feeling of stunned. Taken aback. Then I said "SHIT" out loud.

Deirdre: And what was happening in your body?

Sandy: (Pauses.) Gosh a lot was happening. It hurt. I want to say I saw stars but I don't know if that was a thought or it actually happened. (Pauses further.) I guess it's making sense now. So much was happening in that moment of being overwhelmed. You know, I think I had a memory that I was being attacked but right in that moment I wasn't being attacked. (Looks a bit stunned.) Wow. That's intense. In that moment. This is what you call being hijacked by the past? I was in my apartment which is safe but hitting my head opened up the time capsule of other times when I wasn't safe and when I was hit. (Takes a big breath.) That scares me, so I dissociate. Yeah, that's what happens, not just in this situation but others.

Okay! Then how do you stop that from happening? That would be my question.

Deirdre: It takes time. Training the mind, body, heart to be in the here-and-now, knowing it so clearly and becoming aware of the red flags that indicate past material is leaking in. Let's unpack this a bit more. Let's say you have a time capsule of memories when you were hurt by somebody through touch. Now you're in this moment and somebody puts their hand on your shoulder, meaning well. Not meaning to do any harm. The moment that happens you're not in the here and now. This moment is layered with something from the past. All of a sudden the past invades the present, flooding you with thoughts, memories, feelings. Even though you're in this moment, your body is flooded with undigested material from the past. You're time traveling.

Sandy: (Nodding, saying nothing. After Sandy had some time to consolidate, I continued.)

Deirdre: Be kind to yourself. It takes practice. It takes all the things we've been talking about: separating the fact from the feeling, bare noticing, knowing what the present feels like and how your body alerts you to the past.

Sometimes the first skill to practice is mindfulness, saying to yourself, "Oh! I'm triggered." The second important part is compassionate awareness, "If I'm this triggered now, it must be from the past."

Later when you are more in the present moment, you might wonder, "if I'm this triggered now, what was it like for me back then when I didn't have the resources I have now?" A 3- or an 8-year-old can't integrate frozen, scared, disappointed feelings as well as an adult.

This is the big clue: when the feeling is too big to handle in the present, it's probably about the past.

(Slowing it down again.) Even feeling good can be too big. Some of the research shows that infants sometimes find touch too stimulating. Touch can dysregulate them. Toddlers giggle, laugh and make eye contact—then they'll look away to have time to integrate.

This happens for some when somebody says something good. You like it but you "know" good things won't follow because of a memory of something bad happening when something good happened. Wiring the good moment with a bad experience makes an imprint. Learning to tease that apart takes practice and attention.

Sandy: This is really helpful. I want to say one thing. If in that moment you can't even think because that's what happens in the process of dissociation, then you do this after the fact?

Deirdre: It's hard to stay present in the middle of a trigger or dissociation unless you've been practicing a lot—so, yes, practice after the triggered or disso-ciated storm has passed. In the middle of a trigger you might not be able to do much else but hang on tight. If you can you could say to yourself, "Oh my god, it's too much right now. Let me take a break from this."

Practice slowing down. Establishing safety however you can. Separat-ing facts from feelings, repeating to yourself, "Nothing bad is happening right now. Right now I'm in this moment. The fact is I'm here, in this room, with these people, and nothing bad is happening." You work with yourself using whatever skills you can grab hold of in that moment. And then when you have a little space, you reflect on what happened in that moment. What happened into the next moment? What happened in the moment after that? You're trying to untangle those fast moving moments. Have you ever seen a yarn ball, clumped together? You need to tease it apart. That's all you're doing, you're taking that moment, teasing apart, so you can see the individual strands.

Another group member: This is helping me see connections. Like it's okay when I feel this way, that's what's going on. Just trying to recognize what that is and it's okay. So it gets less and less, but definitely it's not even like one lit-tle thing. It's kind of like interacting with people is triggering, for me. Like this past year, simple little interactions, even people who are safe people, it can be triggering. But it's just good to hear about it.

Another example from a group:

Maryanne: If I think about my experience the only thing is I wasn't sure if we were supposed to be able to pull ourselves from the past or just kind of break down what was happening.

Deirdre: Tell me a little bit more what you mean by that and let me see if I can help you with that.

Maryanne: Well I just, I kind of took apart what happened, in terms of the event that triggered me. But I wasn't able to sort of take myself to a bal-anced place.

Deirdre: It felt out of proportion the whole time? It felt too big for your body?

Maryanne: Well I just, I don't know how to, I feel like it took me to a young place that I don't know really how to take myself out of. So I don't know.

Deirdre: As you're saying it now, you're observing the young place even though it feels like a big experience in your body?

Maryanne: Yeah I am able to observe it. Like I'm able to know that this is coming from a child place and even, in some ways, know what the child place is.

Deirdre: It takes a while. Remember our bodies are concrete. When our nervous system gets activated it takes a longer time to calm down. There are more neural networks going from our amygdala up to our frontal cortex than there are from our cortex down to our amygdala to calm down. So once we get triggered, it takes a while to slow the process down.

Maryanne: Can you help me with this?

Deirdre: Sure. Let's start from the beginning of the . . . when did you start getting activated?

Maryanne: As soon as I heard the words.

Deirdre: Let's go slow.

Maryanne: Yeah. My son and I were thinking of going to visit my mom . . . and I already knew I was triggered.

Deirdre: Okay. What was the thought? What was the feeling? What was the body sensation?

Maryanne: Well, this is interesting. Because I was already feeling like . . . I mean when I said let's go visit I was looking forward to spending a little time with my son on the way to visit my mom. Just the two of us. And then before I knew it . . . I, actually, now that I think about it, I got triggered then.

Deirdre: Sounds like there was a spiraling effect? What's happening inside you?

Maryanne: I felt like, I felt, I think I felt angry. I felt unimportant. Like I didn't matter. Hurt.

Deirdre: And what were the sensations in your body?

Maryanne: Yeah that's hard for me. I think I collapsed.

Deirdre: How do you know that?

Maryanne: My body just feels like it's curling in on itself—I'm shutting down and can't feel anything.

Deirdre: Beautiful description. Can we stay with that moment?

Maryanne: It was like I told myself that I'm not going to feel anything.

Deirdre: What happened next? What was the next moment?

Maryanne: I think I said I thought we were going to spend some time alone.

Deirdre: And what was the thought going on inside?

Maryanne: I mean, I think I thought inside of me it's probably, . . . just let, even though I sort of collapse, there is at the same time another part that isn't going to let the plan be changed so I wouldn't have time with my son.

Deirdre: So there is a whole bunch going on, right? And in that moment when you said, "I thought that we were going to spend some time together" what was the feeling?

Maryanne: Anger.

Deirdre: What was the sensation that was happening?

Maryanne: Collapse.

Deirdre: Let's just see what "collapse" is made of.

Maryanne: Collapse is made of . . . no spine, shrinking, feeling little.

Deirdre: Right. What happened next?

Maryanne: My son said okay—we'll do it your way.

Deirdre: Uh-huh. So what did you feel inside then?

Maryanne: Well I felt deflated, and, but I think I tried to say to myself, well try to be nice. It's okay, it'll be okay. But that was me trying to manage what was happening inside.

Deirdre: Well, there again, if we peel it apart, you had the thought to do a lot of self-talk to try to make it okay, but there was an experience inside of deflated, right?

Maryanne: Yeah.

Deirdre: What's the sensation of deflated?

Maryanne: It's like the air going out of my body. Disappearing.

Deirdre: And what's the feeling that you were having?

Maryanne: I think anger.

Deirdre: What's the experience of anger in your body?

Maryanne: I think I don't experience it.

Deirdre: Well let's see if we can slow it down because somehow you were experiencing something. Because you knew, or you had a sense that you were angry, right?

Maryanne: Yeah, but I think that I'm so scared of it that I actually collapse instead? Or something.

Deirdre: Wow, wonderful tracking inside. As you're exploring this what's happening inside you?

Maryanne: Right now?

Deirdre: Yeah.

Maryanne: I am feeling a little scared by the knowledge of how angry I really feel. The collapse makes it so I can't really feel how angry or how scared I am. I'm a little scared about how much anger there really is.

Deirdre: You have this big feeling of anger and this big feeling of collapse competing with each other?

Maryanne: Well, I think it's the collapse that usually shows and the anger probably comes out indirectly.

Deirdre: Again, good tracking. So as you begin to see this cycle that you have, that you hide the anger and the collapse sort of is what shows, what happens in your body now?

Maryanne: I want to disappear. The history with that, if I got angry, I got punished. So I'm scared about my anger.

Deirdre: Well that makes a ton of sense. Deconstructing a trigger and untangling these kinds of things doesn't make it go away—or even make it better—but it organizes all the pieces and helps us feel grounded as we make sense of what happened. What's happening in your body now?

Maryanne: I'm a little anxious.

Deirdre: What's the thought?

Maryanne: The thought? I've taken up too much group time.

Another member: [laughs] We all have that one, isn't it?

Deirdre: Well, I really want to appreciate you for being so honest and open about an experience that was so big.

Maryanne: Thank you.

Deirdre: So, check with your body now.

Maryanne: It's a little calmer.

Deirdre: Take a moment to check what you need right now.

Maryanne: Right now? What do I need? To talk to my therapist.

Deirdre: Okay, well that's true but right now is right now. We're actually in this moment, right now.

Maryanne: I feel warm, warmth inside. Yeah my body feels warm.

Deirdre: What happens to the nervous parts and the scared parts and the ones that are afraid of being punished?

Maryanne: They feel more settled down.

Deirdre: Perhaps if we slow down the moment, eventually we're going to get to some need that we have. And if we really tend to it, like at first she said, "Oh I've got to talk to my therapist." That's an important need and it's not really in this moment. But if we can keep anchoring it in this present moment, and maybe it's small thing. Maybe it's just like I need to take a breath. Or I need to shake it off or I need to do a little jig right now. Then we can actually tend to that need and meet it. Then you begin to know that listening to yourself can bring up a need that you can actually meet.

USING *PRANAYAMA* (BREATHING PRACTICES) TO SHIFT PHYSIOLOGY

When activated, it can be too much to harness the breath. People are afraid to take in more breath, literally afraid if they take in more they will feel more. Instead those with trauma shut down the breath, constricting it. Tiny sips of breath (Fay, 1986, 2007) and Puffing Breath (Weintraub, 2012) work with people who live with activated trauma physiology, encouraging relaxation. In the "early days," before we knew a great deal of how trauma affected the body, yoga teachers and well-meaning therapists would tell their clients to take long, deep breaths focusing on the three-part breath. In the work I was doing with clients who had dissociative symptoms in hospital settings, I realized it was better to take small thimblefuls of breath, sipping the breath in. When clients were tight with anger or fear, the sips of breath worked to gently soften the nervous system. Puffing Breath encourages clients to release the breath in quiet, incremental ways. This gentle pushing out of the breath engages the lungs and belly, inviting on the other end a soft inhalation. One of the *pranayama* practices of LifeForce Yoga is Stair Step Breath (Weintraub, 2012). Taking a few short breaths to slowly fill the lungs, then exhaling in puffs. This has been shown to work well with anxious and depressed individuals.

TAKING A BREAK

There are also times when our clients need a break from the felt experience of being internally assaulted by their own bodies. They need to know they don't have to always be in a process, or dealing with their traumatic material. They absolutely need to learn how to shift out of this state. They need to know that when the triggered material comes up, they can go into that material without getting swamped or shutting down. Perhaps more importantly, they need to learn they can get out of that state. To prompt them, I invite them to try any of the following options as a means to stop the trigger. This is not a complete or exhaustive list. This list is meant to stimulate possible responses, though you could choose to handle difficult triggering moments. They come from the many people who have told me what helped them when they have been triggered. You may find that none of them work for you. If that's the case then I urge you to become curious about what works, to try other options out, and email me at dfay@dfay.com so I can add your additions to this list.

- Turning your attention to something completely different.
- Coloring books – drawing in the lines is a concentration practice many find helpful.
- It's usually helpful if you turn your attention to things that support you or make you feel good.
- Music can be helpful, especially music that fills your heart with joy.
- Calling a friend, not to talk about the trigger, but to make contact can help a lot.
- Send emails to people you love and tell them one thing about them that you are grateful for.
- If you need your PRN medicine, take that.
- Go for a walk.
- Garden, put your hands in dirt or sand which for some is very grounding; build a rock garden.
- Surf the web; look for positive, nuturing material.
- Read something engaging (comic books, spy novels, romance novels, joke books, or whatever you find engaging).
- Watch re-runs of TV shows (many people watch HGTV as a nonstimulating channel).
- Rent a funny movie.
- Read catalogs.
- Play a computer game, card game, crossword puzzles, or Sudoku.

• Notice your environment in detail (see the mindfulness exercises for that!).
• Do something aerobic.
• Use a punching bag.
• Hold an object that has positive meaning for you.
• Get out into nature.
• Write down the trigger, put it in a box and bury it.
• Talk to your therapist about ways to support yourself through this process.

Practices for Work with Triggers

HUMMING: SOOTHING SOUND

Objective: *A simple way to invite a client into the body is through humming, activating the attachment system for protection and reassurance. Many clients do this naturally. Setting it as a practice can be an easy success step for clients. Humming or singing aloud is part of many traditions, making it a simple migration to using sounds for healing.*

The use of primordial sound is one of the earliest ways to focus the mind and calm the nervous system. For this practice we'll explore two different ways. With either direction you choose, the idea is to repeat the sound or phrase. Some research suggests that as we do something over and over again, or hold that experience in our brain for 17 seconds we literally begin the process of re-wiring and forming new neural networks. So often we are bombarded with images, thoughts, and feelings that form a background noise, a virtual soundtrack that follows us, pre-determining our next experience. Mantra is one way to begin shifting the wallpaper of our experience.

Sound vibration can be very calming. Humming and sounding are all ways to evoke neutral calming sounds. Spiritual ballads or chanting is another way to draw on the calming experience of sound. Using words/gratitude phrases from a spiritual tradition or that feel meaningful to us. It helps if the phrase points us toward a more gracious and beneficent experience. In spiritual traditions the mantras tend to be about surrendering our egos will to the divine or greater good. Whatever you choose, the most important thing is to repeat the phrase over and over and over again. Try for five minutes, then extend to ten, fifteen, and even twenty.

YOGA: SHOULDER CRADLE*

Objective: *Easy comfort with emotional and psychological containment.*

Instructions: Place your right hand on your left shoulder, feeling the weight of your right arm. Notice the effect that has on your head, neck. Bring your left hand up to

* (Adapted with permission from Don Stapleton's Self Awakening Yoga practice.)

anchor on your right shoulder. Lower your head down to rest on the right shoulder cushioned by the left hand. Feel the gentle stretch in the left neck. Letting the breath rock you, cradling your head.

Change arms, bringing left hand to right shoulder, wrapping right hand onto top of left shoulder. Lowering head to the left, feeling the gentle stretch, breathing and rocking, cradling in this self hug.

YOGA *PRANAYAMA: KUMBHAKA*

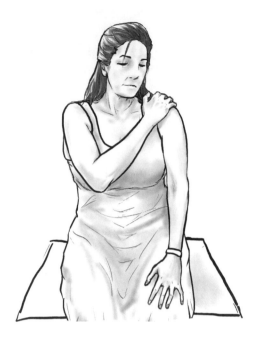

FIG 5.1A   Shoulder Cradle 1

Objective: *This bottom-up practice interrupts procedural patterns that occur when triggered. Retaining the breath is one way to impact the gross levels of patterning in the body as well as harnessing and directing the flow of prana (life force) that flows through the entire system. In training the breath, we create ways for the impetuous nature of externally directed energy to settle. In this quiet Kumbhaka is training to receive the gift of one's own Self energy. The pause we take from all activation is a pause to receive, to fill up, to drink in.*

Instructions: This is not a constriction or a forceful holding. Instead the client learns to meet the breathing pattern with kindness and quietness. Patanjali reminds us this is a form of concentration, focusing on the breath. We can try to control the breath but it's always there like the stream of water flowing down from the mountains to the sea. Kumbhaka, the pausing, resting, harnessing of the breath is a way of receiving oneself. In the pause between inhalation or exhalation there's a chance to meet oneself, to open the gift of oneself.

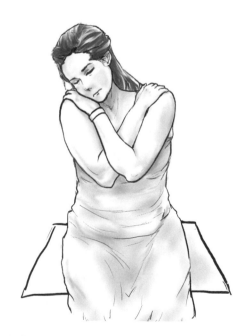

FIG 5.1B   Shoulder Cradle 2

Take a number of normal relaxed breaths

becoming aware of the cycle of breathing. Finding the top of a normal breath. Then feeling into the bottom of the next breath. This is not a time to take long, deep breaths but rather become acquainted with the breath as it is happening in this moment. Noticing every little tingle of the in breath. Then paying attention to the roll over at the top of the breath. Paying attention to every little movement of the exhale. Exploring exactly how the breath ends and a new breath arises.

As you do this for a few times with the softest tiniest pause hold the breath in at the top of the inhalation or very slightly, softly, and gently holding the breath out at the bottom of the exhalation. Without effort, interrupt the habitual breathing patterns.

YOGA *PRANAYAMA*: MODIFIED *KAPALABHATI* – SIPS OF BREATH

Objective: *When triggered the breathing pattern is altered. People hold their breath, or tighten, or their breath speeds up. Training the breath alters the constant pressure of prana seeking movement into the external work. Pausing, resting, harnessing, and harmonizing the breath can, over time, create more quiet and an internal focus.*

Instructions:

Tiny Sips of Breath. Without worrying how much breath someone takes in, accept the invitation to take a tiny sip of breath. It can be a simple breath in and quickly released or a sip of breath that gets held. It doesn't matter the amount. What is important is to orient the person to noticing their breath and inviting breath to cross the threshold from outside to inside.

YOGA: ADAPTED CHILD POSE

Objective: *The traditional child posture in yoga is about resting and taking in nourishment from comfort. This adapted posture addresses the possibility of trauma clients going into regressed states; this modification invites the client to experience letting go of tension by holding onto a large pillow or blanket while sitting. The intention is to calm the mind, allowing stress and fatigue to ease, lengthening the back, letting go of neck tension. It also supports breathing into the back of the torso, the back opening into a dome, lengthening and widening the spine. Leaning over the pillow the client feels the tension letting go in their back without moving them into a regressed position of being curled up on the floor.*

Instructions: Crossing arms in front of the body, hands reaching toward opposite shoulders. Notice any sense of protection. If it feels right tap the upper arms gently, making soft contact. You might have some reassuring or comforting words you'd like to make quietly to yourself as you tap your upper arms. Explore the effect that has on you.

When that feels complete take a large pillow or blanket into your lap. Taking any kind of breath, you like, wrap your arms around the pillow/blanket, letting your body rest, your spine releasing, holding. Notice your breath along the spine. How much does the breath move up and down your spine? With

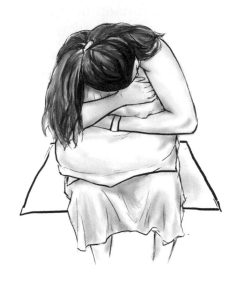

FIG 5.2   Adapted Child Pose

each exhalation, see if you can let go a little more deeply into the holding.

DECONSTRUCTING TRIGGERS: PSYCHOEDUCATIONAL EXERCISE

Objective: *This skill building exercise slows down triggered moments to deconstruct them. Doing so, the client learns what internal pattern from the past is activating the present moment. For this the client needs a pen and paper to help slow the moment, writing specific thoughts, feelings and sensations as a grounding tool.*

Overview: This process has you think of a recent time when you were overwhelmed or shut down and life felt too much or, felt like it was too big for you. Try not to choose something that's so big that you're scared by it. But rather look for something that's about a 5 or 6 on a scale of zero to 10. You want to have something that's big enough but not so big that you can't be curious and interested in it. Then we're going to find ways to untangle all that happened. There are two ways to do this. Neither is "right" or better. Some people find it easier to start from the moment they noticed being triggered, some people find it easier to walk step-by-step toward the trigger. You can either start before you got triggered, meaning you can start when you were calm and easy, walking your way forward into the triggered moment. The other way to do it is you can start when it was way too huge and walk your way back. Either way you do it is fine. There's no right way to do it.

Instructions: For this one, start before the trigger happened. Imagine creating an animated storyboard or graphic novel.

- *What exactly was happening?* Where were you? What were you thinking? What were you feeling? What were the impulses?
- *And then what happened next?* Sometimes I describe this as slicing the baloney really thin. You know when you're at the deli counter and the person asks you "How thick do you want your deli meat?" You get to tell them thick as a steak or paper thin. For this we're going for the really thin. As transparent as you can. You're going to slice each moment so thin that in each moment you can see what you were thinking. What were you feeling? And what was going on in your body? What were the impulses that were getting stirred?
- *Go slow and notice each little piece one moment at a time.* What happened in the next frame? What were the thoughts? Feelings? Sensations?
- *What happened in the next frame?* What were the thoughts? Feelings? Sensations?
- *What happened in the next frame?* What were the thoughts? Feelings? Sensations?
- Remember you can do that from going from when you were calm to when you were triggered or when you were triggered and then walk your way back. This is about exploring what happens at every moment of the process.

One key to help in deconstructing the triggers is you're going to notice that there are some things that feel familiar. It feels "right" and comfortable. You might also have memories or associations that arise, often spontaneously. There might be something that clicks into place which is how some people describe it. That doesn't have to be the case for everything but usually there's some little piece that makes sense of why you're responding the way you are. It's always a good idea to write down or jot down the association and then you can see what's there.

I suggest writing these moment-to-moment experiences down because sometimes we lose track or our mind speeds up and we're trying to process it too quickly. As you're writing, frame what the context was.

- *What was happening outside?* Write a few words about it. What was the thought? What was the feeling? What was the body sensation? What was the next moment?
- *Then, literally like you're going frame by frame.* What was the next context? And the thoughts, feelings, sensations?
- *What was the thought?* What was the feeling? What was the body sensation?
- Walk your way through the trigger this way, breaking it down.

DECONSTRUCTING TRIGGERS

1. *Create safety for yourself.* First things first. If you are in a triggering environment and feel out of control, you might need to leave the situation before you do anything. That might mean going to a bathroom, to a separate office if you're at work, or going for a walk.

   Sometimes we need a little space in order to decompress. Men, in general, need more time than women to lower their physiological arousal. If you can, take the time you need. That might mean telling the person you are with that you will be right back, or back in 10 to 20 minutes.

   If it is a highly unsafe situation you don't have to be graceful, thoughtful, or even considerate in leaving. What's most important in that moment is for you to feel safe. As you practice these skills you will be able to stay in the situation and keep working on yourself without anyone noticing.

   If you're in a situation where you have to be present (or appear to be present) and are still struggling with the triggering material, take a moment for some self-talk. It is sometimes helpful to tell these activated parts that you really want to hear what happened and why they got so triggered, but that you can't be present to them in the way you want to right now. At those times, it's good to let your parts know that you will spend time with them. Let them know when—and keep that promise!

   If you can stay in the situation without increasing the stress to intolerable levels, then explore what else you might need to increase the sense of safety. Do you need to call someone? Talk to a trusted person who is nearby? Take out a piece of paper and write? Talk to yourself? Touch something soft? Or something solid? Grab a special stone you carry?

2. *Explore what happened.* When you are feeling somewhat stable, maybe in

another room or quiet space, you might want to explore what happened. (For some, this means waiting until you are at your therapist's office.) Once you begin to notice where the past is intruding, you'll have a greater chance of deconstructing it.

3. *Deconstructing the triggers:* Take stock of every little thing that happened. Sometimes it's the little things that create the trigger, things we might overlook. We're looking for things in the present which look/feel/smell/sound like something in the past.

   Walk yourself back through time starting from the "before" point. Where were you before you got triggered? What were you thinking, feeling, and what was going on in your body? Go slow and notice.

   Then take the next slice of time. Have you ever seen a storyboard of an animation or a movie? They go frame by frame. That's what we're going to do here. Explore what happened after that first frame. Walk your way through time until the "big bang." What happened? What thoughts/ feelings/ sensations were going on? Is there anything familiar about those T/F/S? A key to deconstructing the triggers is to notice what was familiar about the experience, what pulls you to the past, both internally and externally.

At some point, a memory or association will arise, often spontaneously. For some, having that "click into place" allows them to relax. That doesn't have to be the case for everyone, all the time. Whatever happens, though, it's a good idea to write down the association. Many people keep a notebook with them. Jot down the facts of the situation. And then notice the feelings you had without going into them. Note them on paper (like you did in the bare attention exercise) and bring them up with your therapist to process.

MEDITATION: WIDENING ATTENTION AND GROUNDING ENERGY

Objective: *Narrowing field of consciousness can move client into traumatic schemas. This practice teaches gentle opening of the field of consciousness to receive in here-and-now data points, keeping client more regulated in present moment.*

Instructions:

Instead of moving toward the emotion, in this meditation we relax our attention away from the feeling state.

It's not like the feeling is gone. You know it's there and at the same time you give yourself some distance. It's like you're standing on the shore and a friend is out in a boat out in the ocean. You can see your friend in the boat and you wave from the shore. This meditation gives you space from any intensity.

Start by noticing where the feeling is located in your body. Bring your attention to it without being drawn into it. What will aid you in having some space is to consciously split your awareness. Keeping part of your awareness attending the emotional state while allowing the rest of your attention to expand into sounds around you.

You welcome the feelings while opening your ears. Not in a hypervigilant way but soft. Holding both the internal state and the sounds you hear outside of you.

You might hear birds chirping in the early morning, or a computer humming, or the sounds of the garbage men on the street, or neighbors, or the wind blowing. Let the sounds fill your awareness even as you keep an attentional finger on the pulse of the emotion.

As you do, allow your energy to expand to include this larger field of focus.

Holding both, external sounds keeping you present. Allow the birds, or other sounds, to keep your mind focused and notice the effect this has on your body and your anxiety or depression in particular.

FINDING SUPPORT AND GROUNDING INTO THE BACK

Objective: *Rooted in our core, we have flexibility to move. This supported Tree Pose helps the client feel connected to their back, feeling supported while grounding and relaxing into balancing.*

Instructions: Starting first in a seated position, then move to standing (if you like) with your back against a flat surface. (This can also be done holding onto a chair in front of the client).

Seated Center. Starting in a seated position, move your spine gently. How much contact can you get with your spine? What happens as you reach through the top of your spine? Pressing up. How does that happen? What muscles move to make that happen? What effect does that have on your shoulders, your back, the shoulder blades?

Press down through the bottom of your spine. At the same time you press down press up into your crown.

Assisted Tree Posture. If you feel comfortable move into a standing position. Feel free to stand next to a wall or with your back lightly touching a wall or with a chair nearby. Begin by feeling your back against the wall, touching the wall with various parts of your back to get comfortable with being there. Then feel into the crown and down into the feet.

Just as you did with the seated center posture, reach up through the crown of your head. Notice that as you press through the crown how your chin will slightly drop opening up the back of your neck.

Now at the same time, press down through the bottom of your spine. You'll feel an elongation of your entire spine. What happens to the middle of your back, between your shoulder blades as you do this?

Many people feel some slight adjustment as they do this. There might even be some tension or some pain. Don't try to push beyond what you are comfortable with but take note of the discomfort.

What we're looking for is how you create support and hold balance. Can you feel your feet at the same time you feel up through your crown? Gently move your back, finding your spine.

Being aware of the sensation, allow yourself to ride the sensations, letting them rise, crest, and fall, over and over again.

Bring your attention to the bottoms of your feet. Move them around and find the edges of your feet. How do you feel most comfortable standing? Where do you feel the most balance? Is it on the balls of your feet or the heels? Can you feel the whole of your foot/feet as you stand?

Gently move your balance to your right foot, spreading the toes of your right foot and solidly placing your body on your right foot while your left foot becomes lighter and lighter.

When you are ready lift the left foot lightly keeping your right foot on the ground. Sort of wiggling around and see, feel your right foot. And what is it like to let go of the left foot and be solid on your right, balancing?

Notice all the little tiny movements that take place to keep you balanced on one foot. Remember there's no way to do this right. This is about exploring support and balance. If you can keep focusing your mind on those little tiny micro movements.

And if you want, then bring your left foot up either to your calf or to the inside of your knee. Keep focusing, pressing down through the right foot and up through the crown of your head, so you can keep some balance there. You'll notice how important it is to have these little micro movements to keep you balanced. It also keeps your mind focused.

Let your left foot back down and let relax and feel what it's like to have that release.

Then we're going to rotate over to the other side.

When you have balance and feel grounded bring your hands together in prayer position. Offer yourself a blessing or set an intention for the rest of the day.

Here again, letting yourself notice sensations, how they rise, crest and fall. Hold the posture as much and as long as you can. Breathing along as you surf the waves of sensations, becoming more and more familiar with how sensations move through your body.

And then letting everything go.

Whenever you feel ready try this on the other side, at your own pace and in your own way.

Rotating your balance, feeling your left toes spreading beneath you. Feel the balls of your feet and then the heels of your feet. Rolling easily around on the whole left foot. And press down and up at the same time. Feeling the connection to the earth, down through the floor, even deeper than that, into the earth itself. At the same time pressing up through the crown of your head and lengthening your spine.

When you're ready, begin to let go of your right foot, taking your time to find your balance as you slowly lift off onto the left foot.

Now focus your mind on all those little tiny movements that come.

Finding ways to balance. Noticing while you're doing this that one side might be easier to balance on than the other.

And then bringing the sole of your right foot onto your calf or the inner left thigh. Not trying to do it *right*. Not trying to get to the right stance, in any way. Just feeling the balance and focusing the mind.

Keep focusing, pressing down through the left foot and up through the crown of your head, so you can keep some balance there. You'll notice how important it is to have these little micro movements to keep you balanced. It also keeps your mind focused.

Then let the right foot go. Releasing both feet, maybe shaking your legs and torso before moving on taking time to feel what it's like to have that release.

CHAPTER 6

Develop Boundaries

Nick was on a rampage in my office, furious at what his brother-in-law had said, disgusted with himself for being such a ★★★★ that he hadn't stood up for himself. Nick's self-hatred was florid today. The last few months we had been working on cultivating a more compassionate force field to hold the toxic self-hatred that could envelope him at a moment's notice.

Today, it was worse than ever. I felt like I was psychically wrestling Nick to get him present in the room instead of enacting the painful moment over and over again. "Nick," my eyes steadfastly pulled him into this moment with me. "We're here. We're here in my office. Jeff is not here with us." Even as Nick's eyes continued to dart around a bit, he took a breath. He practiced what we had gone over time and again, slowing his breathing, holding the breath on either the inhalation or exhalation, finding his spine. Gradually his eyes grabbed hold of mine, then filled with tears.

"I'm here with you, Nick. Right here. I see. Let me feel the heat and pain with you." Nick's body rolls down into a ball. "Nick—stay here with me. We can find our way out of this. It's harder if you collapse into it." Using his established toolbox of body practices, he takes a sip of breath, then another one, and another. Nick sits back up, having practiced this a number of times previously. Calibrating his body Nick lands in this moment. He nods, "Okay... I'm here—thanks."

The best boundary in the world is being in the present with the past and the future in their rightful places. Being in the present is where all the choices are. To solidify him being here, I ask, "How much are you here? On a scale of zero to a hundred, what's your SUP (Subjective Unit of Presence)?" Sixty percent, Nick tells me. Presumably the other 40 percent is still writhing in the pain of that moment with his brother. On another occasion I might have explored with Nick where the other 40 percent was, but today I wait a minute until Nick's eyes focus, then ask Nick to discriminate and establish a self-other boundary, "How much of this pain is yours and how much is Jeff's?" Jeff is a bully, consistently demeaning Nick, and unfortunately also Jeff's wife, which distresses Nick enormously. Nick's energetic permeability makes him susceptible to leaky negative energy. This creates a painful convergence point when Jeff's undigested and disowned self-hatred leaks looking for a scapegoat which Nick has an unconscious pattern of accepting and becoming a receptacle of.

Teasing all this apart is a skill we work on consistently. Nick takes this boundary work seriously. He is determined to establish himself as an individual, separate, unique from others in his world. Becoming aware of the self/other distinction has been the bulk of his therapy with me. As Nick sorts out the question, how much of what he is feeling is his versus how much are feelings/energy coming from others, I see Nick "landing" more in his own skin.

Boundaries are generally defined as physical, regarding touch and proximity, and process boundaries, comprising thoughts, feelings, and beliefs (Katherine, 1994; Ogden, Fisher, 2015). Even as trauma violates physical and sexual boundaries, clients often experience a more complicated boundary, which is the focus of this chapter. For those with insecure attachment styles, the rupture of this Self/Other boundary, left unrepaired, creates enormous turmoil.

This psychic boundary between people acknowledges that we are separate from others, allowing us to stay connected without fusing. Without this boundary, a client can reel in psychic disarray when their attachment needs emerge. The anxiously attached person is always aware of the other person, tracking them, noticing flickers of feelings, intentions, motivations, always assessing and interpreting the other person. On the other hand, the dismissively attached person has closed and tightened their boundaries to avoid being caught up in any psychic invasion of another. Their more rigid boundaries provide some solace, yet also keep them from experiencing interactions that could be nourishing and comforting. Those prone to the disorganized styles tend to ricochet from one pole to the other, or to hold multiple realities at the same time, creating internal confusion—hence the term, disorganized. This loss of self-connection happens outside of consciousness, splitting the client intrapsychically and with others interpersonally. Jeremy Holmes (2001) writes of the horizontal and vertical splits that occur in a person. Horizontal splits, in the parlance of psychoanalytic tradition, keep the unconscious out of the conscious mind. "Vertical" splits are ways in which parts of the self are projected out into the world.

What complicates this further with trauma and attachment wounding is the confused time boundary between this present moment and the past (that which has already happened, but is still psychically active). Despite how effectively compelling the past is, we can only attend to the past from the present (van der Kolk, 2015). Fluidly wrapped in evading, or being invaded by the other's experience, those with attachment wounding "time travel" between past and present, or contort themselves into Picasso-like poses, in order to deal in some way with whatever emotions or dissonance is happening around or in them; dismissing, becoming overly permeable, or rapidly switching between the two, trying to get it "right." A person in this situation lives life looking in the rearview mirror, becoming disoriented and upset when life doesn't look different in the present than in the past. Intrapsychic and interpersonal boundaries are erected to keep out distress, and perhaps more importantly, to keep out the enormous disappointment of not being protected, cherished, respected, seen and known as unique and special with separate needs. Those with complicated histories take on either pole of the attachment boundary spectrum, becoming permeable with very little separation between self and other. Defending against being too permeable a person can become rigid and hyper solid; or rapid-fire vacillating between the permeable/rigid poles with different parts taking on different attachment styles. This doesn't happen for those who grow up in a secure environment. By the age of two, Hobson (2002) explains that a child,

> "comes to appreciate the force of the world-according-to-the-other with a new kind of sharpness and definition. She does not simply react to a person's perspective as shown in the person's bodily actions and expressions. She seems to *understand* what a perspective, or even what a particular individual's perspective, really amounts to." (p.79).

This perspective taking allows the child to understand that others are separate, with motives, intentions, experiences and feelings about the world.

Boundaries Allow Appropriate Gating of Information

Developing intrapsychic and intersubjective boundaries allows the client to reclaim their right to be here, to think what they think, to move the way they do, and be exactly as they are. They can take in whatever sensory information they choose, and keep out what they don't want (Adler, Olincy, Waldo, Harris, & Griffith, et al., 1998). They have appropriate gates between themselves and the world, and with themselves and their nervous systems. Gating irrelevant sensory input protects the nervous system from being overloaded with too much data (Braff, Grillon, & Geyer, 1992). Sensory data can be gated out to reduce or stop irrelevant stimuli, or it can be gated in, allowing shifts with incoming or ongoing stimuli (Boutros, Zouridakis, & Overall, 1991). There appear to be two main stages in processing sensory data: identifying the stimulus and then evaluating it (Freedman, Waldo, Bickford-Weimer, & Nagamoto, 1991). Either way, the person can control and modulate the stimuli to a pace that fits them. Grounded in the present moment, it is easier to consolidate a sense of their own Self, which helps them lead from an inner security instead of looking outside or barricading information that could be helpful. This, in essence, is the Internal Family Systems model.

With attachment wounding, the person's intersubjective needs are to be attuned to and validated (Cortina & Liotti, 2014, 2005; Stern, 1985) as a separate being, without losing connection or skewing the gating of sensory and relational data. The imperative to distinguish self from another fights with the need to survive and belong. When there isn't a secure base, clients become afraid of being rejected, shamed, or humiliated. To manage toxic feelings, they create personas and erect masks, developing strategies and parts (Schwartz, 1994) to shield and survive. This is done in the hope they will be able to garner love, attention, and approval.

This perceptual filter makes it difficult for the person to accurately see what they see, or hear what they hear. "Reading" the other's behavior, motivations, and intentions, normally a natural aspect of intersubjectivity, gets muddied as the person picks up mixed messages. Dissonance ensues, making life confusing. The person has trouble distinguishing between the feelings she is having and whatever feelings are active around her. Her sense of self is either permeable, easily affected by others, or locked down, gating information out. The nonconscious evaluation assumes that whatever is floating around must be their own. Consequently, the person morphs into who she thinks she is supposed to be, "exiling" in IFS language, her true nature. Alone, disconnected, worried about being found out as a fraud, she lives her life behind masks and behind the parts she constructed to keep herself safe.

REPAIRING INTERSUBJECTIVE BOUNDARIES

Attachment treatment orients us to look for reconnection, to repair, to join, and to connect. This is the ground that yoga and attachment share. Yoga urges us to remember who we are beyond the wounds that cloud our perception in order to return to the sacred experience of who we are. Attachment theorists have a similar focus in establishing a route for clients to gain an earned secure attachment style. The attachment theorist Karlen Lyons-Ruth (1999) finds that "collaborative communication" for mother and child builds that steady ground. The four components of the collaborative communication framework are: an inclusiveness of what needs, wants, beliefs, and desires the child is experiencing; a willingness to initiate repair when there's disruption; providing an active "scaffolding" of developing efforts which allows the child to find and take small steps forward; and a willingness to be in the struggle of learning while making mistakes, giving the child a way to stay positively connected even while in conflict. With adults safe intersubjectivity is formed where the people "want to be known and to share what it feels like to be them" (Stern, 2004, p. 97). Intersubjectivity, in this context, is a basic motivational system (Cortina & Liotti, 2005; Stern, 2004) that humans have in which intentions, goals, emotions, and sensations are shared. Gallese (2001) coined the phrase "the manifold of shared intersubjectivity" to include joint intentionality. A mature intersubjectivity includes similarities and differences in how people understand each other (Benjamin, 1992; Agazarian, 1997).

In this way, intersubjectivity develops a "third space" between two people (Jennings, 2013) to communicate psychological states (Trevarthen & Aitken, 1994). We know this in the therapy hour when our clients fear there isn't enough time to share themselves fully, fearing they won't be seen and known in a nuanced, responsive way that repairs what they didn't have growing up. Those with trauma and attachment wounding live with an inner reactivity that comes from feeling unknown and invisible. Pilar Jennings (2013) writes:

"Many adults see themselves in this helpless way when the third space in a relationship collapses—who hasn't, at some point, been involved with someone who seems impervious to our subjectivity? What is harder to see are the ways through which we protect ourselves from a collapsed third space. Rather than suffer the terrible sense of being done to, we may opt to be the one who controls space by dominating interactions within that relationship, opting to make others feel helpless instead of being on the receiving end of their efforts at control. There is no such thing as two people—whether baby and mother, two lovers, or teacher and student—being perfectly in sync with each other's needs and wishes. Real intimacy arises from an ongoing process of connection that at some point is disrupted and then, ideally, repaired. I think of this as an interpersonal crochet stitch: connection, disruption, repair, over and over again, until a fabric is created with enough strength and flexibility to endure the war of any two people attempting to know one another."

From a neuroscience point of view, Gallese (2003) proposes that the sharing of meaningful intersubjective space comes through embodied simulation formed by the presence of a "shared, multi-modal, we-centric, blended space" (p. 519). Different from empathy (Stern, 1985), the resonance of the intersubjective space allows us to decode the meaning of others without going through a complex internal computation. We know the shorthand we use to respond to others, whether reactive or attentive. We seldom have the time to thoughtfully explore the nuances of felt experience, translating the sensations, feelings, and thoughts into a coherent whole. Most of the time we respond in a "reflex-like" way (Gallese, 2003, p. 520), translating sensory data into meta-representations in an automatic fashion, which Gallese (2003) calls a "disembodied perspective." In his words:

"There can be no other persons out there independent of us. When we try to understand the behavior of others, our brain is not representing an *objective external personal reality*. Our brain *models the behavior of others, much the same as it models our own behavior*. The results of this modeling process enable us to understand and predict what the behavior of others is.

I propose that simulation, that is, how we model reality, is the only epistemic strategy available to organisms such as ourselves deriving their knowledge of the world by means of interactions with the world. What we call the representation of reality is not a copy of what is objectively given, but an interactive model of what cannot be known in itself. Of course, this also holds for the social interpersonal reality in which we spend all our lives" (p. 521).

We know our clients come to therapy wanting to be known. They want help dealing with the despair of their needs not getting met. Stuck in the patterns formed early in life (Bretherton & Munholland, 1999), our clients cross the vulnerable boundary of coming to see us for help. They want to be understood (Fonagy, 2001), but not just cognitively. Our clients with attachment wounding are at a loss in dealing with the implicitly embedded experiences forming unmet needs and wishes concretized in painful connections and patterns. Making the implicit explicit (Fosha, 2011, 2000) organizes disorganized life experiences. John Bowlby (1984), during his videotaped lecture *Attachment, Separation, Loss* in London, told the audience that ". . . as long as we hide our history from ourselves we are likely to see our present and future in terms of our past." The more clearly you focus on the ways you were treated in the past, Bowlby wrote, "the less likely you are to imagine it in the present." Facing the painful truth is key to healing. Bowlby bluntly tells us, "No one wants to think the mother didn't want them. That's painful. Yet if it's true, it's true. They're better off recognizing that it did happen in the past so it doesn't have to keep happening in the future."

When something painful happens to a child, and they don't have the support to integrate that experience, it becomes encapsulated. A time boundary is erected (Fay, 1997), psychically concretized to keep the past from invading the present moment. Although this radically important strategy keeps the child safe at the time it happens, it later leaks into the present through painful enactments. The Parallel Lives Model described in Chapter 4 (Fay, 1997), helps clients understand this warping of time and space in which they automatically filter the present with the past, losing connection to the reality of the moment, losing connection to who they are located in this time and space, and being left disconnected from others. Confused and disoriented, disconnected from the intersubjective contact that grounds them, people swirl in unconscious projections of the past while living as if that projected past is real in this moment (van der Kolk, 2015). In order to help it make more sense, we orient clients to the felt "reality" of the moment to understand the psychological puzzle pieces swirling in the present moment.

Manfred came to see me on the suggestion of his therapist friend. He had been working with a well-meaning therapist who wasn't trained in trauma and dissociation. Their connection, however, was compelling. The therapist wanted to help, and the client wanted a mother who finally cared. His therapist treated him as a wounded child. Relieved to have his subjective experience seen, Manfred obliged—falling down the dissociative fault line into primitive states of his undigested history. Unfortunately, the therapy he was in made his emotional world worse; he felt he was losing his "grip on reality." In order to cope, Manfred took a long-term disability when he was no longer functioning well in his daily life. As a binge eater, Manfred used food to soften the blow of his aloneness. His friend, observing his decompensation, guided Manfred to come for a consultation, take a break from that therapy and enter into therapy based on the sound principles of trauma and dissociation treatment.

What was obvious from the beginning was how Manfred's felt experience of aloneness didn't square with his external reality. In his everyday life, Manfred is a thoughtful, gracious, considerate, enjoyable person, leading spiritual retreats with large crowds of attendees. He described, however, a childhood where nobody cared about his emotional and psychological world. The few times he couldn't contain his emotions as a child, his mother and father would laugh at him and call him a crybaby. He has no memories of being comforted or having anyone say kind things to him. After the initial few appointments where Manfred "reported" his life, he fell into this cocoon of body symptoms. He stopped being able to speak, sitting through sessions trembling, unable to describe what was happening. For almost a year he would come and I would sit with him, interpreting his gestures, his intersubjective world, attuning to him to translate his world into words. To help him learn about himself I sensed and felt whatever feeling I was having, feeling and feeding it back to him—wondering if the feeling I was having was similar to what he was feeling. I'd ask him, "Can you give me a slight shake or nod of the head if I'm anywhere close to what's happening inside you?" In time words came, plunging him into the well of grief he had at having to end his previous therapy even as he knew it wasn't particularly effective and perhaps even harmful. That opened up the utter and complete loneliness of his childhood, where he had to sequester himself inside his bones in order not to leak his neediness.

Repairing and healing requires the presence of another, someone who cares, who is interested, who is willing to listen deeply and help us translate these *samskaras* into digestible form. The intersubjective matrix allows clients, including Manfred in our subsequent work together, to consciously explore where physical, psychological, and emotional edges are, or where their sense of self begins and ends. To do this, we first need to help our clients know where appropriate physical boundaries (proximity of sitting, agreements about touch or no touch), context boundaries (we're in the office, the appointment starts and ends at this time, these are the fees and structure we're agreeing to), sexual boundaries, and emotional boundaries. The client then knows what they can do with comfort in the therapy relationship. Without knowing the various levels and forms of boundaries, most clients don't feel held in the structure or have the explicit "right" to rail against that structure. Lyons-Ruth's "collaborative communication" of receptive exploration, repair, scaffolding, and safely held conflict informs the therapeutic boundary.

Ascribing intention is one of the main points of shared space. We "read" through mirror and motor neurons, what Gallese calls "embodied simulation" (2009), "getting" what is happening in others through our own felt sense. Trauma survivors need to learn the skill of discriminating the information they receive in this intersubjective matrix of embodied simulation.

Colleen's experience might offer an example. She often found herself activated in painful stories, confused and disoriented by those stories. In therapy we explored whether she was responding to the here and now or to the past traumatic scheme. We began to track what happened when she was triggered when her husband, Marc, turned away from her. The rage responses in Colleen were making the relationship difficult for both of them. Knowing her triggers and her tendency when anxious to leak her anxiety on him (wanting him to do something without knowing what she herself needs), Colleen has learned to slow down, pause, and practice self-compassion, saying to herself, "I'm here. I'm right here with myself. I need attention. I need help." Doing this, Colleen is interrupting her normal pattern sequence. As she says, "For me, it's about what do I think his intention is. So then I fill in the blanks, like what we did in separating facts and feelings. I think I know what's going on, think I know what Marc's intention is. So I'm telling myself the story to be ready for his anger or that he's going to want to control me or that I'll end up powerless, or whatever. I'm preparing for that to happen. That's what creates a problem for me. It's the story I tell myself as I anticipate the intention, usually negative, of whoever the other person is." Colleen's body is reenacting old patterns, and a past history of experiencing violence, even as Marc has never been violent with her. Now when Marc gets a certain look on his face, which Colleen interprets as anger, she practices slowing down, separating Marc from her past perpetrators. In the past, people would have been violent. In this moment, Marc is not and has not been violent—he just has that look on his face. Over and over, Colleen repeats those facts until her mind clears, separating this moment from past moments, releasing the triggered response in her body, acknowledging the boundary that's appropriate for the here and now.

Appropriate, intersubjective boundaries give clients essential ways to explore themselves in some safety, knowing the therapist is willing to initiate repair, break down relational skills into bite-size pieces, all the while willing to struggle with them. Learning to trust the collaborative intersubjective matrix, clients develop separation while connected, trusting themselves or the other won't lose themselves in the process. This freedom to psychologically explore without overexposing themselves to potential shame, embarrassment, or humiliation builds structure and an internal safe haven to which to return. Over time, people shift from expecting painful responses to being open to finding more nourishing responses.

WHERE DO YOU BEGIN AND END? THE BENEFIT OF INTRAPSYCHIC BOUNDARIES

Asking a client, "Where do you begin and end? Where do I begin and end?" is one of the most difficult yet important inquiries. Boundaries function to provide a way to filter information, provide containment, and to protect; yet this function is most often warped in clients. Boundaries give the client the capacity to land inside their own skin, help them know what feelings and thoughts they are having, and discern what emotional and psychic energy is theirs versus what they are picking up from others. They also facilitate tolerating differences inside and outside themselves with appropriate filters on what needs protection and what doesn't. Without boundaries, clients find it difficult to know they are distinct from others, not knowing who they are, what they want, what they value, or how to make a decision, and allowing others to decide for them or influence what they think or feel; conversely they erect impermeably solid boundaries, keeping themselves distinct from others. Appropriate psychological boundaries indicate the edges or limits that define and separate, letting the client know, "This is me. I am not you." In a session, we can raise the exploration with a client, asking them, "Where do you begin and end? Where do I end?" "Do we meet between us?" "How and where is the connection between us?" "How do you know what goes on inside you?" What gives you this information?" This is especially important when someone is triggered or lost in confusion. Distinguishing what gates are open internally, between various parts and self, and what gates are open interpersonally, creates a measure of clarity, ultimately building a sense of self.

These questions establish the here and now intersubjective reality, grounding the client in the present moment. When we ask a client to establish their Subjective Unit of Presence (SUP) on a scale of 0 to 100 or simply asking "How do you know you are here?," we're asking the client to turn inward, discovering how they know they are physically present in this moment. It also invites them to explore their psychological self in the present moment. "How do you know you're connected to me? How do you know you're separate from me?" "What is similar between you and me? What's different?"

The "skin boundary" is one of the essential definitions of the client's physical self; yet it is something to which most clients aren't present. Many clients have learned to retract inside themselves, pulling their sense of self into their bones or viscera as a way of becoming energetically or psychically safe. When a client is rattled we can ask them to become aware of their skin first with mental contact, imagining their skin boundary. Orienting to their physical boundary establishes a psychological reality, an intrasubjective boundary. They are here, in this body, held in this skin. If the client feels comfortable it is then possible to have the client experiment with making contact with their skin. Do they have a felt experience of their skin holding them, demarcating the boundary between inside and outside? Can they feel their own hands on their arms, on their skin? "What's it like to feel yourself within your skin?" I often suggest to clients to fill up within their skin, just like a balloon filling up, then inquiring with them what that is like. When an energy or emotion feels too much, it can be helpful to invite the client to let the rattled energy expand outward to meet their skin, giving it more room and bringing more ease to the system.

In the intersubjective world in which therapy takes place we are co-creating with the client a new possibility, one in which the client can more safely abide, and over time, internalize themselves and their experience with you. Those with insecure status have Internal Working Models (IWM) invariably complementary to the IWM of those with whom they were raised (Brown, Elliott, et al., 2016; Cortina & Liotti, 2005). Despite that, developing an earned secure attachment is possible (Brown, Elliott, et al., 2016; Cassidy & Shaver, 1999; Iyengar, Kim, Martinez, et al., 2014; Saunders, Jacobvitz, et al, 2011). Even though the client will deny having had a "real-life" experience of a secure attachment, we can help them reorganize (Iyengar, Kim, Martinez, et al., 2014; Toth, Rogosch, & Manly, 2006) their attachment representations. Underneath our clients' rejecting connection, or despairing not having the relational connection they wanted, they continue to long for that very relationship even as they doubt it's possible to have. What we see in our offices is the Internal Working Model projected into the current moment. Nick, described at the beginning of the chapter, and Marsha, described later, are certainly two of many examples.

Our clients come into our offices with every variation and strategy for psychological survival, reliving easily triggered trauma schemas that they act out or implode with on a consistent basis. Those with avoidant or resistant histories are drawn to dominance and control (Cortina & Liotti, 2005). Working with establishing safe physical, sexual, and emotional boundaries is vital. Yet, there still remains another level, reestablishing a safer, intersubjective matrix which is a primary theme of this chapter.

Without a secure internal base, the gating of sensory data can inadvertently allow nonconscious absorption of other's intentions, feelings, and thoughts, mingling with their own. An intersubjective therapeutic stance includes listening to both the content the client is sharing as well as feeling into the nonconscious felt expressions. Holding both, we parse out and attune to the nascent, inchoate longing of needing us, the therapist, to affirm, validate, and digest their inner experience with them, help them sort out the sensory data, and organize and normalize experience before they are able to more comfortably take the next step. As we walk with them gently, kindly holding for and with them the possibility of secure connection, our clients find a steady, kind, and consistent connection they can internalize.

INTRAPSYCHIC CONTACT BOUNDARIES

Yet, beyond the physical, sexual, and emotional boundaries that are frayed in our clients, it is the intrapsychic contact boundaries that are most often confused for our clients: the horizontal boundaries between the client and anyone else, and the vertical boundaries that exist internally between various parts of the client (Holmes, 2001; Schwartz, 1994). Somatically, I often remind clients that there is turbulence in crossing from outside to inside or even between parts of oneself. Yvonne Agazarian, in Systems Centered Therapy (1997), attends to the boundary crossing in groups by exploring the similarities and differences. What can you connect to and where can you find similarity? Where is there separation and distance? Agazarian would consistently remind us in her training groups to look for the similarity in apparent differences and the differences in apparent similarities.

Emotional contagion can complicate intrapsychic contact boundaries. Relying on nonverbal communication, a listener can "pick up" an emotion or be triggered by another's emotion instantaneously (Hatfield, Cacioppo, & Rapson, 1993). This kind of implicit emotional contagion happens automatically and unconsciously; it's a precursor to empathy. Tania Singer, a researcher in social neuroscience at the Max Planck Institute for Human Cognitive and Brain Sciences in Leipzig, Germany, illustrates emotional contagion with infants (Singer & Klimecki, 2014). In a hospital setting, when one baby starts to cry, all the babies nearby start crying. This kind of "contagion" happens long before there is a self-other distinction. We also see it with yawning or laughing. We are intersubjective beings, and "catch" what others are experiencing through mirror and motor neurons, most of this unconsciously.

Depending on the attachment style, some people are prone to separation and distance, others toward merging. It's in bringing these unconscious movements and patterns of psychic data into awareness that they can be shifted. On September 11, 2001, I was sitting in my office with a client who had been made CEO of the company she had long been involved in. She was feeling guilty that she was feeling proud and self-satisfied while so many were suffering. Upset with herself for wanting to hold onto feeling so good when the whole country was in shock, we made positive use of the self-other distinction: she felt good for her good luck *and* she felt horror and distress for others impacted.

Becoming aware of others and their response is part of "perspective taking" from the mentalization point of view (Allen & Fonagy, 2008; Liotti & Gilbert, 2011). Instead of merging with another, mentalizing begins the process of knowing where one begins and ends, how one person is separate from another, while noticing what happens inside when others have response/reactions to them. As Jill described in a group, "It's amazing to see how there was a lot of my mind and body being separate, and trying to escape where I was, kind of energetically, while I was still in the situation. Now I can practice staying there even when someone else is different or scaring me. I'm starting to see how I leave the situation so that I can be myself but what I really want is to stay here, with others, connected without losing myself." Her body was there, held in the physical boundaries of environment and external realities, but her heart, body, and mind were trying to escape the intersubjective connection.

Although Bowlby didn't relate to the idea of a "map" to describe the inner attachments realms (Bretherton & Munholland, 1999), the concept of a map helps our clients have concrete, step-by-step navigational tools. Having a set of psychological maps to represent the internal world helps when traversing the internal terrain where the past and present moment are often merged. The Becoming Safely Embodied™ skills (Fay, 2007) provide a concrete, simple, accessible stepping stone to organize a disorganized body/mind. With a sense of a separate self, the client has perspective to access self-compassion, bringing mindful self-compassion into daily practice.

EMBODIED CYCLE OF NEEDS

Ideally, when securely attached, we interact in the "intersubjective matrix" (Stern, 2004), which has a positive interpenetration of minds that, as Stern writes, "permits us to say, I know that you know that I know' or 'I feel that you feel that I feel'" (p. 75). Being in this intersubjective creation, we feel known, seen, connected, and understood in a way that surpasses any logical frame. Clinically we can describe this as a secure base. The felt experience is one of safety, comfort, ease, and letting go. This is the state of being that our clients ultimately come into our offices to return to, saying they haven't had it and they doubt very much that they can have it. It's the longing for that state despite the despair that has them come to see us. This is the benefit of attachment theory and repair, making it possible to repair and reorganize one's attachment status. From an embodied, yogic psychology perspective, secure attachment happens in reminding the client that what they long for is actually a native, natural longing for secure connection that got warped through difficult life situations. What endured, sheltered behind protective intrapsychic boundaries, was their heart continuing to long for this connection whether they had actually had it or not.

A securely attached child, when distressed, reaches for soothing and comfort and then returns to play (Bowlby, 1969, 1988; Holmes, 2001). Somatic therapies (Ogden, Minton, & Pain, 2006; Miller, 2015, 2010; Aposhyan, 2007, 2004; Gendlin, 1978) and yoga (Stapleton, 2004; Miller, 2010) invite us into the bell curve of the introceptive world where something is initiated, rises, crests, and falls. When we are thirsty, we reach for water and are replenished. This cycle of life occurs over and over throughout the day, often in the background of our physiology and mind. In the same way, attachments are intrinsic to humans (Holmes, 2001; Stern, 1985, 2004), not something present only in babies. Consistently turning toward an internal safe base is a need that occurs throughout life (Bowlby, 1988; Holmes, 2009, 2001). Any need produces a longing. We reach for that longing, grabbing it, pulling it in, hopefully letting it replenish. This Embodied Need Cycle is almost always broken in our clients with attachment and trauma wounding. Said simplistically, clients with insecure attachment status reached for what they wanted and needed, but that need didn't get met. That natural cycle of a need/want rising, cresting, and falling was disrupted. When this happens chronically, our clients enter shame cycles, believing they are the problem, and that something is wrong with them.

YOGIC MODEL OF PHYSICAL AND ENERGY BODY

The yogic model of energy bodies, discussed earlier in Chapter 3, can be helpful for clients to distinguish the many layers of boundaries they are subject to and working with at any one time. These energy sheaths, known in Sanskrit as *koshas,* form layers of an interacting participatory system in which one sheath informs every other; simultaneously processing sensory/psychic data. The food or drink we take into our physical bodies (*annamaya*) affects our energy levels (*pranamaya*) which in turn interacts with thoughts and feelings (*manomaya*) all of which are shaped by perceptions that filter experience. Cultivating (*vijnanamaya*) opens wisdom, witnessing what's occurring without being entangled, becoming acutely aware of what we are doing and thinking. The bliss body (*anandamaya*) is always beaconing from beyond the filters that obscure experience, unfolding the vast spaciousness of being. No longer living in a dualistic experience there is only bliss (Klein, 1990; Kṛpālvānanda, Svāmī, 1977; Feuerstein, 2013; Miller, 2010; Stapleton, 2004; Weintraub, 2003, 2012).

When Energy Boundaries Are Out of Balance	
Koshas	**When the *koshas* are out of balance**
Annamaya physical	Physically there but psychologically absent
Pranamaya life force, vital energy, chi	Rattled, irritated, unable to soothe, comfort
Manomaya mental, emotional, beliefs	Ruminating, obsessive thinking, emotionally hyperaroused or shut down, negative self-talk, destructive beliefs
Vijnanamaya Perception, witness, wisdom	Prematurely transcend suffering and the pain of being human; entering power roles of one up or one down; dismissive of importance of connection; dismissive of relational needs and vulnerabilities
Anandamaya bliss body	Unable to feel good, receive pleasure, contribute and be contributed to

For most of our clients, however, these energetic bodies are out of balance. Marsha began to notice her various body layers as we explored what her girlfriend, Sara, called her dissociation. Although tentatively agreeing with her girlfriend that there was "something wrong with her" (which was part of Marsha's Internal Working Model), that her "dissociating" interfered with their relationship, Marsha didn't feel "right" about being told that she was "not present." Exploring the feeling of 'not being present' Marsha noticed a protest inside herself that she felt in her body but wasn't able to verbalize to her partner. In therapy we slowed down her process, studying what thoughts, feelings, and sensations were going on. Doing so, Marsha noticed she had a vertical boundary between herself and Sara keeping her protest unverbalized but present nonetheless. As "homework" I asked Marsha to be aware of her Subjective Unit of Presence (SUP), noticing in what circumstances she felt present, when not, when she felt safe, when not safe. A careful log allowed Marsha to see that when she felt criticized or judged she froze up and cut herself off from her body (*annamaya*). Over time as we sat with that frozen shut off place in therapy, she brought attention and life force into those areas (*pranamaya*), realizing that she had thoughts and feelings of protest and upset (*manomaya*).

Knowing this Marsha realized *(vijnanamaya)* that while she was present to herself she had erected an interpersonal boundary between her protest and expression, externally shutting off expression, terrified of Sara's criticism. Putting these pieces into place gave Marsha a measure of ease and a sense of freedom in the present moment. As we studied the relief, she described a pleasurable sense of spaciousness, relief, and ease *(anandamaya)*.

Marsha's childhood Internal Working Model (Bowlby, 1969) had "programmed" her to accept criticism and judgment from emotionally abusive parents. What was being labeled as dissociation was a vertical boundary Marsha was erecting inside herself to keep herself safe from outside criticism. This intra-psychic boundary shielded Marsha from knowing what she was experiencing. As this pattern became clear, Marsha realized she had, in IFS language, "exiled" this part to keep it safe. It served her well as a child but was now keeping her trapped in a relationship that wasn't nourishing. The more Marsha became aware of her pattern the more she was able to make her implicit protest explicit, dealing with her fears that verbalizing the protest would create a relational rupture. More connected to herself, Marsha found it increasingly difficult to no longer address these issues with her girlfriend. The vertical boundary eased, her horizontal boundary cracked open with Sara, revealing relationship dynamics about conflict which they are still sorting out.

Without knowing where they are distinct from others, and what makes them unique and special, clients can allow others to push their boundaries, lean into them, or break a boundary out of fear of confrontation or fear of the consequences of putting their own needs first. Instead of dealing with the issue, clients with a dismissive orientation often bottle up resentment, anger, or frustration at not being able to act in a self-protective, self-enhancing way. Those clients with an anxious/preoccupied orientation might have a hard time tolerating the turbulence that comes from being different. The inquiry at these times might be, "Where do you go inside your body when you're with this person? How do you hold onto yourself? What are the thoughts, feelings, and body sensations?" "How do you tend to lose yourself? How exactly do you crumble? Is there a place in your body or psyche that seems to be more porous or defended?" Setting up experiments (Ogden, Pain, & Minton, 2006) are used to explore how this happens in the body.

Further questions and somatic explorations to engage the client in their body awareness are attachment questions of proximity: "Where is close enough? Or how far away do you need to be from this person/place? When someone gets too close without your permission what happens in your body? What does your body want to do? How do you respond?" I often initiate a conversation about boundaries by asking what it's like to have the sense of a physical boundary, with walls and doors marking the physical boundary. How does the client experience being with those physical boundaries? What thoughts, feelings, and body sensations are there? Is it new for them to be aware of that physical boundary? Many clients will want to sit where they can see the door so they can be aware if the door were to open. Another woman in a group described, "Having the door closed completes the container we're establishing of being here together, for a common purpose. It makes me feel safer, also I'm less distracted. I noticed when the door was open a bit earlier and someone was outside I found my attention was drawn to them." Certainly in groups, when it's time for a meditation, I would let the group know that I'll be watching the door so that they don't have to, and if someone walks in late I'll gently mention to the group, ". . . and welcome so-and-so as he/she settles into his/her seat."

PUTTING BOUNDARIES INTO PRACTICE

To make this concrete, explore what happens on a plane or in a subway when sitting next to someone you don't know. The physical proximity is one issue to explore but there are the other less well explored and discriminated intrapsychic contact boundaries between self and other or internally between various parts and self. What's similar? What's different? How do you respond? The situation might dictate a certain way of being but what happens inside your body and mind? What thoughts are there about you, about them, about the situation? What feelings do you have? What sensations? Do you draw into your body more? Expand energetically? Do you make sure you have your elbow on the arm rest? All these are simple ways we respond whether on the plane, in public transportation, or in meetings.

It can be helpful to ask a client if they feel safe or not in those situations. If not, how do they form a boundary? Is it energetic? Physical? Do they bury their head in a book? Put on headphones? In your office you can ask them to build a boundary between you through pillows, indicating with their hands, or by expanding their energy out to push against you. The Somerville, Massachusetts therapist and qi gong teacher, Michael Robbins teaches a Luminous Egg practice which I adapt to use with clients to establish this sense of energetic boundary. In a group I led on boundaries, one of the members who had a trauma history with a lot of physical violence became aware of how she held herself in the group: she told us that "My egg is pretty tightly around me." With her permission we explored what happened if she allowed her Egg to stretch open, become more solid. I invited her to get a felt sense of being in her Egg, feeling where she energetically ends in the world, pushing out against me, pushing me away energetically, noticing what happened when she didn't need to retract into her bones, sucked inside in order to have space.

Keeping themselves physically, psychologically and energetically safe is paramount for our clients. Without grounding in a separate sense of self, clients can vacillate between creating space with impervious energetic boundaries that end up isolating them or merging with others in an attempt to not feel alone, inadvertently opening themselves to being flooded with energy. Afraid of being shaken by emotional and physiological tsunamis people actively manage life. A great deal of stress occurs when boundaries (and *koshas*) are too permeable, creating internal emotional contagion where the person feels constantly flooded by distressing emotions, memories, and felt experience. To be able to watch and feel the cycle of sensation rise, crest and fall, an internalized boundary is needed between self and experience. To allow empathy to flourish into compassion the client needs to develop equanimity; a self distinct from the experience without dissociation (Fisher, in press; Fay, 2007; Schwartz, 1994). As an internalized boundary is established the client is better able to separate from the feared felt experience. IFS provides a step-by-step model which helps clients organize their psychological world into parts, continuing to point them toward their Self energy. In a similar way, the *koshas* urge us to remember that the bliss of integration and connection is always shining behind the clouds. We access the bliss body by softening the edges of the boundaries instead of solidifying them.

Making these internalized environments concrete helps establish both external and internal self-distinction. In a group, Jill cowered from others, never feeling quite safe. To support her in having a felt experience of safety, I had Jill use pillows to create a physical manifestation of internal boundary. As a group we explored what that was like. Exploring her internal response, she propped herself up against the wall with the pillows in front of her about 6 feet away. I asked her to energetically fill up the space behind the pillows. She was confused by the question, uncertain what I meant. Slowing down the inquiry I suggested she fill up her body, getting a felt sense of her skin, filling up her body like a balloon with her energy. Once she was able to have that felt sense she then "filled" up the space outside her body within the physical pillow boundary. Getting a felt sense of herself located in that space Jill was able to separate from the cowering energy placing it outside the door. Having Jill engage with the space in this experiential way allowed her to land in the here and now more solidly. Other clients often need to draw a representation or write a phrase ("memory") on a piece of paper to make it concrete before locating it outside of their physical skin boundary, somewhere in the room or outside the room, in order to have space.

Another concrete way to do this is to have clients use a string to indicate a boundary around them so they can get a visual sense of space and a felt sense of themselves within that space. This can be especially helpful for clients that have a porous sense of self. As with the pillows, clients can explore what parts can be within the string boundary and what parts they want outside the string. That sets up an inquiry process of what those parts are (inside or outside) and why they want those parts in that proximal space. This explores the IWM of the client as they represent their parts in external ways. I did this in a group I led on boundaries. Vicky took home the red string she used in the group. She literally draped the red string around the entire edges of her bedroom. As she did so Vicky reported a sense of power, claiming the room. "This is my space. I have the say about what happens here." In an email to me after the group she wrote, "It feels like a stupid thing to do but it helps me remember that I can take up space. When I'm in my room seeing the red string protecting me I can feel my muscles open and expand. I know I'm safe here."

Once a client is located in their body they have a sense of their own self; then they can read what happens inside them. Holding onto that in the presence of others is where it becomes more complicated and where the self-other distinction can get warped. Gallese's fascinating inquiry into "the Shared Manifold of Intersubjectivity" (2003) gives us insight into what is mine and what is yours as we share the space together. Experimenting with the space between is necessary to sort out what is happening inside the client and what is happening in the other person in which the space is shared. This also gives us information about the client's attachment style. Someone with a more dismissive style will feel relieved when the therapist orients away from the client while someone with a more anxious style might easily feel rejected. As Colleen said when someone is annoyed at her and turns away, she gets triggered into feeling abandoned. Her work has been to distinguish herself from others and to identify the intention that she is inferring, then being able to check out her mind-reading of others, finding out what their intention/ motivation is and how that fits with what she feels inside.

Clients often use different protector parts as a boundary or shield. Doing this consciously helps them realize the importance of the previously implicit strategy. They learn to honor why the pattern/part/strategy was developed in the first place. Other clients use headphones or sunglasses as external boundaries as they go out into the world. In yoga and meditation, we invite a softening of these boundaries. Jack Engler has eloquently said we have to "have a self in order to let go of a self." When a client is aware of their self-boundary then can explore gating sensory data, knowing when to ease the boundary open, when to shut it, when to have a flexible boundary.

An easy meditation practice for this is to have clients in a safe space become aware of their skin boundary (as I did with Jill in the example above), then expand beyond that, flowing around other people and objects, moving into and through space instead of fighting or pushing or withdrawing from. "Meeting, being with others, noticing the moment when your skin tightens, your muscles constrict. See what happens as you move more fluidly, without changing yourself, or the other person, not closing up or shutting others out? Can you expand to touch the walls on every side? The ceiling? Floor?" As I remind clients, there's room for all of them. They're welcome to be here as fully as they like. From an attachment perspective I'm inviting them to fill up with themselves in the very best way, which promotes self-confidence, pride, and self-worth (Brown, Elliott, et al., 2016). This exploration also allows the client to notice where they hold, restrict, or are too porous in their energy field. Sometimes it's important to have a stronger boundary on one side (the front, back or sides of the body) while opening up more on another side. Clients begin to notice the differences around them, developing ways to distinguish where they have energetic lacunae. With time and practice clients say this practice "returns my energy back to myself, creating relief and even a sense of contentment." "Instead of draining my energy I seem to be able to fill up. Kind of like learning to be aware of my breath, it comes in and out, without effort." This can also be done with sound, allowing sound to fluidly move through them, letting the sound occur inside them as well as outside (see below for more on the practice).

Practices for Boundary Development

MEDITATION: FILLING UP SKIN / CONTACT BOUNDARY

Objective: *The first part of this meditation is to get a felt experience of filling up the body; letting the skin hold your energy. Once there is a certain comfort with that, the inquiry moves beyond the skin boundary, practicing being with a larger space without tightening or shutting down or grabbing at others.*

Instructions: Gently tapping or touching the skin, get a sense of what it is like to be in your body in this moment. (pause) What sensations do you notice as you sense into the edges of the body perhaps lightly moving your hands along safe edges of the body. Can you feel the warmth of your own hands? Dropping any thoughts or stories you have about your body or being touched as you turn your attention to the felt experience in this moment.

Some people find it helpful to bring their attention to the spine noticing the breath flow up and down the spine. (pause) Flowing next to your heart taking a moment to comfort and reassure yourself that all is well, that you are here in this moment, in a safe place. (pause) Continue to let go of any thoughts as you explore expanding from the inside out toward the edges of the skin where your hands are on the edges of your body. (pause) What sensations are there as you make contact from inside you with the edges of you?

Continue to move fluidly, acknowledging any parts that come up, reassuring them, welcoming any feelings, thoughts and sensations. (pause) Welcoming how your body responds, your skin (pause) and your muscles (pause).

Imagine being in the space with a safe other; (pause) what are you aware of? Flowing, staying connected to your spine, your belly, your heart (pause) what is it like to make contact with others? Fluidly moving around others, no needing to change them or alter yourself or shut anything down. (pause) Imagine taking up space (pause). Expanding to touch the walls (pause) and the ceiling and the floor, (pause) filling up space with your light (pause), your presence (pause).

EXPLORING SELF-OTHER DISTINCTION

Objective: *Explore the self/other distinction, developing an internal locus of attention. This inquiry looks at beliefs, thoughts, feelings, decisions, choices, experiences, wants, needs, and sensations within the body as well as noticing intuitions and unconscious patterns by concretizing internal experience in drawing and writing or using pictures from magazines.*

Instructions: *Have paper, magazines, writing or drawing pencils/crayons nearby*

1. On one side of the paper draw, write or use pictures from magazines to represent who you present to the world, maybe different parts of you that show up with different people, in different roles.
2. On the other side, draw, write, or use pictures from magazines, to describe who you are inside, the "you" that may not often be shared with others.
3. After you're done, compare the words and pictures inside the circle with those on the outside of the circle. What do you notice?

EXPLORING ATTACHMENT BOUNDARIES THROUGH THE *KOSHAS*

Objective: *This inquiry invites exploration of the felt experience of each of the koshas through writing and drawing, expanding the client's idea of what it is to be in a body with boundaries that are just right for you.*

Instructions: Using writing or a journal, take time to explore each layer of the body. Some of these can be done alone, some are best practiced with another person. Be creative and inventive as you play with the questions, welcoming what opens up inside you.

Annamaya / Physical: *Notice the physical experience of being here in this room with me. We're here together. Take a look around the room, letting your eyes orient to colors and shapes that you like. Perhaps aware of how your eyes make contact with objects, shapes, and colors, reaching out, making contact, then shifting. Experiment with seeing, then closing your eyes. Opening, looking, then closing your eyes. You're here, right here. (pause) Perhaps touching the floor or seat of your chair, maybe feeling your arms. Using touch to ground and connect you to this present moment. Yeah, here you are. (pause) feel your head, full of hair or with no hair. This is you in time and space. (pause) physically located right here. Your legs(pause) Your feet (pause) This is you—the physical presence of you. As you attend to your physical body, explore what kind of contact would feel just right with your physical skin boundary. (pause) That's right, (pause) letting go of thoughts as you sense what would feel just right. (pause) It could be a soft, gentle touch. It can be a more solid rub. Or perhaps tapping [pause.] What helps you feel comfortable and safe with the edges of you?*

Pranamaya / Breath - Energy: *Now play with rubbing your hands together feeling your hands heat up then slowly moving your hands apart, noticing what that's like. Can you feel the energy between your hands? Does it feel tight? Pulsing? Warm? Cool? Thick? Tingling? Radiating? (pause) Now placing your hands on your arms explore what happens as you first sense the skin, the edges of your body boundary then lifting your hands up off the skin creating space between your hands and the edges of your body. What do you notice? (pause) If you're comfortable with it continue sensing this energy in your hands moving your hands with this energy to other areas of your body sensing (pause) exploring what effect that has on different parts of your body. Imagine this energy flowing from outside to inside, fluidly interacting with bones, muscles, viscera, organs. Flowing, moving around them, through them. Do your bones respond? What happens when you bring this energy to a muscle? Are there places you want to linger? Maybe even places you want to avoid? No right way to do this, no wrong way, open spacious interest. (pause) Play with moving the energy from inside your body moving it outside (pause) then outside in (pause). shifting back and forth from outside in then inside out.*

Now imagine being with a safe other, letting your energy move from inside your body flowing fluidly outside (pause) Noticing any tendency to tighten, constrict, pull in, shut down or grab onto the other (pause) Sensing, exploring, learning about yourself [pause.] Imagine feeling so safe and at ease that energy moves without complications, finding relaxation in exploring outside of your skin (pause) at ease (pause) comfortable (pause) relaxed (pause) taking space (pause) filling up space.

Manomaya – Feeling/Thoughts: *Orienting now to any feelings that happen as you bring attention to your physical body, to being here in the room with me, bringing attention to left over feelings from the day or week. Maybe noticing feelings or thoughts that sprint around, welcoming them, inviting them to slow down, welcoming parts that demand attention, including them (pause) present to feelings and thoughts relaxed and comfortable (pause) Attuned to thoughts and feelings without letting them take over (pause) giving them so much room (pause) expanding into your entire body, comfortable with having enough space. (pause) Making contact, welcoming what feelings and thoughts are there(pause) exploring what other nourishing feelings and thoughts you would like to have. Inviting those in (pause). Room for all of you (pause).*

Taking time to imagine being with a safe person who welcomed your feelings (pause) knowing intuitively what you were feeling (pause), so attuned to you that your body rested, comfortable in exploring all parts of you (pause), this other comfortable with the many sides of being human. (pause) In this safe space you feel known and seen (pause)

Vijnanamaya – Wisdom, Perception: *Resting in this moment as you listen ever more deeply to what you need (pause) developing your capacity to perceive what would feel just right in this moment. (pause) How can you open to receive even more? What needs to soften to include even more goodness? Imagine feeling so incredibly safe that any feeling that opened up could rise, crest and integrate with ease. (pause) Imagine being so at home in your skin that you had no reason to fear any thoughts or feelings or any external person? (pause) Imagine welcoming whatever longings you have with grace, knowing the longing invites you to move gently toward receiving. (pause) Instinctively listening. You might notice a need for comfort (pause); for contact with another person (pause) something to give yourself some ease.*

Imagine being with someone who really got your wisdom (pause) see them fascinated with how you put things together (pause) they're intrigued with the way your mind works (pause) how your heart makes sense of things (pause) What is it you see in them that has you know they are being with you authentically? How does that translate into a felt experience inside? (pause) You know somehow (pause) how is it you know that in their safe and comforting presence you feel connected, valued, respected. (pause) If you were with the most ideal person who knew you thoroughly and always saw the best in you, what kind of blessing would they offer you? What words of wisdom would they give you that would meet you in just the right way? Breathing in whatever way feels right, see if you can take their words in five percent more (pause) then another five percent. (pause) Finding a way to fill up with their words of wisdom (pause) letting your view of yourself be altered (pause) shifted (pause) changed. (pause) Meeting yourself with self-compassion at all the places where you numb out (pause) shut out goodness (pause) reject kindness and goodness. (pause) All is well. (pause) Wisdom arises from mistakes (pause) from being imperfect (pause) welcoming your common humanity (pause) we are all one (pause) none of us are free from suffering. Offering yourself a blessing that feels exactly right.

Anandamaya: *letting that impulse, movement, tendency, need arise and express itself in whatever way it feels most comfortable? Perhaps allowing a simple sound to emerge, encapsulating the felt experience ----letting your sound just float out, be present, resonate, mingling with all the sounds in the room, outside the room.*

YOGA: MODIFIED WARRIOR (SEATED AND STANDING VERSIONS)

Objective: *To feel the strength of protection. This version of reaching is a "stop" gesture, a gesture of No, stop, not allowed. Just as with reaching for what is wanted, the modified warrior posture is a means of developing the strength to set boundaries.*

Instructions for Standing Warrior option: This strength posture empowers the client to move forward while holding on to his/her ground. Starting with feet together ask yourself, where do I want to move? What parts of me are ready to take a step forward? Then with arms overhead take a step forward with one leg while the other leg grounds in a forward stance. Step legs together again. Bring awareness to your core. See what other parts are feeling hesitant or ready to move. Take another step reassuring any hesitant part that you will be there for every step. Check to see if the part is listening and trusts you.

Instructions for Seated Warrior version: Sit close to the front of the chair so that you have room behind you. One hand is extended in front. The hand can be fingertip extended as if a sword, or the hand can be in a fist or palm facing outwards. The other arm is extended, shoulder height, cocked behind the ear in either the archer position or with a flat palm extended or with a fist.

PSYCHOEDUCATIONAL: STRING BOUNDARY EXERCISE

Objective: *To have a concrete experience of external boundaries so that it can be internalized.*

Instructions: To imagine someone that's difficult for you. See them there in front of you. Then take some yarn or string and wrap it into a circle how-

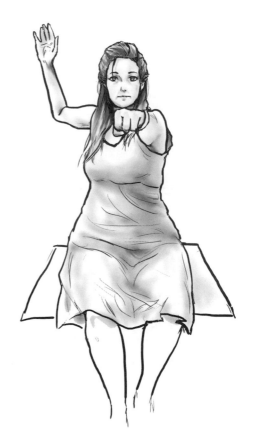

FIG 6.1   MODIFIED WARRIOR

ever far in front and around you that feels right. Stay in contact with what feels good and right. Now stand in the string circle. What's that like? Do you need more space? Less space? From inside the circle see the person out there. What do you want to say to them? What do you imagine they want to say to you? How would you respond?

Self/Other Distinction and Attachment Boundary Inquiry

- Dismissively attached, rigid: Sitting with me, know what happens if you put a palm up to block out your vision of my face. What do you notice in your body? T/F/S? Is it different if you spread your fingers open? Or put a pillow or book up between us blocking out my face and/or body? Imagine piling pillows or chairs around yourself, or maybe turning your back on me. What do you notice in your body? T/F/S?
- Preoccupied/Anxiously Attached, Collapsed: With your hands in front of you, between us, what happens as you let your hands collapse, maybe even flopping, still being able to see me but with your hands collapsed. What T/F/S are you aware of?
- Compare the two. What feels more comfortable? Normal? Familiar? Might there be some advantages to one versus the other? Would one boundary work better for certain circumstances?
- Using magazines, pictures, and drawing find ways to illustrate attachment boundaries.
- How do you know there is an internal you versus an external world? Who is inside? What comprises outside? And who/what part of you is the bridge between these two worlds?
- Where do you end? Where do you notice I end? Do you have a sense of where you begin? Is there a place we meet between? Or do we stay isolated from each other? Does it make it easier to put a hand on your heart as we do this? Or on your belly? Do you need me to look away as you pay attention to this?
- What do you imagine is going on in me as we do this together? Can you sense me separate and different? What's that like for you? How comfortable are you with this experience? Is there anything you need to acknowledge to yourself in order to be more comfortable?

• Can you fill up with you? Allowing your skin to fill up full? Perhaps you're feeling an emotion, can you fill up with that? Letting your skin hold you. Then maybe letting your energy move through that skin boundary. Would you feel comfortable knowing you can affect me? What's that like? If you're comfortable, experiment with virtually pushing me away, taking up all the space in the room, or maybe fluidly moving around me, through me? What happens in you? What thoughts, feelings, body sensations do you have as you do this?

SELF/OTHER DISTINCTION ART EXPLORATION

Objective: *This exercise is helpful in externalizing the often intangible intersubjective boundaries.*

Instructions: Draw a front and back picture of yourself in the room with me (or with another person). Don't worry about trying to do this in a lot of detail. Notice what happens inside your body, taking a felt snapshot of what your internal experience is. Use colors to indicate any variety of feelings and emotions including comfort/discomfort, harmony/disquiet, maybe green to indicate pleasure/enjoyment/ease, blue to indicate neutrality.

Guided Meditation: As you're doing this explore what's important to you right now as you're doing this? What do you care about? What do you believe? What do you hate? What do you love? Who are you? What is attractive to you? What repels you? What do you value? What do you think about? What are you really like? What feels right to have inside you? What are you uncomfortable with and what outside you? When it's outside you, how does that interact with me, or with others? What's that like for you?

REACTING VERSUS RESPONDING

Objective: *With healthy boundaries, we don't have to live in a rigid system of beliefs. Our bodies don't have to be held with intensity or rigidity. We begin to feel safer inside our own systems. We trust we will be able to protect ourselves if need be. As a result, our defenses can be softened and become more permeable. Yet, things will happen beyond your control that scare you. People do things that are wrong and offensive. When that happens, we can either react or respond.*

When we're reacting we're usually in a habitual mode created when we were younger and out of control. Reactions tend to be ways we have to protect by shutting people out, blasting them away, or trying to keep us safe by removing ourselves away from what's happening. Responses on the other hand are current moment determined action resulting from clear boundaries, knowing you are safe with your thoughts/feelings/space and having a sense of knowing yourself.

EXPLORATIONS IN THERAPY SESSION

- Tell about a time in your life when someone said or did something that left you feeling confused about what to think, feel, or do.
- How did you resolve the confusion?
- How do you typically resolve confusion?
- Is there someone recently who has pushed your boundaries?
- What did he/she do?
- How did you respond?
- Looking back now, were you reacting or responding?
- If you were reacting, what defenses did you use? Are these typical for you?
- How did the other person respond to your reactions?

YOGA POSTURE: YES/NO

Objective: *To give a somatic experience of Yes and No*

Instructions: Rolling head left to right, up and down, and all around. Coming to a still place, notice the impulse to nod your head, how the head rocks gently forward and slightly bounces back. Hang out with this movement for a minute, experiencing the rhythm it creates inside.

Now rotate your head from right to left and back again. Let it free wheel on its own, your nose leading your head as you look back across your left shoulder and then back across the right shoulder.

Does one of them feel more familiar than the other? Does one of them feel uncomfortable?

There are lots of variations that can be played with this simple movement depending on the various clinical needs. See the experience below for more ways to practice. Play with them and let me know how they work out for you!

EXPERIENCE: YES/NO

Instructions: While setting up the experiment with your client, let the client lead, control, and be in charge of the play of this experiment. As you're doing this with the client, attune yourself to their comfort level, finding the right "scaffolding" to engage the client with, repairing if there's disruption, reassuring if there's discomfort, normalizing the turbulence of trying something new. You're helping the client monitor their internal experiences, attentive to when the experience is too much while also looking for an optimal level of engagement to help them encounter and stretch this exploratory engagement.

1. One person takes the role of saying "Yes" or "No" either out loud or silently. The partner who is "listening" has an active role of exploring their inner experience. If the client wants, also try to switch roles.
2. Another option is to have the client extend their palm out to indicate STOP. Breathe. Relax. Ground.
3. When, and IF it feels right to switch partners or explore further start up again.

EXPERIENCE: PICTURE YOUR BOUNDARIES THROUGH THE *KOSHAS* VERSION 1

Equipment: Twine or string at least 25 feet long; pens, paper, magazines, coloring pens, and similar items.

Objective: *To explore the various energetic/subtle bodies*

Instructions:

1. *Put the twine on the floor so that it makes a circle.* Let your body be the guide in gauging how big the circle could be. Stand in the middle of the circle. Imagine that everything outside the circle is not you. Imagine that everything within the circle is you. This is your space. What does it feel like to be in this space? How much can you fill up the space inside the circle?
2. *Think about what fills up your circle.* What do you care about? What do you

believe? What do you hate? What do you love? Who are you? What is attractive to you? What repels you? What do you value? What do you think about? What are you really like?

A million things make you distinct from everyone else. What do you value about yourself? What would you want to cultivate?

3. *Write, draw, or use pictures from magazines to describe the external you, the you that is presented to the world.* Who do you present to the world? What does she look like? How do you feel being her? What do you relate to? What are the typical defenses you use to keep yourself safe? Who would you rather show? What do you think you would need to heal in order to feel safe to show her to the world? What do you imagine is outside the circle? Make it as concrete as you like, drawing, writing names, qualities, etc.

4. *Fill one side of a piece of paper with these expressions.*

5. *Then draw, write, or use pictures from magazines, to describe who you are inside, the you that may not often be shared with others, exploring the internal through the koshas:*
    a. *Annamaya:* physical movements, sensations, impulses, action tendencies
    b. *Pranamaya:* energy, breath
    c. *Manomaya:* thoughts, feelings, beliefs, needs, wants, yearnings, longings
    d. *Vijnanamaya:* decisions, choices made, choice points you have, unconscious patterns you're becoming aware of
    e. *Anandamaya:* what allows you to feel pleasure, bliss, ease, contentment

6. *After you're done, compare the words and pictures, what is similar, different, unusual, interesting, compelling?*

7. *Write down to bring into therapy.*

EXPERIENCE: EXPLORING ATTACHMENT BOUNDARIES THROUGH THE *KOSHAS* VERSION 2

To help explore these various attachment boundaries, we can play with how they occur, especially using the *kosha* model. In broad strokes, a dismissive attachment boundary tends to have dualistic, black/white thinking, keeping nourishment out, isolated inside, distancing and dismissing the need for connection or compassion. Pushing back the body tends to be armored, muscles solid, rigid. Anxious/preoccupied attachment styles orient to the outside world without attending to who is perceiving this outside world. Often it's hard to know the thoughts, feelings, beliefs or needs that are there. Asked a direct question the client will ask you to tell them. Their eyes tend to be seeking, pulling you toward. As a therapist you get the sense there's never enough no matter how much you give. It can feel like the client wants to climb into your skin with you.

1. *To open up the exploration, ask your client to feel into their body, skin, chair.* Have them notice you across from them. What happens in their body? Are there any internal movements? Any impulses and action tendencies? Without making anything right or wrong, we're inquiring into whatever attachment boundary is present at the moment. Perhaps there's a strong No! occurring, spoken or unspoken. Or is the client's posture rigid, defending against anything coming in? Or perhaps the client is orienting to you, to doing it right, uncertain of what the client thinks, feels, wants, or needs, looking to you for direction.

2. *As the therapist, you're doing the same exploration inside yourself at the same time.* You're gathering information, about yourself, and any "embodied simulation" going on with the client and between you in the intersubjective field. To explore the intersubjective matrix, you could invite them to notice what happens as they notice that you're there being with them, aware of them. What happens in their physical body? Energy body? Thoughts, feelings and beliefs?

3. *Explore with the client where their preferred way of boundaries are located in space?* Where do they end? Where do they begin? Where in their perceptual world do they experience you beginning and ending? How do they know this? Is it a body "knowing," energetic? Emotional or mental? Is it a concept?

4. *If they feel comfortable, have them either draw or write or use their hands to mimic what they are picking up inside their bodies.* What does that boundary look like? Feel like outside them and inside them? Do they get a sense of rigidity or like there's nothing there?

5. *Invite them to discriminate, exploring, moving from one to the other, fluidly resting in one kosha, moving on to the next.* If they feel "stuck" in one form, invite them (ex: body or feeling realms) to explore another (energy, or pulling back away from it).

6. *When and if it feels right have them explore the opposite.* For example, if they're feeling a rigid, solid, concrete boundary what is it like to feel a softer, more permeable boundary? They can do this in their imagery, through writing, through drawing, sound or through using their hands to mimic the felt expe-

rience. If rigid what is it they are wanting to keep out? Is it a physical sensation, a thought or feeling, or an energy?

7. *What's it like to have both attachment styles at the same time?* Can they hold both together? For this I often have them do the Anjali Mudra or a variation on that.

EXPLORING ATTACHMENT BOUNDARIES WHEN OTHERS ARE INVOLVED

Objective: *This experience may be more advanced for some people as it replicates, and may stimulate relational wounding. The objective is to feel the internal experience in relationship to others noticing the boundaries, felt and concrete between people.*

Instructions: Choose someone specific to explore boundaries with. Imagine them outside the boundary. Come up with some situation that you want to practice crossing a boundary: talking to a boss/co-worker/friend, etc. Inside your space notice what you're thinking, feeling, and what sensations are going on in your body. Take the time to breathe and feel.

1. *What do you want to say to this other person?* Is there a protest going on inside you? What do you need to say to make sure both of you know that boundary is there? When would it, if ever, be okay for you to let this person in? What would you want them to say to make it okay for you to have the boundary?

2. *Explore the similarities and differences between you and the other.* What do you see that is similar to you in the other? What is different? If you didn't know this person, what would you assume is similar? different? What do you want to be the same? different? When you imagine them being similar how would that make things easier inside you? Would there be ways it would be harder for you? When you explore how different they are from you how does that make it easier or harder for you?

CHAPTER 7

Establish Trust: Prana as Guidance

"The storm has passed. For the most part anyway," Rahima told me as she walked to the couch and settled in. She had sent me a frantic email asking to meet. A long term Sufi practitioner and client we had talked a couple times on the phone before she was able to come in person. Knowing I wanted to hear more Rahima continued, "I don't really know what the trigger was, but I found myself eating things I know aren't good for me, drinking more than usual, gaming obsessively. There was this relentless, agitated drive to get out of myself, seemingly without reason. The terrified anxiety was too much to handle, maybe because I couldn't figure out what it was about. I don't even know. So one night before I had yet another glass of wine, I heard your voice telling me to pause, to try and put a wedge in all this reactive behavior. God, it's so hard at those times. I stood there in the kitchen, bent over the counter trying to listen, to pay attention, to do all the things I've learned from you that have helped over the years. It's amazing how hard it is to do this, when I'm caught up in this cycle. Once I paused, though, I felt a shaking in my core. What is that? What on earth happened to make me shake like this now? I tried to find what part was holding the shaking but all there was was the sensation, no storyline. I heard you in my head reminding me if it's out of proportion to the moment it's probably about the past. It's not about now. Okay, that helped. Then I had these—I can't call them memories—more like the imprints you talk about that flash through,

of times in my life when I was alone and scared, but never let myself be, cuz what was the point. there was no comfort, no one to make it okay."

Rahima looked up at me, tears welling in her eyes. "Actually I haven't been able to cry about this until now. Thanks for being here." She knows I'm glad to be there. We've gone through a great deal, in the spiraled journey of her healing. "Getting those imprints didn't stop the anxiety. I think I was waiting to come be with you. That night in the kitchen, I was able to take a thimbleful of the panic and be with it. Let it burn in me. I did all the things we've been practicing. I found the panic in my body, in the small hidden corner of my diagram." Rahima put her hand on the left side of her belly. "I made contact with the color, shape, sounds, the felt experience of it. It really helped to know there wasn't anything catastrophic happening now. That I was safe. I have enough money. I have a couple people that love me. I have a good job. Nothing bad is happening right now. Reminding myself of that helped me open to the frantic panic. Whew, it's still there a bit. (She pauses.) I'm so glad I'm here with you." Tears carved paths down her beautiful skin. "I don't really have any memories per se, but this place in me, it seems like a grieving, enormous sadness of being scared all the time. I can't even say it's a part of me. It's weird. There's no storyline, but something is definitely still there."

Capable as always, Rahima was in charge of the session, while grateful to have our relationship holding her while she did the work. "I'm going to let it burn, okay?" I nodded, admiring how much Rahima was with herself, inspired by her commitment and dedication to her healing, seeing all she learned coming to benefit her in the moment. All the years of practice allowed her to be in this moment, freshly contacting inner experience, without description, without needing to explain. Now she is with herself, letting me feel with her, swim in the intersubjective matrix of her felt suffering. With her eyes closed, held in the safe container of our long-term therapy, Rahima continued the deep sensate contact. Under the story, under the explanations of why she's in pain, is the sensate imprint, the pattern. Yoga invites us, under all the explanations, into the felt experience of the present moment, making contact with the samskara. Patanjali writes of the burning that happens, as the kernels of karmic seeds are removed. That is the intimate experience, touching the place without story, holding attention with equanimity while the swelling of internal sensation moves and shifts and flows, until it, or that piece of the pattern, eases in some way. This is the promise of yoga. As Rahima later said, "The more I put the pieces together, the better I could hold the panic, which eased and then diminished."

In the summer of 1988, Yellowstone National Park had a huge forest fire. That summer National Park Service officials did something controversial that they hadn't done before—they let the fires burn. Businesses in the park complained that letting the fires burn would disfigure and blacken the park and ruin tourism. It did not. Yellowstone received more visitors in 1989 than in any other year that decade.

"Fire is destructive, yes. It's also historic and regenerative. Scientists said the Yellowstone ecosystem needed periodic fires to remain healthy. Burned pine bark proved nutritious for elk. Grizzlies prospered. Aspen seedlings appeared everywhere. And over the next eight years, white bark pine seedlings appeared in all 275 study plots monitored by the NPS." (Heacox, 2015, p. 299). This is the same process yoga advocates: Be with what is. Instead of putting out the fire, or finding strategies to avoid it, let the inner fire burn away that which isn't you, clearing the perceptual lens for consciousness (Singer, 2007).

The question, of course, is how to do this? How do you know what to do? How do you listen to your body, when you're racked with conflicting signals? The theory is relatively easy to understand: being in the transformational fire burns away the stuck patterns of life. Putting that into action is what we all resist. No matter how skilled we are at being in the fire of transformation, resistance is inevitable, until we get close to the root (or get near the root) of the pattern. There always is turbulence moving close. In yogic terms, the beehive of *vrttis* lets loose thunderous sensations, feelings, and thoughts. Tossed into the tumult, we always struggle, not wanting to go near "it." To enter the fire of any transformation—and healing trauma is most definitely a transformational journey—we need navigational tools.

All the skills we've explored so far in this book bring us to the point of knowing, expecting, anticipating, and surfing this turbulence. Ultimately learning to shift, from suffering, being alone with the pain, to having a measure of freedom, is the hardest transformation. Navigating the fiery cauldron of suffering burns away that which isn't one's true nature, so that the essence of who is there, which can never die, can emerge. This is the vital key—finding and knowing we are more than just our suffering, so that we can enter that felt experience. Encountering turbulence in any form, making contact with the pattern, in order to re-pattern from within, and pivot to a more nourishing experience.

THE DEVELOPMENTAL TASK OF BECOMING A SELF

Trauma creates a milieu where it's easy to get lost, and it's hard to trust there's inner guidance. Every child longs to be seen, to have their inherent worth be cherished, for no other reason than that they are there. Not getting this, the heart is plunged into darkness, and the sure knowledge of being unwanted and worthless becomes excruciating. The child's developmental task is to get this value, a worth and a sense of self, from the outside, from caring others who should help to instill it. When that doesn't happen, a different developmental task emerges for an adult: that of listening to the needs, wants, and longings we all have, and responding in such a way that they somehow get met. Living life from the inside out establishes a sense of Self able to tolerate the natural arising of needs and wants, while finding appropriate ways to explore beyond what's comfortable, soothing and reassuring. whenever tension and distress arises from inside. The developmental task of an adult is to learn to live from the inside out, while being mutually and collaboratively related to others, and to life situations.

The key to changing course is held in the protest, which when heard, reassured, and valued, eases and calms the whole system. From an attachment perspective, resistance is the expression of a protest, "It shouldn't be like this!" "It should be different!" "This isn't fair!" "I don't like this!" We've all had those moments. Our clients come to us when they feel stuck in them, unable to pry themselves out. When we're in it, we believe that's all we are. Over time, the connection to the original, free, native expression of being fully ourselves, is lost. For most of us, when protest arises, we clamp down out of fear of disappointment, or we immediately recite the evidence of the multiple times when those needs weren't met. Yoga and attachment theory train us to experience protest differently. The power of the protest is in pointing us toward the direction of getting those needs met, of listening to our inner guidance urging us down a different path. If we shut down, we miss the signpost that our heart is pushing us to see. By this I mean that our longing to be known, seen, understood, cared about, comes through as a need unmet. In essence, our "neediness" links up with where we want to go. If we shut down our needs, shut down that "neediness," we shut down our inner compass, the guidance that continues to push, prod, and urge, that compels us to go toward, and to reach for more, in order to become more fully ourselves, to become a full, uninhibited expression of our true nature. In yoga, we call this drive to return to ourselves *prana*—it's the life force, the energy that animates everything.

We all have different ways of shutting down, when we don't get the response we need or want from others. Each of us has different strategies to deal with the disappointment, the loss, the distress. The pain gets too much and we don't want to deal with it —so we shut it down. It's hard to fathom that the root of our suffering can be integrated into something more wonderful, yet behind that protective barrier, behind the corrosive rust that seals our hearts shut, we continue to seek or yearn for a long, cherished wish to belong, to be loved, and to love freely, safely, and with total abandon. The protest is both an upset with the existing external circumstances, and the way we rail against the constrictions in which we feel caught.

As the protest is both revealed and honored, gradually, over time, you come to know the equanimity that glows behind the protest. Something luminous, gentle, and radiating. As Sharon wrote me, one day after a session, "I was happy to hear you say I did a good job today. Mostly because I could actually hear it without feeling the need to swear at you. And because I felt good about it as well. It amazes me that when I can tap into what I have come to know as truth about myself, I can speak with such clarity and an appreciation of what I've learned about myself, decisions I've made. There is no doubt, no second guessing. I speak from the truth of who I am. It's so hard to remember this when I'm in the struggle, pulled back into the past, as you say, flooded by all of the competing parts within me. So hard to remember when the days and weeks go by without having a glimpse of this wise and wonderful person that others see in me; when all I can focus on is the sad, scared, confused, shameful person, who spends her time either hypervigilant or completely shut off from the here and now.

Tonight, I'm grateful for this view within; grateful that the shame isn't clouding my vision, trying to keep me from gathering up these bits of truth. And I'm grateful for your assurance that you won't let go of the pieces that are waiting to be seen—because of course that's their biggest fear, right? That finally they are coming out into the light and they'll be pushed back into the darkness. (I didn't realize that until I heard you say it today, and I right away knew it was exactly what they needed to hear) Anyway, I've got to get to bed. Just wanted to share where I am, and to take one more step toward making it real."

Our heart knows and reminds us of why we shut down to begin with. Our inner conflict, sensing the longing, and pushing the longing away, can literally bring us to our knees. We either cave, and revert to our old strategies, bottling up the longing once again, closing off, and rejecting our needs and wants, or finally give in to the longing to know our Self, and what we long for. Hopefully (and this might sound odd) but at some point, crippled in we-know-not-what, we can't hold on anymore, can't keep the longing down that we had let go of. We surrender the strategies, the protection. We open the door to transforming our inner world. The protest wants more, different, better. Within the protest, is a longing encapsulated, protected from being felt, even as we know at some point that the protection itself no longer serves us.

Caught in this conflict, we still know we want more, yearn for more. Long desperately for more. All while we cut off that longing out of the fear of not surviving. So, before we do anything, we need to deal with the reality of this. We didn't get what we wanted back then. That's absolutely true. You wouldn't have this scar on your heart if you had been met in exactly the way you "needed" back then. But you weren't met in that way. You didn't receive what you needed. So what you did back then was exactly right, you developed stunningly perfect strategies to keep going, to manage, to survive. You safely packaged up the pain. As a child you did that, to get through, perhaps never to return.

Your heart has a different need. It needs for you to return to it, to not leave it, to not abandon it. Your heart is the pulse point of your life; it needs you. And *prana*, the life-force, urges you to listen, to not forget. To return. For many people, despair is real, healing uncertain, even as hope still fires their longing to trust Joseph Campbell's iconic words, "Follow your bliss." Protector parts urge us not to trust in this possibility, as compelling as it is, advocating that good things are really meant only for other people. The past keeps intruding, erecting hurdles, making it hard to see the path forward, a way around the mountains. They come into our offices, needing a guide, a midwife, or in Diana Fosha's words, a Transformational Other (2011, 2000). This is, in fact, the purpose of this book, and all the practices—helping people to access their own inner wisdom, and trust it in action.

On a very concrete level, learning to be with sensation instead of getting caught in the storyline releases the person into the present moment. When the winds of turbulence are raging inside a nervous system, it's hard to trust that, as with everything in life, everything rises, crests, and ultimately falls. It's hard to trust that the hurricane whipping inside can ever ease. The inclination is to do whatever is possible to stop it, divert it, avoid it. The chapters and practices in this book have laid the groundwork, leading to this final chapter. In order to trust, there has to be a foundation of organizing a disorganized inner world, of practicing easing control, of releasing the attachment wounds of clinging or a determination to be alone, of learning how to be with one's inner world. Yoga reassures us that, in learning to trust one's own inner wisdom, we will be guided into deeper connection. That maybe everything so far is foundational to trust. Learning to trust, to be reassured, to have a felt sense of comfort, that all will be well.

That is one of the essential components of attachment theory, of providing a secure base to return to, in times of stress and distress. It's like the good parent who reassures the child who wakes scared from a nightmare, "It's okay, sweetheart. It's just a dream. I'm right here." Now as adults, we can do what Kristen Neff and Chris Germer suggest: practice offering self-compassion in the midst of our suffering.

Yogic philosophy opens the door for the body/mind/heart to yield into what is, instead of railing against it. We know this from watching infants, whose bodies start out in the primary position of yielding. I'm sure you have the experience of holding an infant, or small child. Their bodies offer no resistance, their muscles yielding, and allowing your hand in. They haven't learned to be tight, armored, defended. This is the first developmental "movement" we start life with; yielding. Without muscle strength and movement articulation, the infant can only yield and wiggle on their back. They then learn to push, to reach, to grab, to pull (Aposhyan, 2014, 2015; Bainbridge-Cohen, 1994; Gundersen, 2013). For many people who have difficult histories, yielding is hard to remember. Bonnie Bainbridge-Cohen writes,

"Babies move toward experience but as you get older you withdraw more and more as a rule. Like when a baby is crying and you do something new, they're happier; whereas adults have the tendency to hold back more in a new situation than in the familiar one. In working with the baby change is a positive experience, depending on how you do it. What I feel strongly is that it's not to go against their will but to help them be successful in what they want. For example, if a baby sees something beyond its kinesphere perceptually, but its movement is retarded so that it can't get to it, there's a frustration. When the baby realizes there's something out there, it means they almost have the ability to go after it. If they're limited in some way, inhibited, they you can help them. Often people tell me after I've worked with their baby that the next day the child does the thing on their own that I helped them do the day before. I try not to do anything that the child isn't ready to do. I know that from my experience and my nature. So I'm not teaching the child something; I'm really helping them manifest what it is that they would do if they weren't blocked, and to get what they want. That's hard to explain." (1994, p. 111)

If we look at the developmental movements of a child, we watch the cycle of yielding, reaching, pushing, grasping, pulling. These organized movements or patterns are preceded by and follow a developmental progression that allows a gradual integration into purposeful, pleasurable, and communicative movement (Aposhyan, 2014, 2015; Bainbridge-Cohen, 1994; Gundersen, 2013; Polatin, 2014). Yielding, as Susan Aposhyan so profoundly teaches, is different than collapsing (2014, 2015). Yielding is about staying within oneself while also releasing into another person or object; this is the natural state of an infant before developing the strength to reach, push, grab, or pull. The developmental shift into earning secure selfhood as an adult comes from being able to yield once again. It means letting go of willfully pushing one's way through life, avoiding whatever is disturbing and emotionally distressing. Instead, we learn to soften and yield into what arises, despite how painful it is. Maybe everything up to this point is to guide us, to teach us to remember how to trust, to follow instinct, to be able to receive from inside, and from outside.

We can map this onto attachment theory. Yielding is about allowing in, letting others affect us. Pushing teaches us to leave something behind to move toward. It also pushes things we don't want, away, develops protective boundaries, provides appropriate separation when needed. Reaching is about exploring, moving toward, asking, wanting, needing. To grasp is to draw toward, or to cling to when scared. Pulling brings others to us, providing connection in a physical, emotional way.

Yielding requires trust. Without fundamental trust we have to re-teach our hearts and bodies to yield, to remember how to trust this present moment, this life and the others that are part of our life. To yield, we interact with something, making contact, and then release into it. When twin fetuses move within the womb, there is a slight slowing down, as they encounter one another, a consciousness of there being another there (Castiello, Becchio, et al., 2010). This is different when we touch ourselves. We don't have that momentary delay or slowing down. Perhaps this indicates a primordial self/other distinction that we are instinctively aware of, a boundary between "me" and "you." But it also speaks to contact and connection. In knowing that someone else is proximate, there is an intuitive respect in making contact, and understanding of the Self/Other boundary.

Take a moment, and attend to your own body. Bring your attention to one of your arms, for example. Let it collapse into your lap, or onto a pillow. What is that sensation like? Does your arm immediately become a dead weight? Most of us hold onto the tension, letting go of the arm with fits and starts. We find it hard to let that go, the tension within it that armors and protects us. What is it like to yield your arm into your lap or a pillow? What's different, what is similar? Yielding, as an adult, Susan Aposhyan informs us, is the experience of being present in ourselves, and letting go, trusting that the other (the pillow, or another person, or our lap) will receive us and not cause harm. In one of my Trauma, Attachment & Yoga training sessions, the group explored the difference between yielding and collapsing. Almost everyone agreed that they found it hard to just let go and "relax." The group described a predominant body experience of clenching and being tight. I suggested that we inquire if maybe the goal isn't to relax? What if the intention is to have contact and yield around you. I saw the quizzical look on everyone's face. Perhaps you have a similar question as you read this.

Think of an ice cube melting in your hand—what happens? Your hand starts getting too cold, and you want to pull away, right? Whether you stay with the experience or put the ice away the ice continues to melt, moving, flowing, around the resistance. While the tendency to pull back is happening, the ice melts, and water flows around you. What if that's all that it's about? Moving, flowing around resistance, instead of reacting to it. Perhaps that's the basic element of trust—of being with something. Moving, flowing without resistance or around any resistance. This is the power of trusting *prana* to guide us through the rocks, hurdles, and barriers of the *samskaras* of life. (Of course, I hope it goes without saying that there are situations and life circumstances where it is imperative to stop something, to not yield, but to instead protest vigorously, and push against.)

In the famous interview Bill Moyer had with Joseph Campbell, Moyer asks,

"Do you ever have the sense of . . . being helped by hidden hands?" Campbell's response informs us what is possible, "All the time. It is miraculous. I even have a superstition that has grown on me as a result of invisible hands coming all the time—namely, that if you do follow your bliss you put yourself on a kind of track that has been there all the while, waiting for you, and the life that you ought to be living is the one you are living. When you can see that, you begin to meet people who are in your field of bliss, and they open doors to you. I say, follow your bliss and don't be afraid, and doors will open where you didn't know they were going to be." (Campbell, J. & Moyers, B., 1988, p. 150). This is the promise of learning to be with one's inner world, of being awake to sensations, and guided from within.

Yet, as Campbell also tells us, this is a heroine's journey, spiraling in and out of hidden pockets of our psyche. Despite all we have learned as therapists, every therapist new to the inner chaos of trauma and attachment learns this side-by-side with every client who opens the door for us. Arabelle is the client I cut my teeth with. No matter how much we know about trauma and dissociation, it isn't until we meet that one client, who introduces us to the chaos, disorganization, and primitive overwhelm, that we put any theory into clinical knowledge. Arabelle first came to me when she was in her teens, a recovering addict, straight out of detox. She described her trauma history without emotion or upset and, as with every trauma survivor, she wanted to get better, faster. Her frequent request let me know that I was bound to fail her.

As I worked with her over the years, it became clear that she had a diagnosis of Dissociative Identity Disorder; her complex history slowly began to emerge. From her and with her, I experienced how primitive rage and unmet attachment needs can leak, spilling over into time outside of the therapy hour. I learned intersubjective boundaries. There was a period of close to three years where she came consistently, but wouldn't talk to me. She silently fumed that I wasn't rescuing her. Despite this, on the occasions when she would talk to me, she advocated for herself to be in one of my groups. Finally relenting, she started the Becoming Safely Embodied™ group, but would barely interact.

One day, I came into the group room. Arabelle's back was to me as she was teaching those who weren't there the week before with beautiful clarity how to distinguish a thought from a feeling from a sensation. That finally broke the ice between us, as she allowed me to see how much she had been learning and putting to practice, yet was terrified to let me know in case I would tell her she didn't need therapy anymore. She was fascinated with my having lived in an ashram and my years of meditating, and began developing her own practice. Laying the foundation inside her mind/body/heart gave her a sense of freedom—until the next fault line opened. This is the journey that we begin to ease around: our "stuff" comes up (sometimes too fast to handle), rises, crests, and with practice and skill building, it then falls and integrates. Our strategies to prematurely transcend our humanness never really work long term. It's in learning to be with this unending cycle that spirals through our life that we find our freedom.

Yoga, like Mindful Self-Compassion, reminds us that we are not separate, that we are not alone in our suffering. Similar to Hansel and Gretel in the Grimm's fairytale, we have to realize that we are lost, look for the breadcrumbs, and follow the often imperceptible trail home to our true nature. This is the path of healing trauma. First, not identifying with the traumatic events, recognizing the suffering inherent in what happened, while most of all orienting to the internal push inside, to remember who we are. In yoga, as in psychotherapy, we discover that we are not the composite of our personality traits alone. That there is more. In the practice of yoga, we follow *prana*, acknowledging the pain, listening to the protest (the "it shouldn't be like this"). To look wider than the pain, orienting to a nascent something else. Reaching for that new possibility, pulling the horizon of our lives into our present, we learn to ride the restless surf of sensation, releasing *samskaras*, relaxing around *vrttis*, to find ourselves reunited with who we are. Joseph Campbell's wisdom reminds us:

"Now, I came to this idea of bliss because in Sanskrit, which is the great spiritual language of the world, there are three terms that represent the brink, the jumping-off place to the ocean of transcendence: sat-chit-ananda. The word 'Sat' means being. 'Chit' means consciousness. 'Ananda' means bliss or rapture. I thought, 'I don't know whether my consciousness is proper consciousness or not; I don't know whether what I know of my being is my proper being or not; but I do know where my rapture is. So let me hang on to rapture, and that will bring me both my consciousness and my being.' I think it worked." (Campbell & Moyers, 1991, p. 149).

Jane, a long-term client, with incredible heart and wisdom, wrote about her own experience in navigating this process.

"I became attached to myself after a long, and at times difficult journey. Only when my therapist began to frame the blast site of my inner world as an attachment wound did things really begin to change for me. Where other therapists tried to manage my symptoms and sorrows by attention and attunement, the holes in my inner bucket doomed 'refill and refuel' models for me. A pattern of relational disappointments and glorious, game-changing authentic encounters with my therapist helped me begin the process of trusting my feelings, and attaching to my experience of myself. While the disappointments were confusing, and at times distracting, they proved to be as important as the moments of risky trust and love. Coming to see the imposition of my inner world onto that relationship helped me see it at last for what it was: my repetition.

Externally, my experience of being professionally shut down intensified and over time. I came to see that there, too, I was replaying an old attachment drama. I was loyal to a withholding institution, in hopes it would eventually come to recognize me as worthy and give me a sense of myself. I overlaid past circuitry on a present-day situation: I endowed the institution with the power to give me the self I had always wanted: shiny and new, acceptable and accepted.

I left that job, that career, and that twenty-plus-years storyline. I started a new story. This time, I'm at the center, shakily at times, but I give myself meaning and value. The practice is to feel what I feel, in my body and mind, and then to deepen into it. Then do it again and again, each time with a growing sense of trust and earned inner security."

Most of us rebel against letting go of what is known, even if it is painful. Our evolutionary drive is first to be safe, then to explore. It's in meeting life as it is, that we develop trust and cultivate this earned security. Stress builds character, Ed Tronick (2007) writes, describing the interactive mismatches of being an infant. "These mismatches stress the infant by generating negative emotions, but the infant has coping behaviors for repairing them to turn a mismatch into a match and the negative emotions into positive emotions. Developmentally, the experience of repairing these mismatches has several positive benefits for the infant. First, the infant's sense of effectance or mastery is increased. Second, his coping capacities are elaborated. And third, following Spitz's formulation, with the reiteration and accumulation of the experience of successfully repairing mismatches in his daily interactions with his mother, the infant internalizes a pattern of interactive coping that he brings to interactions with other partners." (p. 156).

Integrating and shifting the order of the infant coping behaviors put forth by Tronick, Beebe, and others, we see a path forward for adults.

- Signals, sensations, feelings, and thoughts act as signals to draw our attention, asking us to modify something, to intervene in the pattern, not to become caught in the story of despair and worthlessness. As our clients learn to be in relationship with their thoughts, feelings, and body sensations, as signals rather than as indications that something terrible is happening, these signals become a call for energy and for emotional regulation. It's a call for action, though not necessarily toward destructive action. Feelings can be signals to do something, to repair, to integrate, to listen, to pay attention, whether with our internal parts, or with other people. This fosters learning about our own state, as well as that of others, respecting the whole relationship, horizontally and vertically. As Beebe, Jaffe, and Cohen (2002) write, "I change you as you unfold and you change me as I unfold."
- *Withdrawal* – The act of taking a break, slowing down, not engaging, withdrawing from external stimulation is akin to the yogic practice of pratyahara, withdrawing the senses from outside, in order to explore the inner world.
- *Alternative focus, averting, and scanning* – This consistent training to turn toward the Nourishing Opposite instead of fixating on what's painful shifts our Internal Working Model into one of an internal secure base.
- *Self-comfort* – In a world full of stimulation and constant demands, we find the practices of self-compassion, simple mindfulness, and concentration are practices of exploring sounds, movements, words, and behaviors that provide ease.
- *Escape* – We learn to value times of solitude, filling up with this contact with the Self, reframing dissociation into other creative, positive forms.
- *Avert/scan* – Involves exploring the larger world beyond our comfort zone for ways to reinforce a positive path forward.

Filled with contentment, after a session where Jessie withdrew from old patterns, and found more Nourishing Opposites and qualities, she reflected, "This is the shift—remembering this moment, the awareness of that connection, showing up there with my son. At this point I feel, whatever arises in the relationship, the timing will be right. This is amazing—all stuff flowing in, moving through me." I acknowledged with her all the work that she has done in her life, that set her up to cherish this moment of grace and guidance. "I need to pay attention to that. The other day I realized I needed to keep slowing down. The more I feel better, the more I want to grasp, and get on top of things. All the things I haven't been able to do, because I haven't had the energy. Staying slow. Spend time sitting in the open guidance. Taking quiet time, more than usual, to allow the guidance. It's really about trusting, and letting go of pushing or struggling. I want to learn more of how to be. I feel like I'm heard by you, understood, you get it. When you said this flow is "entering the divine stream" I had this felt experience, solid inside, knowing I'll be okay. I can stay in that sense, being held, cared about, in a sort of global goodness that is also uniquely connected to me."

YOGIC MAP OF EMBODIED THERAPY FOR SAFE TRAUMA RECOVERY

Perhaps stating the obvious, healing trauma requires a huge toolbox for therapist and client, as they shuttle through the cycles of excavating history as well as cultivating a nourishing force field that ultimately makes it easier for traumatic memory to be integrated. Yoga offers both, a map grand enough in which to reframe protest, despair, and detachment, using suffering as pointers to a new direction. Patanjali wrote that, in yoga, the posture of life should be steady and easeful (YS 2:46), accompanied by a relaxation of tension, and being open to the Infinite (YS 2:47), out of which arises the pair of opposites (YS 2:48). Those simple phrases can be unpacked. We are where we are, feeling whatever we feel. If we're happy and content—great. Often, however, we're not. We're disappointed, upset, irritated—and sometimes those moments can feel frequent in our busy and stressful lives.

Rather than going down the old, familiar rabbit hole of the past, perhaps with thoughts grumbling, or feeling annoyed, with sensations of tension, yoga asks us to feel this upset as a way to orient ourselves to what it is we really want. Riffing from Patanjali's Sutras, urging us to explore the opposites (YS 2:48), I started calling the "Nourishing Opposite." My greatest teacher in this is the geranium in my office, given to me by the master gardener, Amy Murphy. Every time I turn the geranium around, away from the window, so its leaves face me, the geranium, my teacher, would consistently and persistently turn back toward the light. It knows what it needs—light and warmth to grow. I realized how much we could learn from this simple plant. How might I consistently and persistently turn toward what is nourishing? What happens to most of us, however, is that life intervenes. We get caught in the *samskaras* and forget what nourishes us. We forget to consistently turn toward that nourishment. Why is this?

As we've explored in other areas of the book, navigating turbulence is not easy. We are disoriented by the pain and suffering, yet also by the good that happens. We've so trained our bodies, minds, and hearts to protect, that when good things happen, we're at a loss. We've forgotten how to receive, to yield into this nourishment. We've filled our bodies and storybooks with memories of disappointment, rejection, and humiliation. Exploring and remembering what we've forgotten—that our essence is good, that we are worthy of goodness and kindness—can be very confrontive. Parts of us hold on tight to the protective armor of hurt and anger, making it hard to move toward what there is that calls us forward. It requires clearing the debris—the pain, the wounds, the distress, the upset along the way. For this, we need the concentration practice of equanimity, to ride the bell curve of sensation, allowing the sensations to heat up, and burn themselves out. We need all of the skills outlined in this book, and more, practiced repeatedly. We need to have ways to find ease, such as the profound practice of iRest Yoga Nidra, resting, and letting the nervous system calm.

This gives room for *prana* to guide us, move us toward self-integrating. Without those preliminary practices, our body, heart, and mind aren't softened to shift. As *prana* continues to insistently propel through us, it gets contorted by the knots and tensions in our physical and energy bodies. The beauty is, when we find ourselves contracted, we can look for the Nourishing Opposite thought, feeling, or body sensation. We reach for the nourishing quality that would antidote the distress inside. Even better, as we hold both sides of the polarity, we sit in the seat of the Self. The more we yield, the more we fill with *Sat-cit-ananada*, and find the One no longer separated into two. From this perspective *Prana* offers guidance. We learn to trust *prana's* singular agenda, to remove obstacles keeping us from Oneness, the unifying connection with Self. Like a rushing stream surging down the mountains, to the sea, *prana* cannot be stopped. It will move around, over, and through whatever is in its way. This torrent of energy is always pouring through us, making it difficult to concentrate and draw inwards. Our task is to harness this energy, learning to contain it, so that we can use it and direct it.

In a state of self-acceptance ". . . prana is freed from the habitual and often unconscious patterning in your body and is released, activating hidden potentials and new capacities. Awakened prana is a healing and integrating intelligence. Something in your being will shift. It will not be something you plan, wish for, or cause to happen through your will and actions" (Stapleton, 2004, p. 45). From this perspective, uncovering trauma actually opens the door to hope, possibility, and healing. It's the invitation to return to your Self, of remembering the inherent innate qualities of who you really are. Don Stapleton continues, "Nurturing your relationship to self through expanding awareness is a means for taking refuge from the dynamic and changing circumstances of life, refuge in infinite self-love. On this journey there is no failure, even when the landscape turns desolate and strange. The knowledge that this is your unique and personal journey provides its own comforting peace.

Ultimately, is it our innate intuition of *Samadhi*, the unity and interconnected-ness with all things that guides us away from mistakenly identifying the flocculat-ing realities of the moment as being absolute. Self-Awakening Yoga presents a method for moving beneath the surface appearances of reality to witness the underlying unity. This quest is something that we must discover within ourselves. Until we make this quest our life's purpose, we will always be living against the flow of the universe." (p. 303)

As adults, people with complicated histories need to learn the skills to navigate mismatches and develop mastery. This book encourages learning the skills of slow-ing down, of identifying the basic building blocks of internal experience, knowing the body's signaling and information flow, separating facts from feelings and inter-pretations, exploring sensations, drawing energy inside instead of avoiding internal experience, knowing what is needed or wanted, identifying choice points, and turn-ing toward more nourishing internal or external sources. These are skills that trauma survivors can practice on their own. Building this internal foundation opens the door for someone to ground in their own Self-knowledge, and be guided from within, into a fuller, more nourishing life. An example of this was reported in *Vanity Fair* (October 2015), on an article about Pope Francis, and his decision not to live in the papal palace. "It is still the most telling thing he has done. He said the decision was simple: 'Inside my self I distinctly heard a 'no.'" With that decision Pope Francis aligned with his own values and purpose as a human being.

What this does is repair and develop internal Self capacity. Shown here (See Figure

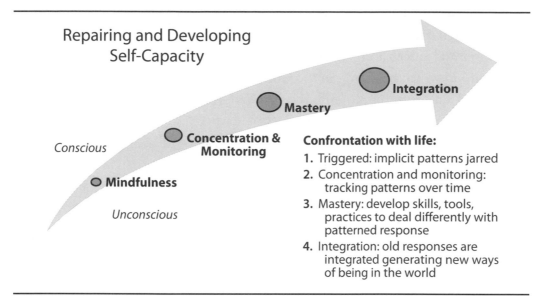

FIG 7.1   REPAIRING AND DEVELOPING SELF-CAPACITY

7.1) as an ascending arrow, this is just one cycle of a spiral, moving us in an upward, unfolding path. Never complete, always learning, developing, growing, changing, becoming. Our capacity to be present and live a full and satisfying life is often buried inside, unawakened. It's generally through some kind of confrontation that our implicit patterns are jarred—or, in the case of trauma, when those implicit patterns and memories erupt, sometimes violently, into our consciousness. Mindfulness gives us the capacity to notice what is, without judgment, welcoming thoughts, feelings, sensations, and behaviors, just as they are. Becoming familiar with the pervasive and persistent patterns that mark our reactive cycles to life we need non-judging mindfulness to hold us from the brink of being lost in the muck of it all.

As we name and identify what is happening, we need the skill of concentration to stay focused instead of getting distracted. This level of concentration opens an inherent non-hypervigilant monitoring, exploring sequences, tracking patterns, behaviors, and intentions, over time. Monitoring the ways a person gets affected and how they affect others creates organization of mind. Exploring under the story to see the deep patterns brings a sense of mastery, as the person develops skills, tools, and practices to deal differently with implicit patterns. This includes developing the ability to intervene in non-verbal, non-narrative body experiences that often herald nascent implicit patterns. Sensitivity to one's own inner world simultaneously encourages an active interest in the hearts and minds of others and their internal experiences, intentions, and motivations, free from negative valences. Integration and internal organization occurs, as the old responses are released or woven into new ways of being in the world. Life begins to make sense as the arising "stories" and patterns ping the Internal Working Model and reactivity is lowered. Feelings and interpersonal reenactments become mirrors to see oneself, instead of tools of self-torture. Life has a felt experience of being in perspective.

Sharon's example gives a glimpse of this process during an online Trauma, Attachment and Yoga seminar. She had been struggling with the idea of yielding and trusting, yet she was committed to at least being open. At first she wrote to the group, "Although I've listened to the videos about a dozen times, I've been very resistant to do the meditations. I think, partly because they start with assuming a relaxing position, which apparently I'm reluctant to do these days, even on vacation at the beach! I guess this month has been more about engaging my mind in understanding the content, which was helped by your handouts—thanks for them."

Two or three weeks later Sharon wrote us all, "As I prepare to go visit my family for a few days, I've been so appreciative of others' reflection of their own family visits. Many experiences are so similar to the way I feel when I am with my family. I often feel disoriented. It feels as if I have this alternative reality that they're unaware of; it's hard for me to live in their reality, their 'hall of mirrors' but I'm afraid of what I can and can't share of my own reality. So I feel like I'm invisible, out of it, unable to connect with them and unable to connect to myself, for fear of everything spilling out causing me to 'fall apart.' As I prepare for the visit I try to remember the times I've been able to connect in some way—usually with people on a one-on-one encounter keep my expectations simple—to just be able to see and be seen by the other. I try to remember that I've been successful in doing that in the past—and it always feels good, and real. But it's something I rarely allow myself to yearn for. And it's definitely something I have to reach for. And that feels scary most of the time.

Now about this month's content, I've been having a hard time setting aside time to listen and read and really pay attention to what's presented this month. Perhaps it's because I'm on vacation, but my level of concentration is pretty low. However, I've spent the past nine days living a mile from the beach and have managed to get into the ocean most days. I'm up in Maine where the water is still cool enough that you can feel it on your skin, and as I've reflected on it today, I've realized how wonderful it's been to have the felt experience of being wrapped in the salt water. I taught my son to float and together we practiced 'yielding' to the waves, knowing that even though they felt like they were going to crash over us, if we just floated, we would either stay above them, or pop right back up on top of them. I thought of your words, and the folks in this group, as I, a lifelong swimmer, allowed my body to yield to the amazing experience of water enveloping me, and realized I may not be getting the words, but the concept is so alive in my body's memory of the soothing water.

And then, today, as I floated through the calm inlet, it was so quiet, I could hear my breathing. The gentle *So Hum*, made louder by hearing it under water. And I didn't have to do anything but float and listen. I felt like I could've done it all day. And instead of my regular panic at the thought of being mindful or still or quiet, I felt the peace of just being. I am grateful—for the awareness, the connection, and the feeling of being alive!"

Remembering that the healing journey is a spiral, with unending waves of rising, then falling, and integrating moments, we learn to flow, to yield into life, allowing *prana* to move us organically toward the life we really want to live. Accessing what we love, what we long for, what we yearn for, while being grounded in the here and now, we awaken wisdom and guidance, directing us in our own unique way home.

Glossary: Key Terms from Yogic Philosophy

asana. A posture to integrate the physical body with the intellectual, emotional, and spiritual dimensions of consciousness. Asanas are the third building block of the Eightfold Path of Yoga.

Brahma Viharas. In Theravada Buddhism, the Brahma Viharas are the heavenly abodes of the mind: May I be happy. May I be at peace. May I live with ease. May I be free from suffering.

citta. The perceptual field holding all; also known as consciousness.

dharana. This is the sixth limb of the Eightfold Path of Yoga. *Dharana* is the practice of concentration, slowing down our inner world to focus single point-edly on one object to the exclusion of all else.

dhyana. Meditation and contemplation is the seventh limb of the Eightfold Path of Yoga in which the yogi has an uninterrupted flow of quiet stillness without fluctuations of the mind.

gunas. The three *gunas* are particular combinations of energies that interact on a fundamental level to evolve into physical forms, present in every moment, in everything, everywhere. Together the energy of fire *(rajas),* solidity *(tamas),* and serenity and lucidity *(sattva)* shift and move through all interactions, emotional expressions, and attachment patterns.

Hatha yoga. Hatha yoga is the overarching term used to describe most forms of yoga as practiced in the West. The building blocks of the Eightfold Path of Yoga have ethical and character foundations of the *yamas* (integrity) and *niyama* (character and spiritual support), and the practices *(sadhana)* of *asana (*postures to balance the physical body), harnessing breath to integrate life force energies (*pranayama*) and to clear the energy body, *pratyahara* (developing an internal locus through withdrawing senses), concentration (*dharana*), meditation (*dhyana*), and *samadhi* (dissolving of separation). Together, *yamas, niyama, asana, pranayama, pratyahara, dharana,* and *dhyana,* and *samadhi* are the limbs that form the Eightfold Path of yoga.

koshas. The many layers of the physical, energetic and spiritual body.

metta. Loving kindness. *Metta* practice is to cultivate the qualities of loving kindness despite other energies being activated.

niyamas. The second limb of the Eightfold Path of Yoga are the ethical and characterological foundations called *niyamas.* They're manifested in the qualities of purity (*sauca*), contentment (*santosha*), self-discipline (*tapas*), self-study (*svadhyaya*), and surrender (*Ishvarapranidhana*). Character and spiritual support come from the *niyamas,* which are the practices that build wise character. Together, *yamas* and *niyamas* form the first two limbs of Patanjali's Eight Limbs of Yoga. The five niyamas are *sauca, santosh, tapas, svadhyaya,* and *Ishvarapranidhana.*

prana. The Sanskrit word for "life force" whose vital energy animates everything, everyone, everywhere. This intelligent life force actively participates in every moment and aspect of life.

pranayama. The art and science of breathing practices, harnessing and training the breath. Used to remove obstacles in the flow of the body's life force. *Pranayama* is the practice of tuning in and aligning ourselves with the positive benefits of *prana* to physiologically activate the parasympathetic nervous system, shifting the fight-flight response, giving energy when we're depleted. *Pranayama* is the fourth limb of the Eightfold Path of Yoga.

pratyahara. The fifth limb of the Eightfold Path of Yoga, *pratyahara* is the practice of withdrawing the senses and developing an internal locus of attention.

sadhana. Yogic practices.

samadhi. The final, eighth stage of the Eightfold Path of Yoga is the dissolving of separation.

samskaras. Imprints of life experience made on consciousness

sattvic. (adj.) Characterized by serene and balanced energy. The *sattvic* energy of compassion and kindness eases the intense vulnerability of suffering alone.

vasana. Habit patterns developed over time through repetition of actions, thoughts, feelings, and predispositions.

vrttis. Beliefs, feelings, sensations, and memories (both helpful and detrimental) that form the perception of what we see and know. In yogic philosophy, we are conditioned by previous experience, and the *vrittis* arise out of that conditioning. The detrimental *vrttis* are ignorance, ego, grasping, aversion, and resistance. Helpful *vrittis* include *metta* (loving kindness) and *karuna* (compassion).

yamas. An ethical and characterological foundation of hatha yoga, as manifested in the qualities of integrity, nonviolence, truthfulness, energy management, and openness. The *yamas* provide skills for positively restraining the full force of *prana,* organizing and training the mind, heart, and body to a balanced way of living in the world. Together, *yamas* and *niyamas* form the first two limbs of Patanjali's Eight Limbs of Yoga. The five yamas are nonviolence (*ahimsa*), truthfulness (*satya*), nonstealing (*asteya*), energy management (*brahmacharya*), and letting go (*aparigraha*).

Acknowledgments

IN RETROSPECT, I HAVE been in training to trust the invisible movement of *prana,* the life force that moves through everything, everywhere, all the time. *Prana* pushed me to first visit and then become a resident of Kripalu Center for Yoga and Health in the mid-1980s for six-plus years. There the practice of yoga taught me to appreciate how *prana,* when we trust it and flow with it, will guide us on the journey to wholeness. This became personal when my trauma history erupted. I was catapulted into the transformative process of healing.

Who I am is formed by those Kripalu connections indelibly imprinted into my heart. Thomas Amelio has been a teacher and a soul friend as we traveled through vast inner and outer spaces. His spiritual wisdom and Advaita classes introduced me to the yoga that grounded my heart's rhythm and body's energetic experiences. Our excursions to retreat with Jean Klein, the humble Advaita teacher, opened realms I longed for as Jean led us into mind-bending body explorations that are still etched in my mind, heart, and body. Jean's presence continues to radiate in my life, giving a solid platform for easing the nervous system and dissolving into vast spaciousness.

Don Stapleton, cofounder of Nosara Yoga Institute and early formulator of Kripalu yoga, opened the first doorway through which I fell in love with yoga, finding a safe way to enter the body. I continue to learn from Don through the incredible movement inquiries of Self-Awakening Yoga. Don's leadership has guided how I encourage safety in groups.

Anna Pool's steady friendship, then and now, helps me navigate the complications of life. Dinabandhu (Pat Sarley) was an early teacher and mentor challenging and guiding me to trust *prana*. Vasanti and Umesh Baldwin gifted me with safety and laughter.

Through Kripalu I deepened a connection with Amy Weintraub and the Life-Force Yoga Institute which I'm proud to have been trained in. Thank you for continuing to push me to write, Amy, and for suggesting me to Andrea Dawson Costello at W. W. Norton. Andrea first invited me to write this book, then spent a year formulating the content with me. I was sorry when Andrea left Norton, yet glad to have Ben Yarling's capable hands in guiding and completing this book.

During an internship at McLean Hospital, while at Smith College School for Social Work, the staff at the dissociative unit asked whether I would teach yoga and meditation in the evenings to the clients on the unit. That opportunity, and the clients I worked with there in the 1990s, helped hone my heart and skill for translating the ancient teachings to help those who suffer.

I'm grateful for my personal therapy with Rachel Brier, Rachel Harris and to Jack Engler, who helped me find my way as a contemplative psychotherapist in the unfamiliar world of Boston still fresh out of ashram life.

I'm grateful to Bessel van der Kolk for inviting me to join his team so many years ago when I left Smith. Those years formed the solid foundation of my professional life. The important learning environment Bessel creates is enhanced by the team of thoughtful, respectful professionals, many who have become an enduring part of my life. Sarah Stewart opened the door for that opportunity, a long-lasting professional and personal relationship that thrives today. Janina Fisher continues to be a mentor and friend, someone I learn from and have healed with through these many years. Thanks to Patti Levin for guidance, friendship, and early reading and feedback on chapters. Jodi Wigren's clinical consultation and feedback not only guided me over the years but helped me shape ideas not yet fully formed.

When Bessel brought Pat Ogden to Boston for one of his yearly conferences I found a bridge from practicing yoga to body-centered psychotherapy. Teaching for Pat, in what was then known as Hakomi Somatics and is now Sensorimotor Psychotherapy, solidified my understanding and use of body-oriented therapy. I'm immensely honored to have been there in those early years as SPI became the contributor it now is in healing trauma. Celia Grand, another fellow trainer who became a great friend, has made walking the psychospiritual path of life much easier. I appreciate her reading of various chapters, giving me feedback and courage to make the book better.

Richard Schwartz, and the Internal Family Systems model that he founded, have been important in my personal therapy and professional development, giving a framework not only for "parts" but for the visionary inclusion of Self in the field of mental health.

Chris Germer is a human being with a heart of gold. His compassionate kindness has walked with me through some knotty client consultations. Our monthly group has come to be compassionate ground. Thank you, Chris, for reminding all of us that the heart is the true ground for a professional practice.

It was while taking a workshop with Daniel Brown that a missing piece felt into place for me: attachment. Dan taught us weekly, then monthly, about the spectrum of attachment and human development, carving distinctions out of the huge literature. The book, *Attachment Disturbances*, with Dan and David Elliott at the helm, came to completion as I was in the midst of writing this book.

Frank Corrigan, M.D. has a unique combination of intelligence, friendship, and humanity that steered me through complicated research and gave me the basis to understand dissociation from an attachment perspective. My time with Diana Fosha's consultation group provided reassuring relevance for therapy as I love to do it.

I'm grateful to Paul Gilbert and the Compassionate Mind listserv whose members I've learned and benefited from on a regular basis. That the listserv exemplifies compassionate exploration is the direct transmission of Paul Gilbert's extraordinary generosity and compassion.

It has been one of the greatest delights of my life to enter the intersubjective matrix with those of you who trusted the impulse to join the first Trauma, Attachment and Yoga Training: Amanda Peacock, Angela Carini, Barbara Henricks Dugan, Barbara van Zoeren, Beryl Minkle, Caitlin Williams, Elisa Elkin-Cleary, Elizabeth Spencer, Heidi Berke, Jeri Schroeder, Laura Fasano, Laura Fisher, Maureen Bryne, and Ray Howard.

There are so many clients I have been privileged to work with whose contributions are indelibly imprinted in every line in this book. I'm moved to tears reflecting on your life, your courage, your commitment to yourselves. Thank you for the honor of walking with you on this journey as you flowered into who you are today. Thank you for teaching me how to be a better therapist, for working through mishaps and mistakes so that we would both emerge as better people.

My parents, Dorothy and Michael, encouraged adventure and exploration, most certainly in the external world. For that I am immensely grateful. They also graced me with siblings—Sheila, Mike, Pat, and Dan—providing a secure basis, to move through thick and thin. That they have spouses that extend my sense of family is something I'm enriched by. The friendship my sister Sheila and I have formed over these many years, working through intense relational knots, has taught me the power of attachment repair.

Research indicates we can shift insecure attachment. For me this has crystallized in Jack Volpe Rotondi, providing a felt internal security with a validating external love. Thank you for bringing out the best in me, for being such a delight and support, for gifting me with secure intimacy. Then, of course, thank you for editing and reviewing each word and chapter of this book before I handed it in. Your feedback made for much better organization, as you well know!

Writing is humbling. First there is the research, reading as much as I could of what others have written, weaving threads of influence into my explorations. I wish I had the mind that retains where every thread of influence comes from so I could offer my deep appreciation for how you all contributed to and shaped my thinking. I have tried to indicate where I learned what I did. If, despite my best intentions, I missed anyone or anything, I apologize for those errors.

References

Adele, D. (2009). The yamas and niyamas: Exploring yoga's ethical practice. Duluth, MN: On Word Bound Books.

Adler, L. E., Olincy, A., Waldo, M., Harris, J. G., Griffith, J., Stevens, K., Flach, K., Nagamoto, H., Bickford, P., Leonard, S., & Freedman, R. (1998). Schizophrenia, sensory gating, and nicotinic receptors. Schizophrenia Bulletin, 24, 189–202.

Agazarian, Y. (1997). Systems-centered therapy for groups. New York: Guilford Press.

Ainsworth, M. D. S., Blehar, M. C., Waters, E., & Wall, S. (1978). Patterns of attachment: A psychological study of the strange situation. Hillsdale, NJ: Lawrence Erlbaum Associates, Inc.

Allen, J. & Fonagy, P. (2008). Mentalizing in clinical practice. Arlington, VA: American Psychiatric Publishing.

Amelio, T. (2015). Personal communication.

Amelio, T. (1989–1994). Advaita Yoga ongoing class. Kripalu Center for Yoga and Health. Lenox, MA.

Aposhyan, S. (2014, 2015). Training in Chicago. Personal communication.

Aposhyan, S. (2007). Natural intelligence: Body-mind integration and human development. Boulder, CO: NOW Press.

Aposhyan, S. (2004). Body-mind psychotherapy: Principles, techniques, and practical applications. New York: W. W. Norton & Company.

Assagioli, R. (1988/2007). Transpersonal development: The dimension beyond psychosynthesis. Forres, UK: Smiling Wisdom/Inner Way Productions.

Bakermans-Kranenburg, M.J., & van IJzendoorn, M.H. (2009). The first 10,000 Adult Attachment Interviews: Distributions of adult attachment representations in clinical and non-clinical groups. Attachment & Human Development, 11(3), 223-263.Bainbridge-Cohen, B. (1994). Sensing, feeling, and action. Northampton, MA: Contact Editions.

Barkow, J. (1989). Darwin, sex, and status: Biological approaches to mind and culture. Toronto, ON: University of Toronto Press.

Barks, C. (1995). The essential rumi. New York: HarperCollins.

Beckes, L., IJzerman, H., & Tops, M. (2015). Toward a radically embodied neuroscience of attachment and relationships. Frontiers in Human Neuroscience, 9, 266.

Beebe, B. (2003). Brief mother–infant treatment using psychoanalytically informed video microanalysis. Infant Mental Health Journal, 24(1), 24–52.

Beebe, B., & Lachmann, F. M. (2014). The origins of attachment: Infant research and adult treatment. East Sussex, UK: Routledge.

Beebe, B., & Lachmann, F. M. (2002). Infant research and adult treatment: Co-constructing interactions. New York: Analytic Press.

Beebe, B., & Lachmann, F. M. (1994). Representation and internalization in infancy: Three principles of salience. Psychoanalytic Psychology, 11(2), 127–165.

Beebe, B., Jaffe, J., Markese, S., Buck, K., Chen, H., Cohen, P., Bahrick, L., Andrews, H., & Feldstein, S. (2010). The origins of 12-month attachment: A microanalysis of 4-month mother-infant interaction. Attachment & Human Development, 12, 1, 3–141

Beebe, B., J. Jaffe, & and Cohen, P. (2002). Support groups and video-bonding consultations for mothers and infants of 9–11. Manuscript, NYSPI, April, 2002. FEMA Liberty Fund; Robin Hood Foundation.

Benau, K. (2013). Podcast on www.dfay.com.

Benjamin, J. (1992). Recognition and destruction. An outline of intersubjectivity. In Skolnick, N. & Warshaw, S. (Eds.). Relational perspectives in psychoanalysis (pp. 43–9). Hillsdale, NJ: The Analytic Press.

Boon, S. (1997). The treatment of traumatic memories in DID: Indications and contraindications. Dissociation, 10, 65–80.

Boutros, N., Zouridakis, G., Overall, J. (1991). Replication and extension of P50 findings in schizophrenia. Clinical EEG and Neuroscience Journal, 22, 40–45.

Bowlby, J. (1969). Attachment and loss, Vol. 1: Loss. New York: Basic Books.

Bowlby, J. (1973). Attachment and loss, Vol. 2: Separation. New York: Basic Books.

Bowlby, J. (1979). The making and breaking of affectional bonds. New York: Brunner-Routledge.

Bowlby, John (1980). Attachment and loss, Vol. 3: Loss, sadness, and depression. New York: Basic Books.

Bowlby, John. (1984). Attachment, separation, loss. London, UK: Lifespan Learning Video.

Bowlby, J. (1988). A secure base: Parent-child attachment and healthy human development. New York: Basic Books.

Braff, D. L. & Geyer, M. A. (1990). Sensorimotor gating and schizophrenia. Human and animal model studies. Archives of General Psychiatry, 49, 206–215.

Braff, D. L., Grillon, C., & Geyer, M. A. (1992). Gating and habituation of the startle reflex in schizophrenic patients. Archives of General Psychiatry, 49, 206–215.

Braten, S. (Ed.). (2007). On being moved: From mirror neurons to empathy. Philadelphia, PA: John Benjamins Publishing Co.

Breines, J., & Chen, S. (2010). Self-compassion increases self-improvement motivation. Personality and Social Psychology Bulletin, 38(9): 1133–1143.

Bremner, J. D. & Marmar, C. R. (Eds.). (1998). Trauma, memory, and dissociation. Washington, D.C.: American Psychological Association.

Bretherton, I., (1992). The origins of attachment theory: John Bowlby and Mary Ainsworth. Developmental Psychology, 28, 759–775.

Bretherton, I. & Munholland, K. A. (1999). Internal working models revisited. In J. Cassidy & P. R. Shaver (Eds.). Handbook of attachment: Theory, research, and clinical applications (pp. 89– 111). New York: Guilford Press.

Brewin, C. R., Gregory, J. D., Lipton, M., & Burgess, N. (2010). Intrusive images in psychological disorders: Characteristics, neural mechanisms, and treatment implications. Psychological Review, 117(1), 210–232.

Brewin, C., Lanius, R., Novac, A., Schnyder, U., Galea, S. (2009). Reformulating PTSD for DSM-V: Life after criterion A. Journal of Traumatic Stress, 22(5), 366–373.

Bromberg, P. (2011). The Shadow of the tsunami and the growth of the relational mind. New York: Routledge.

Brooks, D. (2015). The road to character. New York: Random House.

Brown, D. (2012). Peak Performance Workshop. Harvard University Continuing Education Conference notes and handouts. Boston.

Brown, D. (2005–2015). Attachment seminar (ongoing). Newton, MA.

Brown, R. & Gerbarg, P. (2012). The healing power of the breath: Simple techniques to reduce stress and anxiety, enhance concentration, and balance your emotions. Boston: Shambhala Publications.

Brown, D. (2005–2015). Attachment seminar. Newton, MA.

Brown, D., Elliott, D., et al. (2016). Attachment disturbances in adults: Treatment for comprehensive repair. New York: W. W. Norton & Company.

Brown, D. (2013). Workshop: Meditation & visualization practices for everyday living & well-being and to enhance peak performance. Boston, MA: Harvard Medical School Department of Continuing Education

Bryant, E. (2009). The yoga sutras of Patanjali. New York: North Point Press.

Bucci, Wilma. (1997). Psychoanalysis and cognitive science: A multiple code theory. New York: Guilford Press

Buck, R., (1994). The neuropsychology of communication: spontaneous and symbolic aspects. Journal of Pragmatics, 22, 265–278.

Cacioppo, J. & Patrick, W. (2008). Human nature and the need for social connection. New York: W. W. Norton & Company.

Campbell, J. & Moyers, B. (1991). The power of myth (p. 149). New York: Anchor Books.

Campbell, J. & Moyers, B. (1988). The message of myth. The power of myth, Episode Two. Public Television. http://www.jcf.org/new/index.php?categoryid=31.

Cassidy, J. & Shaver, P. (1999). Handbook of attachment: Theory, research, and clinical applications. New York: The Guilford Press.

Castiello, U., Becchio, C., Zoia, S., Nelini, C., Sartori, L., Blason, L., et al. (2010). Wired to be social: The ontogeny of human interaction. PLoS ONE 5(10), e13199.

Cheung, M. S. P., Gilbert, P., & Irons, C. (2004). An exploration of shame, social rank and rumination in relation to depression. Personality and Individual Differences, 36, 1143–1153.

Chrisholm, J.S. (1996). The evolutionary ecology of attachment organization. Human Nature-An Interdisciplinary Biosocial Perspective, 7(1), 1-37.

Chu, J. (1998). Rebuilding shattered lives: The responsible treatment of complex posttraumatic stress and dissociative disorders. New York: Guilford Press.

Corrigan, F. (2014). Shame and the Vestigial Midbrain Urge to Withdraw. In Lanius, U., Paulsen, S., & Corrigan, F. Neurobiology and treatment of traumatic dissociation: Toward an embodied self. (pp.173-191). New York: Springer Publishing.

Corrigan, F., Wilson, A., & Fay, D. (2014a). Attachment and Attachment Repair. In Lanius, U., Paulsen, S., & Corrigan, F. Neurobiology and treatment of traumatic dissociation: Toward an embodied self (pp. 193–212). New York: Springer Publishing.

Corrigan, F., Wilson, A., & Fay, D. (2014b). The compassionate self. In: Lanius, U., Paulsen, S., & Corrigan, F. (Eds.). Neurobiology and treatment of traumatic dissociation: Toward an embodied self (pp. 269–288). New York: Springer Publishing.

Cortina, M. & Liotti, G. (2014). An evolutionary outlook on motivation: Implications for the clinical dialogue. Psychoanalytic Inquiry, 34(8), 864–899.

Cortina, M. & Liotti, G. (2005). Building on attachment theory: Toward a multimotivational and intersubjective model of human nature. Rapaport-Klein Study Group Annual Meeting. June 11, 2005.

Cory, G. & Gardner, R. (2002). The evolutionary neuroethology of Paul MacLean: Convergences and frontiers. Westport, CT: Praeger Publishers.

Damasio, A. (1995). Descartes' error: Emotion, reason, and the human brain. New York: HarperCollins.

Depue, R A. & Morrone-Strupinsky, J. V. (2005). A Neurobehavioral model of affiliative bonding: Implications for conceptualizing a human trait of affiliation. Behavioral Brain Science, 28(3), 313–350.

Dickerson, S. S. & Kemeny, M. E. (2004). Acute stressors and cortisol response: A theoretical integration and synthesis of laboratory research. Psychological Bulletin, 130, 335–391.

Duschinsky, R. (2015). The emergence of the disorganized/disoriented (D) attachment classification 1979–1982. History of Psychology, 18(1), 32–46. http://doi.org/10.1037/a0038524.

Ekman, P. (2003). Emotions revealed. New York: Owl Books/Henry Holt & Company.

Elliott, S. & Edmonson, D. (2005). The new science of breath. Allen, TX: Coherence Press.

Emerson, D. (2015). Trauma-sensitive yoga in therapy: Bringing the body into treatment. New York: W. W. Norton & Company.

Engler, J. (1993). Becoming somebody and nobody: Psychoanalysis and Buddhism. In Walsh, R. & Vaughan, F. (Eds.). Paths beyond ego: The transpersonal vision. New York: G. P. Putnam's Sons.

Falconer, C., Slater, M., Rovira, A., King, J., Gilbert, P., et al. (2014). Embodying compassion: A virtual reality paradigm for overcoming excessive self-criticism. PLoS ONE 9(11): e111933. Doi.10.1371/journal.pone.011933.

Falconer, C., Rovira, A, King, J., Antley, A., Fearon, P., Ralph, N., Slater, M., & Brewin, C. (2016). Embodying self-compassion within virtual reality and its effects on patients with depression. British Journal of Psychiatry Open 2, 74–80.

Fay, D. (2015). Trauma, attachment, & Yoga training manual.

Fay, D. (2007). The Becoming Safely Embodied skills manual. Boston: Heartfull Press.

Fay, D. (1986). The Becoming Safely Embodied skills handouts. Watertown, MA.

Feiring, C. & Taska, L. (2005). The persistence of shame following sexual abuse: A longitudinal look at risk and recovery. Child Maltreatment, 10, 337–349.

Ferentz, L. (2014). Treating Self-Destructive Behaviors in Trauma Survivors: A Clinician's Guide. New York: Routledge.

Feuerstein, G. (2013). The psychology of yoga: Integrating Eastern and Western approaches for understanding the mind. Boston: Shambhala Publications.

Fisher, J. (2017). Healing the fragmented selves of trauma survivors: Overcoming internal self-alienation. New York: Routledge.

Fisher, J. (2015). Dissociative phenomena in the everyday lives of trauma survivors. Paper presented at the Boston University Medical School.

Fisher, J. (2013). Overcoming trauma-related shame and self-loathing. Eau Claire, WI: CMI Education-PESI Workshop.

Fisher, J. (2010). Psychoeducational aids for treating psychological trauma. Cambridge, MA: Kendall Press.

Fisher, J. (2000). Ongoing training. Watertown, MA.

Fonagy, P. (2001). Attachment theory and psychoanalysis. New York: Other Press.

Fonagy, P., Gergely, G., Jurist, E., & Target, M. (2002). Affect regulation, mentalization, and the development of the self. New York: Other Press.

Fosha, D. (2011). AEDP Immersion (training). New York.

Fosha, D. (2000). The transforming power of affect: Model of accelerated change. New York: Basic Books.

Freedman, R., Waldo, M. C., Bickford-Weimer, P., & Nagamoto, H. (1991). Elementary neuronal dysfunctions in schizophrenia. Schizophrenia Research, 4, 233–243.

Gallese, V. (2001). The 'Shared Manifold' Hypothesis: From mirror neurons to empathy. Journal of Consciousness Studies, 8(5–7), 33–50.

Gallese, V. (2009). Mirror neurons, embodied simulation, and the neural basis of social identification. Psychoanalytic Dialogues, 19, 519–536.

Gallese, Vittorio. (2003). The manifold nature of interpersonal relations: The quest for a common mechanism. Philosophical Transactions of the Royal Society, 358, 517–528.

Gendlin, E. (1978). Focusing. New York: Bantam Dell.

Gerhardt, S. (2004). Why love matters: How affection shapes a baby's brain. London, UK: Routledge.

Germer, C. & Neff, K. (2014). Mindful Self-Compassion (MSC) Teacher Guide. San Diego, CA: Center for Mindful Self-Compassion. Germer, Christopher. (2009). The mindful path to self-compassion: Freeing yourself from destructive thoughts and emotions. New York: Guilford Press.

Germer, C. K. & Neff, K. D. (2013). Self-compassion in clinical practice. Journal of Clinical Psychology, 69, 856–867. doi: 10.1002/jclp.22021.

Gilbert, P. (1997). The evolution of social attractiveness and its role in shame, humiliation, guilt and therapy. British Journal of Medical Psychology, 70, 113–147.

Gilbert, P. (1998). What is shame? Some core issues and controversies. In P. Gilbert, & B. Andrews (Eds.). Shame: Interpersonal behavior, psychopathology, and culture (pp. 3–36). New York: Oxford University Press.

Gilbert, P. (2003). Evolution, social roles, and differences in shame and guilt. Social Research, 70, 1205–1230.

Gilbert, P. (Ed.) (2005). Compassion: Conceptualisations, research and use in psychotherapy. London: Routledge.

Gilbert, P. (2007). Psychotherapy and counselling for depression, 3rd Ed. London: Sage.

Gilbert, P. (2009a). The compassionate mind. Oakland, CA: New Harbinger Publications.

Gilbert, P. (2009b). The nature and basis for compassion focused therapy. Hellenic Journal of Psychology, 6, 273–291.

Gilbert, P. (2009c). Introducing compassion-focused therapy. Advances in Psychiatric Treatment 15, 199–208.

Gilbert, P. (2010). Compassion focused therapy: The CBT distinctive features series. London, UK: Routledge.

Gilbert, P. & Choden. (2014). Mindful Compassion: How the science of compassion can help you understand your emotions, live in the present, and connect deeply with others. Oakland, CA: New Harbinger Publications.

Gilbert, P. & Irons, C. (2005). Focused therapies and compassionate mind training for shame and self-attacking. In, P. Gilbert (Ed.). Compassion: Conceptualisations, research and use in psychotherapy (263–325). London, UK: Routledge.

Gilbert, P., McEwan, K., Matos, N., & Rivis, A. (2011). Fears of compassion: Development of three self-report measures. Psychology and Psychotherapy: Theory, Research and Practice, 84(3), 239–255. doi:10.1348/147608310 X526511.

Gilbert, P., McEwan, K., Catarino, F., Baião, R., & Palmeira, L. (2014). Fears of happiness and compassion in relationship with depression, alexithymia, and attachment security in a depressed sample. British Journal of Clinical Psychology, 53, 228–244. doi: 10.1111/bjc.12037.

Gilbert, P, Miles, J. (Eds.) (2002). Body shame: Conceptualisation, research and treatment. Suffolk, UK: Routledge.

Gundersen, A. (2013). Podcast on www.dfay.com.

Hallward, A. (2011). Safe space radio. www.safespaceradio.com/category /writing-difficult-stories.

Hanh, T. N. (1999). Walking meditation. Call me by my true names: The collected poems of Thich Nhat Hanh (p. 194). Berkeley, CA: Parallax Press

Hatfield, E.; Cacioppo, J. T.; Rapson, R. L. (1993). Emotional contagion: Current directions. Psychological Science 2, 96–99. doi:10.1111/1467-8721.ep10770953.

Heacox, K. (2015). The national parks: An illustrated history. Washington, DC: National Geographic.

Heffernan, M., Quinn Griffin, M. T., McNulty, S. R., & Fitzpatrick, J. J. (2010). Self-compassion and emotional intelligence in nurses. International Journal of Nursing Practice, 16, 366–373.

Herman, J. L. (1992). Trauma and recovery. New York: Basic Books.

Hobson, P. (2002). The Cradle of Thought: Exploring the origins of thinking. New York: Oxford University Press.

Hollis-Walker, L. H., & Colosimo, K. (2011). Mindfulness, self-compassion, and happiness in non-meditators: A theoretical and empirical examination. Personality and Individual Differences, 50, 222–227.

Holmes, J. (2014). John Bowlby and attachment theory, New York: Routledge.

Holmes, J. (2009). Exploring in security: Towards an attachment-informed psychoanalytic psychotherapy. New York: Routledge.

Holmes, J. (2001). The search for the secure base: Attachment theory and psychotherapy. New York: Routledge.

Holmes, J. (1996). Attachment, intimacy, autonomy: Using attachment theory in adult psychotherapy. Lanham, MD: Rowman & Littlefield Publishers.

Hrdy, S. B. (2009). Mothers and others: The evolutionary origins of mutual understanding. Cambridge, MA: Harvard University Press.

Hughes, D. (1998). Building the bonds of attachment: Awakening love in deeply troubled children. Lanham, MD: Rowman & Littlefield Publishers.

Iyengar, U., Kim, S., Martinez, S., Fonagy, P., & Strathearn, L. (2014). Unresolved trauma in mothers: intergenerational effects and the role of reorganization. Frontiers in Psychology, 5, 966. http://doi.org/10.3389/fpsyg.2014.00966.

Jaffe, J., Beebe, B., Feldstein, S., Crown, C. L., & Jasnow, M. D. (2001). Rhythms of dialogue in infancy: Coordinated timing in development. Monographs of the Society for Research in Child Development, 66(2), 1–132.

Jennings, P. (2013). Spring: A journal of archetype and culture. Tricycle, 89.

Junger, S. (2016). Tribe: On Homecoming and Belonging. New York: Twelve/ Grand Central Publishing.

Katherine, A. (1993). Boundaries: Where you end and I begin. NY: Fireside/ Simon & Shuster.

Karen, R. (1998). Becoming attached: First relationships and how they shape our capacity to love. New York: Oxford University Press.

Kaufman, G. (1989). The psychology of shame: Theory and treatment of shame-based syndromes. New York: Springer Publishing Co.

Keltner, D. (2009). Born to be good: The science of a meaningful life. New York: W. W. Norton & Company.

Klein, J. (1990). Transmission of the flame. Guernsey, UK: Third Millennium Publications.

Klein, M. (1946). Notes on some schizoid mechanisms. International Journal of Psycho-Analysis, 27, 99–110.

Klimecki, O. & Singer, T. (2011). Empathic distress fatigue rather than compassion fatigue? Integrating findings from empathy research in psychology and social neuroscience. In Oakley, B., Knafo, A., Madhavan, G., & Sloan Wilson, D., (eds.). Pathological Altruism. Oxford University Press 368--383.

Kṛpālvānanda, S. (1977). Science of meditation. Kayavarohan, Gujarat, India: Shri Dahyabhai Hirabhai Patel.

Ladinsky, D. (1996). I heard God laughing: Poems of hope and joy. New York: Penguin Books.

Lang, P. J. & Bradley, M. M. (2010). Emotion and the motivational brain. Biological Psychology, 84(3), 437–450. http://doi.org/10.1016/j.biopsycho.2009.10.007.

Lanius, U., Paulsen, S., & Corrigan, F. (2014). Neurobiology and treatment of traumatic dissociation: Towards an embodied self. New York, New York: Springer Publishing.

Lazar, S. W,, Bush G., Gollub, R. L., Fricchione, G. L., Khalsa, G., & Benson, H. (2000). Functional brain mapping of the relaxation response and meditation. Neuroreport, 11, 1581–1585.

Levine, P. (1997). Waking the tiger: Healing trauma. Berkeley, CA: North Atlantic Books.

Lewis, M. (1992). Shame: The exposed self. New York: Free Press.

Linehan, M. M. (1993). Cognitive-behavioral treatment of borderline personality disorder. New York: Guilford Press.

Liotti, G. & Gilbert, P. (2011). Mentalizing, motivation, and social mentalities: Theoretical considerations and implications for psychotherapy. Psychology and Psychotherapy: Theory, Research and Practice, 84(1), 9–25.

Liotti, G. and Gumley, A. (2008). An attachment perspective on schizophrenia: The role of disorganized attachment, dissociation and mentalization. In: Moskowitz, A., Schäfer, I., & Dorahy, M. J. (Eds.). Psychosis, trauma and dissociation: Emerging perspectives on severe psychopathology. Chichester, UK: John Wiley & Sons, Ltd. doi: 10.1002/9780470699652.

Lyons-Ruth, K. (2006). Play, precariousness, and the negotiation of shared meaning: A developmental research perspective on child psychotherapy. Journal of Infant, Child, and Adolescent Psychology, 5(2), 142–159.

Lyons-Ruth, K. (1999). The two-person unconscious: Intersubjective dialogue, enactive relational representation, and the emergence of new forms of relational organization. Psychoanalytic Inquiry, 19, 576–617.

Lyons-Ruth, K. Dutra, L, Schuder, M. R., & Bianchi, I. (2006). From infant attachment disorganization to adult dissociation: Relational adaptations or traumatic experiences? The Psychiatric Clinics of North America, 29(1), 63–86, viii.

Lyons-Ruth, K., Repacholi, B., McLeod, S., & Silva, E. (1991). Disorganized attachment behavior in infancy: Short-term stability, maternal and infant correlates, and risk-related subtypes. Development and Psychopathology, 3(4), 377-396.

Maharshi, R. (1985). Be as you are: The teachings of Sri Ramana Maharshi. New York: Penguin Putnam, Inc.

Main M. & Solomon J. (1986). Discovery of a new, insecure-disorganized/disoriented attachment pattern. In Yogman, M. & Brazelton, T. B. (Eds.), Affective development in infancy (pp. 95–124). Norwood, NJ: Ablex.

Meins, E. (1997). Security of attachment and the social development of cognition. East Sussex, UK: Psychology Press.

Michael, T., Ehlers, A., Halligan. S., & Clark, D. (2004). Unwanted memories of assault: What intrusion characteristics are associated with PTSD? Behaviour Research and Therapy, 43 (613–628).

Mikulincer, M. & Shaver, P. (2010). Attachment in adulthood: Structure, dynamics, and change. New York: Guilford Press.

Miller, R. (2010). Yoga nidra: A meditative practice for deep relaxation and healing. Louisville, CO: Sounds True Publishing.

Miller, R. (2014). iRest Yoga Nidra Level I Training Manual. Given at Santa Monica, CA, Sept, 2014.

Miller, R. (2015). The iRest Program for Healing PTSD: A proven-effective approach to using yoga nidra meditation and deep relaxation techniques to overcome trauma. Oakland, CA: New Harbinger Publications.

Moullin, S., Waldfogel, J., & Washbrook, E. (2014). Baby bonds: Parenting, attachment and a secure base for children. The Sutton Trust (research report).

Muktananda. (1992). I am that: The science of hamsa from the Vijñāna Bhairava. South Fallsburg, NY: SYDA Foundation.

Muni, R. (1994). Awakening life force: The philosophy and psychology of "spontaneous yoga. St. Paul, MN: Llewelyn Press.

Murray. H. (2008). Explorations in personality. New York: Oxford University Press.

Nathanson, D. (1992). Shame and pride: Affect, sex, and the birth of the self. New York: W. W. Norton & Company.

Neely, M. E., Schallert, D. L., Mohammed, S. S., Roberts, R. M., Chen, Y. (2009). Self-kindness when facing stress: The role of self-compassion, goal regulation, and support in college students well-being. Motivation and Emotion, 33, 88-97.

Neff, Kristin. (2011). Self-compassion: Stop beating yourself up and leave insecurity behind. New York: HarperCollins.

Neff, Kristin D. "Self-compassion and psychological well-being." Constructivism in the human sciences 9.2 (2004): 27-37.Neff, K. (2003). Self-compassion: An alternative conceptualization of a healthy attitude toward oneself. Self and Identity, 2, 85 –101.

Neff, K., Hsieh, Y. & Dejitterat, K. (2005). Self-compassion, achievement goals, and coping with academic failure. Self and Identity, 4, 263–287.

Neff, K., Kirkpatrick, K., & Rude, S. (2007). Self-compassion and adaptive psychological functioning. Journal of Research in Personality, 41, 139–154.

Nisargadatta, S. (1973). I am that. Durham, NC: The Acorn Press.

Ogden, P, and Janina F. (2015). Sensorimotor Psychotherapy: Interventions for Trauma and Attachment (Norton Series on Interpersonal Neurobiology). New York: W.W. Norton & Company.

Ogden, P., Minton, K., & Pain, C. (2006). Trauma and the body: A sensorimotor approach to psychotherapy. New York: W. W. Norton & Company.

Panksepp, J. & Biven, L. (2012). The Archaeology of Mind: Neuroevolutionary origins of human emotions. New York: W. W. Norton & Company.

Pennebaker, J. (1990). Opening up: The healing power of expressing emotions. New York: Guilford Press.

Perls, F. (1969/1992). Gestalt therapy verbatim. Gouldsboro, ME: The Gestalt Journal Press.

Peterson, C. & Seligman, M. (2004). Character strengths and virtues: A handbook and classification. New York: American Psychological Association and Oxford University Press.

Polatin, B. (2013). The actor's secret: Techniques for transforming habitual patterns and improving performance. Berkeley, CA: North Atlantic Books.

Porges, S. (2011). The polyvagal theory: Neurophysiological foundations of emotions, attachment, communication, and self-regulation. New York: W. W. Norton & Company.

Robbins, M. (2014). Qi Gong class handouts. Somerville, MA.

Rocha, Tomas, 2014. "The Dark Knight of the Soul" The Atlantic (June 25, 2014). Available at: http://www.theatlantic.com/health/archive/2014/06/the -dark-knight-of-the-so uls/372766/ [accessed September 12, 2014].

Salzberg, Sharon. (1995). Loving-kindness: The revolutionary art of happiness. Boston, MA: Shambhala Publications

Saunders, R., Jacobvitz, D., Zaccagnino, M., Beverung, L., & Hazen, N. (2011). Pathways to earned-security: The role of alternative support figures. Attachment & Human Development, 13(4), 403–420.

Schore, A. (1994). Affect regulation and the origin of the self: The neurobiology of emotional development. Hillsdale, NJ: Lawrence Erlbaum Associates.

Schuengel, C., Bakermans-Kranenburg, M., & van Ijzendoorn, M. (1999). Frightening maternal behavior linking unresolved loss and disorganized infant attachment. Journal of Consulting and Clinical Psychology, 67(1), 54–63.

Schwartz, R. (1994). Internal family systems therapy. New York: Guilford Press.

Schwarz, L. S., Corrigan, F. M., Hull, A. M., & Raju, R. (In Press). The comprehensive resource model: Effective therapeutic techniques for the healing of complex trauma. London: Routledge.

Servan-Schreiber, D. (2004). The instinct to heal: Curing depression, anxiety, and stress without drugs and without talk therapy. Emmaus, PA: Rodale Press.

Shah, A. & Vaccarino, V. (2015). Heart rate variability in the prediction of risk for posttraumatic stress Disorder. JAMA Psychiatry, published online September 9, 2015. Doi:10.1001/jamapsychiatry 2015.1394.

Singer, M. (2015). The surrender experiment: My journey into life's perfection. New York: Harmony Books.

Singer, M. (2007). The untethered soul: The journey beyond yourself. New York: New Harbinger Publications.

Singer, T., & Klimecki, O. (2014). Empathy and compassion. Current Biology, 24(18), R875–R878.

Sivananda, S. (2008). The science of pranayama. Uttar Pradesh, India: The Divine Life Society.

Solomon, J., & George, C. (1999). Attachment disorganization. New York: Guilford Press.

Stapleton, D. (2015 & 2016). Self-awakening yoga teacher training manual. Rochester, VT: Healing Arts Press.

Stapleton, D. (2004). Self-awakening yoga: The expansion of consciousness through the body's own wisdom. Rochester, VT: Healing Arts Press.

Stark, E., Parsons, C., Hartevelt, T., Charquero-Ballester, M., McManners, H., Ehlers, A., Stein, A., Kringelbach, M. (2015). Post-traumatic stress influences the brain even in the absence of symptoms: A systematic, quantitative meta-analysis of neuroimaging studies. Neuroscience & Biobehavioral Reviews, 56, 207–221.

Steele, K., van der Hart, O., & Nijenhuis, E. (2005). Phase-oriented treatment of structural dissociation in complex traumatization: Overcoming trauma-related phobias. Journal of Trauma and Dissociation, 6(3), 11–53.

Steele, K., van der Hart, O., & Nijenhuis, E. R. S. (2001). Phase-oriented treatment of complex dissociative disorders: overcoming trauma-related phobias. In A. Eckhart-Henn & S. O. Hoffman (Eds.). Dissociative disorders of consciousness. Stuttgart, Germany: Schattauer-Verlag.

Stern, D. (2004). The present moment in psychotherapy and everyday life. New York: W. W. Norton & Company.

Stern, D. (1985). The interpersonal world of the infant. New York: Basic Books.

Stone, M. (2008). The inner tradition of yoga: A guide to yoga philosophy for the contemporary practitioner. Boston, MA: Shambhala Publications.

Stuewig, J. & McCloskey, L. (2005). The relation of child maltreatment to shame and guilt among adolescents: psychological routes to depression and delinquency. Child Maltreatment, 10, 324–336.

Taimni, I. K. (1961). The science of yoga: The yoga-sutras of Patanjali in Sanksrit with transliteration in Roman, translation in English and commentary. Madras, India: Theosophical Publishing House.

Tangney, J. & Dearing, R. (2002). Shame and guilt. New York: Guilford Press.

Trevarthen, C. and Aitken, K.J. (2008) Brain development, infant communication, and empathy disorders: Intrinsic factors in child mental health, Development and Psychopathology, 6(4), 597–633.

Tomasello, M. (2010). Origins of human communication. Cambridge, MA: MIT Press.

Toth, S., Rogosch, F., & Manly, J. T. (2006). The efficacy of toddler–parent psychotherapy to reorganize attachment in the young offspring of mothers with major depressive disorder: A randomized preventive trial. Journal of Consulting and Clinical Psychology, 74(6), 1006–1016.

Trevarthen, C. & Aitken, K. (2001). Infant intersubjectivity: Research, theory, and clinical applications. Journal of Child Psychology and Psychiatry, 42(1) 3–48.

Trevarthen, C. (1979). Communication and cooperation in early infancy: A description of primary intersubjectivity. In M. M. Bullowa (Ed.), Before speech: The beginning of human communication (pp. 321–347). New York: Cambridge University Press.

Tronick, E., (2007). The Neurobehavioral and social-emotional development of infants and children. New York: W. W. Norton & Company.

Van der Hart, O., Nijenhuis, E. R. S., & Steele, K. (2006). The haunted self: Structural dissociation and the treatment of chronic traumatization. New York: W. W. Norton & Company.

Van der Kolk, B. (2015). The body keeps the score. New York: Viking Penguin.

Van der Kolk, B. (1994). The body keeps the score: Memory and the evolving psychobiology of post-traumatic stress. Harvard Review of Psychiatry 1(5), 253–265.

Van der Kolk, B., McFarlane, A., & Weisaeth, L., (Eds.) (1996). Traumatic stress: The effects of overwhelming experience on mind, body, and society. New York: Guilford Press.

Wallin, D. J. (2007). Attachment in psychotherapy. New York: Guilford Press.

Waters, E. & Valenzuela, M. (1999). Explaining disorganized attachment: Clues from research on mild-to-moderately undernourished children in Chile. In Attachment disorganization. (Eds.) Solomon, J. & George, C. New York: Guilford Press.

Weintraub, A. (2012). Yoga skills for therapists: Effective practices for mood management. New York: W. W. Norton & Company.

Weintraub, A. (2013). LifeForce Yoga Level 1 Training. Tucson, Arizona.

Weintraub, A. (2003). Yoga for depression. New York: Random House.

Whiten, A. (1991). Natural theories of mind: Evolution, development and simulation of everyday mindreading. Oxford, UK: Basil Blackwell.

Zlochower, A. & Cohn, J. (1996). Vocal timing in face-to-face interaction of clinically depressed and nondepressed mothers and their 4-month-old infants. Infant Behavior and Development, 19(3), 371–374.

Index

Note: Italicized page locators indicate figures; tables are noted with *t*.